Forew KU-736-904

Renal nursing is a wonderful profession where attitudes and actions make a difference. It leads the way in putting patients at the centre of everything we do and, in overcoming interprofessional resistance to team-working, roles in nursing have advanced in many directions. As this handbook shows, one nurse alone cannot cover the whole spectrum and depth of renal nursing care within a single job plan or range of experience. The authors are to be congratulated that the principles which underpin renal nursing stand out as clearly as the detail necessary to practise at the highest level. Renal nurses play a central role in the kidney care multiprofessional team by both delivering direct patient care and listening to patients, their families, and carers. Communication is about listening first. Renal nurses are ideally placed to support individual patients and to identify their real needs. They ensure that colleagues across health and social care, commissioners, and managers understand the requirement for holistic care, balancing psychosocial and bio-medical considerations and individual values, aspirations, and health beliefs. People with kidney disease need support; not only to navigate the complexity of modern health and social care, but to challenge the institutions and practices should they fall short of adding value to individual patient care.

The knowledge, skills, and competencies required to safely, effectively, and efficiently nurse people with kidney disease in a range of healthcare settings provides opportunities that few other areas of nursing can rival: the management of acute kidney injury, choice and preparation for renal replacement therapy, and conservative kidney care in the community, to name but a few. Evidence shows that teamwork in the dialysis unit impacts upon staff and patient satisfaction and translates into improved patient outcomes. Strong leadership is not solely a nursing responsibility; it is a requirement across the whole team but, skilled renal nursing is the building block of a functional team. The camaraderie of kidney care is infectious and is appreciated by our patients. Good care is evidence based and must be firmly rooted in an understanding of biology, health, illness, and the impact of 21st-century healthcare interventions; safeguarding patient welfare. Renal nurses need to measure, evaluate, and report in local and national clinical audit, research studies, and quality improvement projects. Historically, eminent nurses have consistently led innovation and practice. Modern-day renal nursing continues this long tradition; pioneering change and pushing the boundaries of healthcare delivery forward in response to what is really important for people with kidney disease. This handbook provides an introduction to that life; detailed knowledge of kidney care for aspiring renal nurses, packed with a wealth of information that can be used to make a difference.

Donal O'Donoghue
National Clinical Director for Kidney Services, 2007–2013,
Department of Health, England, UK

Preface

It is a privilege to add this book to the portfolio of the Oxford Nursing Handbook series, which has a long tradition of providing practical guides for colleagues across the professional spectrum who are involved in delivering day to day clinical care. In this new handbook, we have focused in depth on all aspects of nursing the patient with kidney disease; from acute kidney injury through to renal replacement therapy and end of life care. The nature and complexity of kidney disease is such that patients with chronic kidney disease develop lifelong relationships with the healthcare professionals on whom they and their families rely for expertise and support. The collective wisdom of the multiprofessional team is essential in responding to their needs and helping them to manage the trajectory of chronic illness. In this book, we have aimed to reflect the unique contribution that nursing makes to delivering patient-centred care to this group of patients within the context of the multiprofessional team. We are grateful to our contributors, who have been drawn from a range of professions allied to medicine; each experts in their own right.

Historically, renal medicine has been defined by innovation and technological advances that have placed it at the cutting edge of modern clinical practice. This has exposed renal nurses to a breadth of experiences, knowledge, and skills, creating unique opportunities for professional development and career progression. First and foremost, this book is designed to support and guide nurses through the range of treatment options and care strategies available for patients with kidney disease, giving them confidence to respond effectively in a variety of clinical situations. As nurses who are committed to working in the field, the authors also hope that this book may, in part, inspire today's nurses to become tomorrow's leaders.

Finally, every book comes with a health warning and this one is no exception. Data and evidence have been sought from the most contemporary sources available at the time of writing but, in such a rapidly progressive area of clinical practice, it is impossible to reflect every aspect with complete accuracy; things inevitably change with the lapse of time. We hope that you find this book useful and accessible.

Althea Mahon
Karen Jenkins
Lisa Burnapp

Contents

Symbols and abbreviations

📖	cross reference
⚠	warning
▶	important
♂	male
♀	female
∴	therefore
~	approximately
≈	approximately equal to
±	plus/minus
↑	increased
↓	decreased
→	leading to
1°	primary
2°	secondary
⏱	online reference
–ve	negative
+ve	positive
α	alpha
β	beta
6-MP	6-mercaptopurine
aAPD	assisted automated peritoneal dialysis
ABD	adynamic bone disease
ABGs	arterial blood gases
ABOi	ABO blood group incompatible
ABPM	ambulatory blood pressure monitoring
aCAPD	assisted continuous ambulatory peritoneal dialysis
ACEI	angiotensin-converting enzyme inhibitor
ACKD	anaemia of chronic kidney disease
ACR	albumin: creatinine ratio
ADC	altruistic donor chain
ADH	anti-diuretic hormone
ADPKD	autosomal dominant polycystic kidney disease
AGEs	advanced glycosylated end products
AIN	acute interstitial nephritis
AiT	antibody incompatible transplantation
AKC	advanced kidney care
AKCC	advanced kidney care clinic

AKI	acute kidney injury
Alb	albumin
ALP	alkaline phosphatase
ALT	alanine transaminase
ANA	antinuclear antibody
ANCA	antineutrophil cytoplasmic antibody
aPD	assisted peritoneal dialysis
APD	automated peritoneal dialysis
APKD	adult polycystic kidney disease
ARB	angiotensin receptor antagonist
ARF	acute renal failure
AST	aminotransferases enzymes
ATG	rabbit anti-human thymocyte immunoglobulin
ATN	acute tubular necrosis
AUC	area under the curve
AVF	arteriovenous fistula
AVG	arteriovenous graft
AXR	abdominal x-ray
B_2m	beta-2 microglobulin
BBV	blood-borne virus
bd	twice daily
BFR	blood flow rate
BGL	blood glucose level
BHS	British Hypertension Society
BKV	BK virus
BMI	body mass index
BNO	bowels not opened
BP	blood pressure
BPM	blood pressure monitoring
BSA	body surface area
BTS	British Transplantation Society
BNU	blood urea nitrogen
Ca	carcinoma
Ca^{2+}	calcium
CAPD	continuous ambulatory peritoneal dialysis
CBT	cognitive behaviour therapy
CCB	calcium channel blocker
CCF	congestive cardiac failure
CHF	chronic heart failure
chol	cholesterol

CIT	cold ischaemic time
CK	creatine kinase
CKD	chronic kidney disease
CMT	conservative management team
CMV	cytomegalovirus virus
CNI	calcineurin inhibitor
conc	concentration
COPD	chronic obstructive pulmonary disease
CPN	community psychiatric nurse
Cr	creatinine
CrCl	creatinine clearance
CRP	C-reactive protein
CRRT	continuous renal replacement therapy
CPR	cardio pulmonary resuscitation
CT	computed tomography
CVA	cerebrovascular accident
CVD	cardiovascular disease
CVP	central venous pressure
CXR	chest x-ray
DBD	donor after brain death
DBP	diastolic blood pressure
DCD	donor after circulatory death
DD	deceased donor
DDKT	deceased donor kidney transplant
DDS	dialysis disequilibrium syndrome
DFPP	double filtration plasmapheresis
DGF	delayed graft function
DoH	Department of Health
DIC	disseminated intravascular coagulation
DKD	domino kidney donation
DM	diabetes mellitus
DMSA	dimercaptosuccinic acid
DNA	deoxyribonucleic acid
DOPPS	Dialysis Outcomes Practice Patterns Study
DPI	dietary and protein intake
DVT	deep vein thrombosis
EBPG	European best practice guidelines
EBV	Epstein–Barr virus
EC	extracorporeal
ECG	electrocardiogram

ECHO	echocardiogram
eGFR	estimated glomerular filtration rate
EMU	early morning urine
EOL	end of life
EOS	electronic offering system
ESA	erythropoietin stimulating agent
ESI	exit site infection
ESR	erythrocyte sedimentation rate
ESKD	end stage kidney disease
EU	European Union
FACS	flow cytometry crossmatch
FBC	full blood count
FH	family history
FK506	tacrolimus
FSGS	focal segmental glomerulosclerosis
GA	general anaesthetic
GBM	glomerular basement membrane
GDPs	glucose degradation products
GFR	glomerular filtration rate
GI	gastrointestinal
GN	glomerulonephritis
GP	general practitioner
H&I	histopathology and immunogenetics
HAART	highly active antiretroviral
HALDN	hand-assisted laparoscopic donor nephrectomy
Hb	haemoglobin
HbA1c	glycosylated haemoglobin
HBeAb	hepatitis B e antibody
HBeAg	hepatitis B e antigen
HBsAg	hepatitis B surface antigen
HBsAb	hepatitis B surface antibody
HBPM	home blood pressure monitoring
HBV	hepatitis B virus
HCl	hydrochloride
HCT	haematocrit
HCV	hepatitis C virus
HD	haemodialysis
HDF	haemodiafiltration
HF	heart failure
HIT	heparin-induced thrombocytopaenia

HIV	human immunodeficiency virus
HIVAN	human immunodeficiency virus-associated nephropathy
HLA	human leucocyte antigen
HLAi	human leucocyte antigen incompatible
hpf	high powered field
hr	hour
HRC	hypochromic red cells
hrly	hourly
HRQOL	health-related quality of life
HSP	Henoch–Schönlein purpura
H_2O	water
HTA	Human Tissue Authority
HT	Acts Human Tissue Acts
HTLV	human T-lymphotropic virus
IA	independent assessor
IBW	ideal body weight
ICS	Intensive Care Society
ICU	intensive care unit
IDH	intradialytic hypotension
IDPN	intradialytic parenteral nutrition
Ig	immunoglobulin
IHD	ischaemic heart disease
IM	intramuscular
INR	international normalized ratio
IP	intraperitoneal
IPHP	intraperitoneal hydrostatic pressure
IS	immunosuppression
IT	information technology
IV	intravenous/ly
IVC	inferior vena cava
IVIg	intravenous immunoglobulin
IVU	intravenous urogram
JVP	jugular venous pressure
K^+	potassium
KDMR	kidney donor matching run
KMR	kidney matching run
KTA	kidney transplant alone
KUB	kidney, ureter, and bladder
L	litre
LA	local anaesthetic

LCP	Liverpool Care Pathway
LD	living donor
LDC	living donor co-ordinator
LDH	lactate dehydrogenase
LDKT	living donor kidney transplant
LDL	low-density lipoprotein
LDN	living donor nephrectomy
LFT	liver function test
LV	left ventricle
LVH	left ventricular hypertrophy
MAOI	monoamine oxidase inhibitor
MBD	mineral bone disorder
MC&S	microscopy, culture and sensitivity
mcg	microgram
MCGN	mesangiocapillary glomerulonephritis
MCH	mean corpuscular haemoglobin
MCHC	mean corpuscular haemoglobin concentrate
MCV	mean corpuscular volume
MDRD	modification of diet in renal disease
mg	milligram
MgCl$_2$	magnesium chloride
MHC	major histocompatibility complex
MI	myocardial infarction
miH	minor histocompatibility system
ml	millilitre
MM	multiple myeloma
MMF	mycophenolate mofetil
MODN	mini-incision open donor nephrectomy
MPA	mycophenolic acid
MPT	multiprofessional team
MRI	magnetic resonance imaging
MRSA	meticillin-resistant *Staphylococcus aureus*
MSU	midstream urine sample
mTOR	mammalian target of rapamycin
Na$^+$	sodium
NaCl	sodium chloride
NAD	nothing abnormal detected
NB	take note
NBM	nil by mouth
NDAD	non-directed altruistic donor

ng	nanogram
NGT	nasogastric tube
NHS	National Health Service
NHSBT	NHS Blood and Transplant
NICE	National Institute for Health and Clinical Excellence
NKF	National Kidney Federation
NKF-KDOQI	National Kidney Federation Kidney Dialysis Outcome Quality Initiative
NLDKSS	National Living Donor Kidney Sharing Schemes
NODAT	new-onset diabetes after transplantation
NORS	National Organ Retrieval Teams
NSAIDs	non-steroidal anti-inflammatory drugs
NSF	national service framework
NTC	non-tunnelled catheter
NTL	national transplant list
od	once daily
ODA	operating department assistant
ODT	Organ Donation and Transplantation
ODTF	Organ Donation Taskforce
ODR	organ donor register
OTC	over the counter
PAK	pancreas after kidney
PAN	polyarteritis nodosa
PCA	patient controlled analgesia
PCP	pneumocystis pneumonia
PCR	protein:creatinine ratio
PD	peritoneal dialysis
PE	pulmonary embolus
PEG	percutaneous endoscopic gastrostomy
peri-op	perioperative/ly
PET	peritoneal equilibration test
PEX	plasma exchange
pg	pictogram
pH	potential hydrogen
PMH	previous medical history
PMP	per million population
PN	pyelonephritis
Po	oral
PO_4	phosphate
post-op	post-operative/ly

PPD	paired/pooled donation
PPI	proton pump inhibitor
pre-op	preoperative/ly
PRN	'pro re nata'; as needed
PTA	pancreas transplant alone
PTH	parathyroid hormone
PTLD	post-transplant lymphoproliferative disease
PTRA	percutaneous transluminal renal angioplasty
PVD	peripheral vascular disease
qds	4 times a day
QOF	quality outcomes framework
QOL	quality of life
RA	Renal Association
RAS	renal artery stenosis
RBC	red blood cell
RCT	randomized controlled trial
re	reference to
Rh	rhesus
RNA	ribonucleic acid
RPGN	rapidly progressing glomerulonephritis
RO	reverse osmosis
RRF	residual renal function
RRT	renal replacement therapy
SBP	systolic blood pressure
SC	subcutaneous
SGA	subjective global assessment
SHPT	secondary hyperparathyroidism
SLE	systemic lupus erythematosus
SMA	superior mesenteric artery
SN-OD	specialist nurse-organ donation
SOB	shortness of breath
SPK	simultaneous pancreas and kidney
TB	tuberculosis
TBM	thin basement membrane
TC	tunnelled catheter
TCR	T-cell receptor
tds	thrice daily
TIA	transient ischaemic attack
TLDN	total laparoscopic donor nephrectomy

TOD	target organ damage
TPMT	thiopurine methyltransferase
TPN	total parenteral nutrition
TPR	temperature, pulse, respirations
TSAT	transferrin saturation
TT	transplant tourism
Tx	transplantation
U&Es	urea and electrolytes
UF	ultrafiltration
UFF	ultrafiltration failure
UFR	ultrafiltration rate
UK	United Kingdom
UKDEC	UK Donation Ethics Committee
Ur	urea
URR	urea reduction ratio
URTI	upper respiratory tract infection
US	ultrasound
USA	United States of America
USB	universal serial bus
UTI	urinary tract infection
UV	ultraviolet
vs	versus
VA	vascular access
VRE	vancomycin-resistant enterococci
VTE	venous thromboembolism
VZV	varicella zoster virus
WBC	white blood cell
WCC	white cell count
WHO	World Health Organization
wk	week
wkly	weekly
yr	year
yrs	years
yrly	yearly

Contributors

Melissa Chamney
Senior Lecturer, Programme
Manager, Adult Nursing, City
University, London, UK

Peter Ellis
Programme Director CPD
Interprofessional Practice,
Strategic Lead Partnerships;
Internationalisation
Senior Lecturer, Canterbury
Christ Church University,
Canterbury, UK

Diane Green
Principal Renal Dietitian,
Salford Royal Hospitals NHS
Foundation Trust, UK; Honorary
Clinical Lecturer, University of
Chester, Chester, UK

Clare Morlidge
Senior Renal Pharmacist
East and North Hertfordshire
NHS Trust, Lister Hospital,
Stevenage, UK

Hayley Wells
Principal Renal, Transplant
& Urology Pharmacist,
Guy's & St. Thomas'
NHS Foundation Trust,
London, UK

With special thanks to all our family, friends and colleagues, in particular Ray James for their support and understanding completing this Oxford Handbook.

Chapter 1

Renal pathophysiology

Introduction

The aetiology of chronic kidney disease (CKD) is multifactorial; the prevalence and causes vary with ethnicity, geographical, and socio-economic factors. The prevalence of CKD stages 3–5 in the UK is 4.1% with a ♀ to ♂ ratio of 1:1.5.[1] Incidence has risen due to increasing rates of risk factors (e.g. diabetes, hypertension, obesity, smoking, age) plus early detection programmes and increased awareness of CKD. There is also a rise in incidence of communicable diseases, e.g. human immunodeficiency virus (HIV), hepatitis B and C, and tuberculosis (TB), and diseases contracted abroad, such as schistosomiasis. Diabetes continues to be the most common cause of end stage kidney disease (ESKD) in the UK (see 📖 pp. 134–5).

UK Renal Registry causes of ESKD in 2009[2]

- Glomerulonephritis (GN): 11.5%
- Pyelonephritis: 7.3%
- Diabetes: 25.3%
- Renal vascular disease: 6.1%
- Hypertension: 6.9%
- Polycystic kidney disease: 7.3%
- Unknown aetiology: 20.7%
- Other causes: 15.5%

There are many causes of CKD which cannot be covered completely in this chapter; some of the less common conditions can be found in the pathophysiology appendix of this handbook.

Nephrotic syndrome

Nephrotic syndrome is not a disease in itself; it is a common collection of signs and symptoms which reflect glomerular injury and can result from a number of diseases. Damage to the glomerulus causes leakage of large amounts of protein due to increased permeability of the glomerular basement membrane (GBM); however, larger molecules such as red blood cells (RBCs) do not pass into the urine.

The main initial goal is to treat the signs and identify the underlying cause to prevent long-term kidney damage.

Causes

- Idiopathic
- Diabetic glomerulosclerosis
- Focal segmental glomerulosclerosis (FSGS), mesangiocapillary GN, or minimal change GN
- Infections, e.g. HIV, hepatitis B and C, malaria, schistosomiasis
- Neoplasm
- Medications, e.g. non-steroidal anti-inflammatory drugs (NSAIDs), tamoxifen, gold, captopril, penicillamine, antimicrobials
- Renal amyloidosis
- Systemic lupus erythematosus (SLE)—lupus nephritis.

Clinical features

- Initially presents with a complication such as a deep vein thrombosis (DVT) (due to hypercoagulable state), infection, or shortness of breath (SOB)
- Frothy urine as a result of proteinuria
- Generalized oedema, e.g. periorbital, pitting oedema to legs, pleural effusion, pericardial effusion, ascites:
  - ↓ plasma oncotic pressure 2° to ↓ serum albumin (Alb) → ↓ circulating blood volume → release of renin → ↑ aldosterone → sodium (Na^+) and water (H_2O) retention → fluid in tissue → oedema
- Proteinuria >3.5g/24hrs or protein: creatinine ratio (PCR) >350mg/mmol
- Lipiduria
- Hypoalbuminaemia <25g/L 2° to protein excretion
- ↑ production of lipoproteins → hyperlipidaemia, ± cholesterol deposits (xanthomas)
- BP can be normal, may be ↑ or ↓
- Rash, e.g. butterfly rash seen in SLE
- Evidence of neuropathy or retinopathy in diabetes.

Management

- Identify and treat the underlying cause, drugs commonly used include corticosteroids, immunosuppression (see 📖 p. 489), cytotoxic (e.g. cyclophosphamide)
- ► Cytotoxics—observe for side effects, e.g. ↓ white cell count (WCC), ↑ risk of infection, nausea and vomiting, haemorrhagic cystitis (usually prescribed oral mesna to protect the bladder and an antiemetic):
  - teratogenic—discuss risks of infertility and ensure ♀ aware not to get pregnant
  - ↑ oral fluids, intravenous (IV) fluids as per medical orders
- Use angiotensin-converting enzyme inhibitor (ACEI) or angiotensin receptor antagonist (ARB) to ↓ blood pressure (BP), aim for BP 125/75mmHg and for their antiproteinuric effect (see 📖 p. 92)
- Fluid management:
  - restrict Na^+ intake <2.4g/24hrs (salt intake <6g/24hrs)
  - ↓ oedema using diuretics, e.g. furosemide, ± IV diuretics if severely oedematous
  - daily weight and monitor input and urine output (medical staff will set a target weight loss, e.g. 0.5kg loss/24hrs)
  - monitor lying and standing BP, observe for any postural drop which may indicate hypovolaemia
  - daily electrolytes to monitor Na^+ and potassium (K^+)
- ± protein restriction—liaise with medical staff and renal dietitian
- Hypercoagulable state caused by ↑ platelet aggregation, ↓ anti-coagulant factors, ↑ procoagulant factors, ↓ intravascular volume,
  ↑ HCT 2° diuretics and ↓ mobility which can lead to:
  - DVT or pulmonary emboli, observe for signs of SOB, chest pain, leg pain /swelling, ↓ O_2 saturation
  - renal vein thrombosis, observe for signs of flank pain or development of haematuria (associated with membranous nephropathy and renal amyloidosis)
  - ± high-risk patients may require prophylactic anticoagulation aiming to keep international normalized ratio (INR) 2–3 whilst nephrotic
- Monitor for signs of infection, e.g. pyrexia, ↑ WCC:
  - more susceptible to infection (occurs in ~20% patients) due to ↓ complement activity and impaired T-cell function
  - treat any signs of infection
  - observe skin integrity as more prone to skin tears → cellulitis (common in the lower limbs)
- Treat dyslipidaemia (e.g. statin and/or low-fat diet) to prevent cardiovascular events
- Acute kidney injury (AKI) is uncommon; however it may occur (see 📖 p. 100).

Acute nephritic syndrome

Nephritic syndrome is a collection of signs and symptoms and is similar to nephrotic syndrome (see 📖 pp. 4–5); however, the damage to the glomerulus allows larger molecules such as RBCs to pass through to the urine. The resulting inflammation to the glomerulus causes reduced kidney function and Na^+ and H_2O retention which leads to hypertension.

Causes

- IgA nephropathy
- Henoch–Schönlein purpura (HSP)
- SLE—lupus nephritis
- Postinfective GN
- Anti-GBM disease
- Small vessel vasculitis, e.g. antineutrophil cytoplasmic antibody (ANCA) +ve
- Idiopathic crescentic GN
- Mesangiocapillary GN.

Clinical features

- Symptoms may be gradual or progress rapidly to an AKI—kidney biopsy to tailor treatment to the underlying cause
- Hypoalbuminaemia
- Haematuria ± RBC casts
- Proteinuria <3.5g/24hrs
- Mild hypertension
- Impaired kidney function, e.g. ↑ urea (Ur), ↑ creatinine (Cr)
- ± azotaemia/oliguria.

Management

- Manage fluid status:
  - accurate daily fluid volume assessment and adjust intake according to urine output and fluid volume
  - ± fluid allowance as prescribed by medical staff, e.g. 1L/24hrs
  - restrict Na^+ intake <2.4g/24hrs (salt intake <6g/24hrs)
  - ± loop diuretic to ↑ fluid removal
  - daily weight
- Lying and standing BP, aim for BP ≤130/80mmHg:
  - ± ↑ BP as a result of ↑ fluid volume
  - if dehydrated may require IV fluids
- Monitor liver function tests (LFTs), urea and electrolytes (U&Es), and full blood count (FBC) daily
- ± haemodialysis (HD) if AKI (see 📖 pp. 116–19)
- Refer to renal dietitian for nutritional assessment and supplementation (see 📖 pp. 202–3)
- Treat the underlying infection if present
- Management of the underlying systemic disease, drugs commonly used include corticosteroids, cytotoxics, and IS (see 📖 p. 489).

Primary glomerular diseases/disorders

Causes

Hereditary
- Alport's syndrome, Fabry's syndrome, and thin basement membrane (TBM) disease.

Primary
- IgA nephropathy.

Secondary to other diseases
- Diabetes mellitus, SLE, bacterial endocarditis.

Glomerulus
- The normal functioning of the glomerulus depends on a structurally intact GBM and adequate renal blood flow
- The glomerulus has 3 layers which together function as a selective filtration barrier preventing large molecules, e.g. proteins and blood, passing into the urine:
  - fenestrated endothelium
  - GBM
  - podocytes.

Glomerulonephritis
GN is the term used for those glomerular disorders that usually involve immune-mediated injury as a result of circulating immune complexes deposited within the glomerulus.
- Exogenous (e.g. bacterial)
- Endogenous (autoimmune, e.g. SLE) as seen in Figure 1.1.
- A 2° response → fibrin deposits within the glomerulus causing glomerular damage and ↑ capillary permeability as a result of:
  - complement activation
  - inflammation with neutrophils
  - T cell dysfunction
  - platelet aggregation
  - activation of the kinin system.

Resultant damage to the glomerulus allows loss of large molecules such as proteins, which would normally be kept in the blood, to pass into the urine. In some conditions, such as anti-GBM disease, there are deposits of anti-GBM antibodies which activate the 2° response. This can result in the basement membranes of other organs being affected, for example, in the pulmonary alveoli in Goodpasture's syndrome (see 📖 p. 580).

Classification of GN
Classification of GN includes the assessment of clinical features, history, histology and/or aetiology. Terms used to describe the extent of the damage to the glomerulus include proliferative, meaning throughout the glomerulus or focal, affecting only one area.

Acute GN
- Kidneys appear normal in size or enlarged and oedematous.

Chronic GN
- Kidneys are normal in size or small and show cortical scarring.

Presentation
- Acutely with nephrotic syndrome or acute nephritis (see 📖 pp. 4–5, 6)
- May be an incidental finding when being investigated for another problem, e.g. proteinuria found on routine urinalysis.

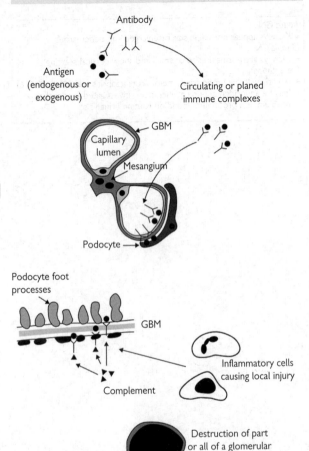

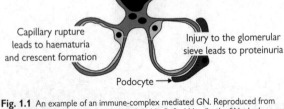

Fig. 1.1 An example of an immune-complex mediated GN. Reproduced from Steddon S, Ashman N, Chesser A, et al. (eds). *Oxford Handbook of Nephrology and Hypertension*, Oxford: Oxford University Press, 2007, with permission from Oxford University Press.

Non-proliferative glomerulonephritis

Minimal change GN (minimal change disease)

Exact pathophysiology is unknown. Fusion of the podocyte foot processes occurs in the glomerulus due to production of glomerular permeability factor. This allows large molecules to pass through the filtration barrier.

- Good prognosis (80–90% remission), affecting 1.3♂:♀ of all ages:
  - accounts for 20% of nephrotic syndrome cases (adults)
  - most common cause of nephrotic syndrome in children (tends to respond well to treatment)
- Diagnosis is made on kidney biopsy.

Causes include:

- Trigger, e.g. allergen, immunization, or viral illness
- HIV
- Drugs, e.g. NSAIDs, lithium, antimicrobials e.g. rifampicin, cephalosporins, sulfasalazines
- Malignancy —Hodgkin's lymphoma.

Clinical features

- Proteinuria ± nephrotic syndrome, severe oedema, i.e. peri-orbital, pleural and pericardial effusions, hypovolaemia → ↓ BP
- Renal impairment (60% in adults, 20% children), ↓ Alb, ± haematuria, lipiduria, ↑ cholesterol, ± localized skin infection, abdominal pain (can lead to spontaneous peritonitis).

Management

- As for nephrotic syndrome (see 🕮 p. 5)
- Corticosteroids and IS with 80–90% remission and 30–70% relapse
- Complications include renal thrombosis, DVT; AKI 2° acute acute tubular necrosis (ATN).

Membranous glomerulonephritis (MGN)

GBM thickening with granular deposits of immunoglobulin IgG → endothelial cell proliferation throughout all of the glomeruli.

- Occurs between ages of 40–60yrs with a ratio of 2♂:1♀ and is the most common cause of nephrotic syndrome (20–30%)
- 1/3rd progress to ESKD in 10–20yrs; 1/3rd have spontaneous remission
- 5% progress to crescentic GN (rapid deterioration in kidney function).

Causes include:

- Idiopathic (75%)
- Solid tumours (10%), e.g. lung, prostate, or bowel
- Hodgkin's and non-Hodgkin's lymphoma
- Hepatitis B and C
- Malaria, syphilis, schistosomiasis, streptococcal infection
- SLE, rheumatoid arthritis, diabetes mellitus
- Drugs e.g. penicillamine, captopril, NSAIDs, heroin, gold.

Clinical features
- Nephrotic syndrome, proteinuria, microscopic haematuria, ↑ BP, ↓ Alb, ↑ low-density lipoprotein (LDL), ↑ cholesterol, ↓ immunoglobulins IgG >IgA.

Management
- Treat and manage the underlying condition or disease
- Treatment as for nephrotic syndrome (see 📖 p. 5)
- Lifestyle modifications (see 📖 pp. 84–5)
- ± corticosteroids, cytotoxics, and/or IS aiming at stopping the progression of kidney damage (see 📖 p. 489)
- Good prognosis if normal kidney function and <4g/24hrs proteinuria
- Poorer prognosis if impaired kidney function proteinuria >10g/24hrs and persistent proteinuria 4g/24hrs >1yr.

Focal segmental glomerulosclerosis (FSGS)

Some of the glomeruli are affected (i.e. focal) with sclerotic changes and hyaline deposits in the capillary lumen. There are no immune complex deposits present.
- More common in men-2♂:1♀
- 50% of patients with FSGS will progress to ESKD
- Diagnosed on kidney biopsy
- Recurrent disease post transplantation (Tx) ranges from 30–90% and tends to be higher if age of onset of the original disease was at a younger age and disease progression is aggressive.

Causes
- Idiopathic
- Alport's syndrome
- Renovascular disease
- Membranous nephropathy
- IgA nephropathy
- Sickle cell disease
- IV heroin use
- Pre-eclampsia
- SLE
- Reflux nephropathy
- Diabetic nephropathy
- Anti-GBM disease
- Infective endocarditis
- HIV nephropathy
- Morbid obesity.

Clinical features
- Proteinuria, ↑ BP or nephrotic syndrome (Alb <20g/L; see 📖 p. 4), less proteinuria in 2° FSGS, microscopic haematuria, renal impairment, ↑ cholesterol, and ↑ LDL
- Alb <20g/L usually progress to ESKD.

Management
- Identify and treat the underlying cause
- ACEI and/or ARBs → ↓ proteinuria and ↓ BP
- ± corticosteroids, IS, cytotoxics (see 📖 p. 489)
- Lifestyle modifications (see 📖 pp. 84–5)
- Treat hyperlipidaemia, e.g. statin and low-fat diet
- Antifibrotic agents, e.g. pirfenidone, rosiglitazone to ↓ progression
- Poor prognosis in young black men with proteinuria >10g/24hrs.

Proliferative glomerulonephritis

Membranoproliferative/mesangiocapillary GN (MCGN)

Deposits of immune complexes in the glomerulus causing thickening of the GBM and mesangial proliferation.

- MCGN affects ♂ = ♀ aged between 8–30yrs
- More common in developing countries
- 50% progress to ESKD at 10yrs
- Investigations are aimed at identifying the underlying causes and include immunoglobulins, protein electrophoresis, hepatitis B and C serology, rheumatoid factor, and cryoglobulins
- 3 subtypes: type II MCGN may recur in a transplanted kidney.

Causes include:

- Idiopathic
- Hepatitis B and C
- Autoimmune, e.g. SLE
- Chronic infections
- Schistosomiasis
- Mixed cryoglobulinaemia
- Chronic thrombotic microangiopathies
- Sjögren's syndrome.

Clinical features

- ↑ BP, ± microscopic haematuria, ± acute nephritis, ± nephrotic syndrome, e.g. proteinuria >3.5g/24hrs, ↓ Alb, ↑ cholesterol, ± rapidly progressive renal impairment
- ± ↑ complements, rhesus (Rh) factor, cryoglobulins depending on underlying cause.

Management

- Treat the underlying cause
- Restrict Na⁺ intake <2.4g/24hrs (salt intake <6g/24hrs)
- ± use of diuretic and management of BP <130/80mmHg
- ↓ proteinuria using an ACEI or ARB
- ↓ cholesterol (e.g. statin)
- Lifestyle modifications (see 📖 pp. 84–5)
- ± corticosteroids, mycophenolate mofetil (MMF) + corticosteroids in progressive renal impairment (see 📖 p. 489)
- ± antiplatelet drugs, e.g. aspirin and dipyridamole trial for persistent proteinuria to slow progression.

Rapidly progressive or crescentic GN (RPGN)

Compression of the glomeruli and Bowman's capsule occurs as a result of increasing numbers of epithelial cells and macrophages. The increased pressure causes damage to the glomeruli and leakage of fibrin.

- Crescent shapes are formed which can be seen under electron microscopy, hence the term crescentic GN

- There are 3 subtypes:
  - type I is anti-GBM antibody disease
  - type II is immune complex RPGN, e.g. lupus nephritis
  - type III is pauci-immune, e.g. renal limited vasculitis or ANCA +ve.
- RPGN affects ♂=♀
- May take only days to progress or longer, e.g. months
- It has a poor prognosis, usually rapidly progressing to ESKD
- Diagnosis is made following a kidney biopsy, ANCA, and presence of anti-GBM antibodies.

Causes include:
- Idiopathic
- Goodpasture's syndrome
- Wegner's granulomatosis
- Polyarteritis nodosa
- SLE, e.g. lupus nephritis
- HSP, post-infectious, e.g. streptococcal infection, infective endocarditis
- Cryoglobuminaemia
- Churg–Strauss syndrome.

Clinical features
- Flu-like symptoms, e.g. fever, arthralgia, myalgia, fatigue, abdominal pain
- Central nervous system (CNS) involvement, e.g. seizures
- Microscopic polyangiitis, necrotizing arteritis, e.g. livedo reticularis
- Allergic asthma, ↑ eosinophils in Churg–Strauss syndrome
- Anti-GBM—respiratory tract symptoms, e.g. sinusitis, cough, haemoptysis
- Macroscopic haematuria (red cell casts), proteinuria
- Renal impairment, ↑ BP oliguria, oedema, and rapidly progressing to ESKD.

Management
- Aim treatment at underlying cause
- Prevent and treat infection
- ± corticosteroids, cytotoxic drugs (see 📖 p. 489)
- ± IS (see 📖 p. 489)
- Plasma exchange (see 📖 p. 416)
- Lifestyle modifications (see 📖 pp. 84–5).

Immunoglobulin A nephropathy

IgA is deposited in the mesangium of the glomerulus causing cell proliferation and the influx of inflammatory cells causes injury to the glomerulus.

- Globally, most common cause of GN, usually presenting with microscopic haematuria:
  - patients often asymptomatic; usually 20–30yrs of age; long-term kidney damage is common
  - more common in Asians and Southern Europeans
- Diagnosis includes ↑ IgA (50%), urine microscopy, PCR, 24hr protein urine collection; if rash present may require a skin biopsy and kidney biopsy to distinguish from other causes of GN.

Causes

- May be idiopathic in nature
- Possible genetic basis and is associated with inflammatory bowel disease or coeliac disease, skin/joint diseases, e.g. psoriasis and HSP
- Liver disease, especially alcoholic liver disease.

Clinical features

- Micro- or macroscopic haematuria, ± asymptomatic
- Usually associated with recent upper respiratory tract infection (URTI) or febrile illness
- ± vasculitic rash
- Proteinuria (usually not in the nephrotic range i.e. <3.5g/24hrs)
- ± AKI if rapidly progressive GN
- ↑ BP.

Management is dependent on severity

- BP ≤125/75mmHg and to ↓ proteinuria to <1g/24hrs, first-line ACEI or ARB (see 📖 p. 92)
- Fish oils to limit progression of disease
- Lifestyle modifications (see 📖 pp. 84–5)
- Corticosteroids if nephrotic
- Crescentic IgAN may require IS and corticosteroids (see 📖 p. 489).

Prognosis

- Dependent on the degree of renal impairment
- ~50% chance of recurrence following a kidney Tx; however, this is not a contraindication for transplantation and does not necessarily lead to graft loss and failure.

Progression to ESKD is more common in those with

- Impaired kidney function
- Heavy proteinuria (>3g/24hrs)
- Difficult to manage BP
- Tubulo-interstitial fibrosis or rapidly progressive crescentic IgA nephropathy.

Secondary glomerular diseases/disorders

Causes include SLE, HSP, tumours, amyloid, diabetes, drug treatment, and infections.

Lupus nephritis

SLE is a multi-organ autoimmune disease which may affect joints, skin, vasculature, nervous system, heart, and kidneys. Immune complexes are deposited along the basement membrane, causing either diffuse proliferative GN, membranous glomerulopathy, or focal proliferative GN (see 📖 pp. 8–10).

* Common in those of non-European descent such as Afro-Caribbeans or Asians and affects 9♀: 1♂
* Onset of symptoms usually age 15–50yrs; no known cure
* Diagnosis by kidney biopsy and presence of autoantibodies
* Transplantation is not contraindicated if lupus is quiescent.

Clinical features

* Proteinuria and/or microscopic haematuria, ↑ BP (20–50%), ↓ kidney function (20–30%).

> ### Management
> * IS agents, steroids, and cytotoxic drugs (see 📖 p. 489)
> * Advise on pregnancy for ♀ child-bearing yrs (see 📖 pp. 544–6)
> * The main aim of treatment is to maintain remission and prevent progression of kidney disease by lifestyle changes, e.g. smoking cessation, ↑ exercise, ↓ salt intake <6g/24hrs (see 📖 pp. 84–5)
> * Maintain BP <130/80mmHg; ACEI or ARB if proteinuric >1g/24hrs
> * Treat lipidaemia (e.g. statin).

Hepatitis C

Hepatitis C virus (HCV) causes hepatitis, cirrhosis of the liver, and hepatocellular cancer.

* Causes MCGN due to cryoglobulin deposits in medium and small vessels of the skin, joints, and glomeruli → inflammation and injury.

Clinical features

* Weight loss, lethargy, ± purpuric rash to legs, arthralgia, heptatosplenomegaly, Raynaud's phenomenon, ± acute or disseminated vasculitis
* Renal signs: haematuria, proteinuria, ↑ BP, renal impairment, AKI.

Hepatitis B

It is estimated that 350 million people are infected by hepatitis B virus (HBV) worldwide. Prevalence is higher in areas such as Africa and South-East Asia.

- In adults, it can cause either membranous GN, MCGN, or polyarteritis nodosa (PAN)
- Diagnosed on kidney biopsy or other tissue for PAN
- Seroconversion from hepatitis B e antigen (HBeAg) +ve to hepatitis B e antibody (HBeAb) +ve ↓ renal impairment

Clinical features
- Heavy proteinuria (nephrotic syndrome), liver disease, ↑ BP, haematuria and progressive renal impairment, PAN is treated with corticosteroids and plasma exchange.

Management
- *Hepatitis B:*
  - refer to hepatologist for treatment—the aim is to clear the virus with drugs such as interferon and lamivudine
  - offer immunization to the family for hepatitis B and the patient requires vaccinating against hepatitis A
- test for hepatitis C infection and HBV DNA
- *Hepatitis C:*
  - interferon and antiviral agents, however they will not reverse kidney damage
  - use ACEI to ↓ proteinuria
- offer immunization to the patient for hepatitis A and B
- *Hepatitis B and C:* patient and family members should be provided with education on:
  - avoiding sharing razors, nail clippers, earrings, toothbrushes
  - practising safe sex, e.g. using condoms
  - minimizing alcohol intake.
▶Transplantation in HBV, HCV, and HIV patients is not contraindicated but is best planned in collaboration with hepatology and virology specialists (see 📖 p. 448).

HIV-associated nephropathy (HIVAN)

HIVAN is increasing due to rises in HIV infection rates i.e. 33 million worldwide. HIV infection of the renal proximal tubular cells and podo-cytes → collapsing FSGS and cystic tubular dilatation. Progression to ESKD occurs within 1–4 months and HIVAN accounts for ~60% of HIV kidney lesions. Other causes of CKD are associated with the following:
- Use of nephrotoxins (e.g. amphotericin), highly active antiretroviral therapy (HAART) causing ATN and AKI (usually reversible)
- Precipitation of crystals in renal tubules, e.g. drugs such as sulfadiazine, aciclovir
- Other diseases, e.g., hepatitis B, C, or syphilis (e.g. membranous GN)
- IgA deposits, postinfectious GN, interstitial nephritis—cytomegalovirus virus (CMV) or drug, e.g. trimethoprim, sulfamethoxazole
- Amyloidosis

- Thrombotic thrombocytopenia purpura (TTP)
- Risk factors include advanced HIV, low CD4 count, black population (genetic and environmental links), presence of other co-morbid conditions (e.g. diabetes), family history (FH) of CKD.

Clinical features
- Proteinuria (nephrotic syndrome, see 📖 p. 4–5), renal impairment, oedema, and normal BP.

Management
- Antiretroviral therapy, using the HAART regimen have been shown to slow rate of progression of kidney disease
- Use of ACEI to reduce proteinuria, ± steroids.

Renal parenchymal disease/tubular and interstitial disease

Pyelonephritis (PN)

Accounts for ~8% of primary kidney disease in the UK; caused by bacterial infection affecting the renal parenchyma usually due to lower urinary tract infection (UTI).

- The most common organisms are *Escherichia coli*, *Proteus*, *Pseudomonas* and *Klebsiella* spp
- Diagnosis is made by ↑ WCCs, ↑ C-reactive protein (CRP), urine and blood cultures:
  - US of the kidneys may show enlargement.

Acute PN

- More common in ♀
- Risk factors include urinary tract structural abnormalities, pregnancy, diabetes, sexual intercourse, post procedure or trauma to the urinary tract, obstructive condition, or with chronic illness
- In ♂ more common >40yrs of age with kidney stones or prostate disease.

Chronic PN

- Nephrosclerosis 2° to chronic repeated infections
- Common complication in adults who as a child suffered from ureteric reflux and repeated infections, or an obstruction 2° to renal calculi, or a structural malformation that causes urinary stasis.

Clinical features

- Loin pain, nausea and vomiting, ± UTI symptoms, e.g. burning, offensive smelling urine, frequency, ± rigors, untreated can lead to septicaemia.

Management

- ↑ fluids, if unable to drink orally IV fluids to maintain hydration
- IV antibiotics
- Reverse obstruction if this is the cause.

Acute interstitial nephritis (AIN)

An inflammatory reaction → inflammatory cells (e.g. T cells and mono-cytes) move in to the interstitial tissue → compression of the renal tubules, ↓ glomerular filtration, and impaired H_2O and solute reabsorption.

- ♂=♀ usually age 50–60yrs.

Causes

- Idiopathic
- Drugs, e.g. proton pump inhibitor (PPI; e.g. omeprazole), NSAIDs, antibiotics (e.g. penicillin, rifampicin, cefalotin/cephalothin), allopurinol, diuretics (e.g. furosemide, thiazide)

- Chinese herbal remedies
- Infections, viral e.g. HIV, TB, hepatitis C, streptococcal, Epstein–Barr virus (EBV)
- Malignancy
- Collagen vascular disease, sarcoidosis, Sjögren's syndrome
- Common cause of AKI 2° to an inflammatory disease.

Clinical features
- ± ↑ BP, renal impairment, oliguria, flank pain, impaired kidney function rapidly progressing to AKI, allergic reactions may be accompanied by a rash, arthralgia, fever, eosinophilia, eosinophiluria, sterile pyuria with a nothing abnormal detected (NAD) urinalysis.

Management
- Identify and stop the cause, e.g. medication with renal impairment resolving usually once drug stopped
- Corticosteroids
- Acute HD if AKI (see 📖 pp. 116–19).

Chronic interstitial diseases
As a result of chronic inflammation, fibrosis and scarring causing the loss of renal tubular function.

Causes include:
- Drugs, e.g. NSAIDs, lithium, Chinese herbal remedies
- Lead poisoning
- Infections, e.g. TB
- Reflux nephropathy
- Sarcoidosis
- Autoimmune diseases, e.g. Sjögren's syndrome
- Sickle cell disease
- Chronic pyelonephritis.

Clinical features
- Polyuria, nocturia, proteinuria, pyuria, glycosuria 2° to renal tubular acidosis, renal impairment.

Management
- Lithium monitoring with annual kidney function check and avoid thiazide diuretics → ↑ lithium plasma concentration
- Treat underlying cause, e.g. infection
- Manage as for CKD (see 📖 p. 126).

Cystic diseases

Cystic disease is hereditary, developmental, or acquired. Not all lead to renal impairment. Simple cysts in the kidney increase with age; incidence ~50% aged >50yrs. Most patients are asymptomatic; the cyst(s) often an incidental finding or diagnosed when a cyst ruptures causing flank pain.
• Kidney function is not affected; but important to scan simple cysts by computed tomography (CT) if US shows abnormally echoic cysts to rule out malignancy.

Autosomal dominant polycystic kidney disease (ADPKD)

ADPKD accounts for ~5–10% of ESKD patients on renal replacement therapy (RRT), occurs in 1:400–1:1000 live births and is an inherited autosomal dominant disease. Cysts originate in the distal tubules and as they grow they compress the parenchymal tissue and cause glomerulosclerosis. Fluid-filled (yellow) cysts ↑ in size → rupture.
• Carriers can be ♂ or ♀ with 50% risk in a child if one parent has defect
• ± FH of the disease; genetic testing available but use uncommon
• Disease may not become evident until age 20–40yrs
• ↑ risk ESKD ADPKD type 1 and early symptomatic presentation
• If the native kidneys causing recurrent infection ± extremely large, bilateral nephrectomy may be recommended prior to transplantation.
• Diagnosis: US or CT scan—enlarged kidneys; multiple cysts throughout.

There are 2 types of ADPKD
• ADPKD 1:
  • mutation on chromosome 16
  • more common type occurring in about 85% of cases
• ADPKD 2:
  • mutation on chromosome 4
  • 15% of cases; present in older age and progresses more slowly.

Clinical features
• Flank pain as a result of bleeding in the kidney
• ↑ BP, renal impairment, polyuria or nocturia due to inability to concentrate the urine, proteinuria (<1g/24hrs)
• Microscopic haematuria, ± macroscopic haematuria at times
• Renal calculi (20%)
• Cysts to liver (10–40%), pancreas, and spleen
• Intracranial aneurysms (ICAs) (4–10%).

Management
- Aim for BP ≤130/80mmHg; 1° ACEI/ARB (see 📖 p. 92)
- ↓ cardiovascular (CV) risk, e.g. statin and low-fat diet, smoking cessation (see 📖 pp. 84–5)
- Ruptured cysts
- Pain control and bed rest
- Observe for signs of infection (e.g. pyrexia, flank pain); treat PRN
- IV fluids
- Prevent ± treat renal calculi (uric acid or calcium oxalate common)
- Screen with cranial magnetic resonance imaging (MRI) if FH of ICAs.

Renal vasculitis

Vasculitis is caused by an inflammatory response which damages the blood vessels and may cause an aneurysm, haemorrhage, ischaemia, or an infarct secondary to an occlusion. Vasculitis may be classified by size, type, and location of the vessels affected and the presence of ANCA antibodies. Causes are either primary or secondary, e.g. infective endocarditis, systemic infection, or paraneoplastic state.

Polyarteritis nodosa

PAN is a systemic vascular condition which involves inflammation of the small and medium blood vessels causing focal, segmental, or necrotizing GN, followed by RPGN, and may be associated with hepatitis B infection.

- Usually occurs between the ages of 40–60yrs and ♂=♀
- Can affect the heart, gut, and CNS
- Renal infarction 2° to ↑ BP can lead to progressive renal impairment
- 5yr survival rate is ~80% with treatment; ↓ when associated with hepatitis B (~73%)
- Risk factors for poor prognosis include age >50yrs, renal impairment, gut or cardiac complications with ↑ prognosis if diagnosed early
- Diagnosis is usually made on angiogram and/or biopsy.

Clinical features

- Arthralgia, myalgia, fever, and weight loss
- Mottled purple discoloration of the lower limbs (livedo reticularis) and peripheral neuropathy
- Gastrointestinal (GI) involvement—abdominal pain or blood-stained faeces
- Renal signs include renal impairment, ↑ BP, haematuria, or flank pain (renal infarcts).

Management

- Corticosteroids, cyclophosphamide, ± methotrexate, IS, e.g. azathioprine and drug choice is dependent on severity of the disease (see 📖 p. 489)
- ACEI or ARB to ↓ BP <130/80mmHg
- Hepatitis B antigen +ve patients may require interferon-alpha and plasmapheresis (see 📖 p. 416).

Other vasculitides

Churg–Strauss syndrome

Multisystem, presents with allergic rhinitis, asthma, and eosinophilia; affects small and medium vessels mainly in the lungs and skin. It can be present for wks or yrs before vasculitic symptoms appear. ♂=♀ with unknown aetiology and causes vasculitis ± focal and segmental necrotizing GN.

- Treatment includes corticosteroids, ± alkylating agents, ± interferon with ~40% relapsing.

Cryoglobulinaemia: 2° to inflammation in capillaries, venules and arterioles from deposits of immune complexes (see 📖 p. 18).

Vasculitis: 2° connective tissue disease/disorders, e.g. SLE, rheumatoid arthritis affecting the small arteries, arterioles and venules, +ve antinuclear antibody (ANA).

Other causes: these include hypersensitivity to a drug, viral infection, e.g. HBV and HBC, CMV, EBV, appear similar to PAN or microscopic polyangiitis.

ANCA +ve small vessel vasculitis

Involves the small vessels, capillaries, venules, and arterioles → a focal necrotizing crescentic GN and associated with ANCA +ve serology.
- In Europe it affects ~20 per million population (PMP) with ♂=♀:
  - ↑ incidence with age peaking at 55–70yrs
- ↑ mortality rate, 90% at 2yrs untreated; 70–80% 1yr survival if treated
- Risk of recurrence, 25–50% within 3–5yrs; more common in Wegener's granulomatosis
- Disease needs to be quiescent prior to transplantation
- Renal limited vasculitis is known as a pauci-immune GN and, although it is ANCA +ve, there is no evidence of systemic disease.
  - No immune or complement deposits are found on kidney biopsy.

Causes include:
- Wegener's granulomatosis—a systemic vasculitis affecting the medium and small arteries, venules, and arterioles. It is rare and commonly causes inflammation of the respiratory system, e.g. nasal passages, upper respiratory system, as well as the kidneys, causing a necrotizing vasculitis (ANCA PR3 +ve)
- Microscopic polyangiitis/polyarteritis
- Renal limited vasculitis.

Clinical features
- Fever, weight loss, malaise, myalgia, and polyarthritis
- Upper respiratory tract symptoms, e.g. nasal discharge, epistaxis, sinusitis, oral or nasal ulcers, otitis media (deafness), cartilaginous involvement, e.g. collapse of nasal bridge and tracheal stenosis
- Pulmonary, e.g. cough, dyspnoea, haemoptysis, pulmonary haemorrhage
- Renal, e.g. asymptomatic urinary abnormalities to rapidly progressive GN and AKI
- Skin, e.g. palpable purpura or diffuse fine vasculitic rash
- Peripheral neuropathy
- Optic, e.g. conjunctivitis, uveitis, optic tract granulomata and proptosis
- GI, e.g. abdominal pain and bloody diarrhoea
- DVT.

Management
- Induction therapy—IV prednisolone (usually pulsed) is used if ↑ Cr >500µmol/L or pulmonary haemorrhage
- Cytotoxic, e.g. cyclophosphamide
- ± plasma exchange 5–7 consecutive days for those with pulmonary haemorrhage (see 🔲 p. 416)
- HD if AKI (see 🔲 pp. 116–19)
- Maintenance treatment usually given for 2–5yrs of oral prednisolone, azathioprine, MMF, or methotrexate.

Renal vascular disease

Hypertensive nephropathy/nephrosclerosis is covered in ☐ Hypertension (see ☐ p. 74).

Renal artery stenosis (RAS)

Stenosis of one or more renal arteries caused by fibromuscular dysplasia (fibrous thickening of artery wall) or atheroma in artery wall.

- ↓ renal blood flow 2° to narrowing of the vessel → stimulates the release of renin and the production of angiotensin II → vasoconstriction, release of aldosterone and sodium retention, ↑ BP, and ↓ glomerular filtration rate (GFR)
- ↑ incidence (~50%) with atherosclerosis or peripheral vascular disease (PVD), compared with ~7% of people >65yrs of age
  - ↑ risk of CV event such as myocardial infarction (MI) or cerebrovascular accident (CVA)
- Diagnosed using renal US, DPTA (diethylene triamine pentaacetic acid) ± MAG3 (mercaptoacetyltriglycine), Doppler ± angiogram.

Clinical features
- ↑ BP ± difficult to control
- ↓ GFR
- ↑ ≤20% Cr or ↓ 15% in GFR post commencement of ACEI or ARB
- Ankle oedema due to fluid retention
- Orthopnoea and pulmonary congestion
- NAD urinalysis
- PVD, abdominal aortic aneurysm (AAA), abdominal bruits
- Loin pain and new haematuria due to renal infarct.

Management
- Conservative: aim for BP <130/85mmHg; do not use ACEI or ARB, e.g. loop diuretic, β-blocker, or vasodilator, ± multiple agents to control BP:
  - ± aspirin for prevention of CV and cerebrovascular events
  - patient education re modifying risk factors (see ☐ pp. 84–5)
- Interventional treatment: either percutaneous transluminal renal angioplasty (PTRA) ± stent (⚠ may recur without stenting) or surgical revascularization if:
  - 70% stenosis
  - bilateral renal arteries are involved
  - disease present in one single functioning kidney.

Renal vein thrombosis

Can be unilateral or bilateral; causes reduced renal blood flow and kidney function. Commonly associated with nephrotic syndrome and malignancy. Diagnosis is made by venogram, CT scan, or renal Doppler.

Clinical features
- Renal infarct—flank and loin pain; tenderness, macroscopic haematuria, renal impairment, and ↑ lactate dehydrogenase (LDH)

- Pulmonary emboli
- Nephrotic syndrome with tumours, e.g. renal cell carcinoma (see 📖 p. 5).

Management
Anticoagulation until non-nephrotic (alb >35g/L).

Fibromuscular dysplasia
Caused by the formation of fibrous tissue within arterial walls. A non-inflammatory and non-atherosclerotic condition, commonly affecting internal carotids and renal vessels.
- Usually affects the mid-distal renal artery and causes a ↓ in kidney perfusion → activation of the renin–angiotensin system resulting in ↑ BP
- More common in younger ♀; usually asymptomatic with ↑ BP
- Diagnosed using renal angiogram.

Clinical features
- Transient ischaemic attacks (TIAs), CVA, and ↑ BP.

Management
- Managing BP using an ACEI or ARB as first line and then adding a thiazide diuretic
- Revascularization either via PTRA or surgery.

Cholesterol emboli
More common in older people, typically post angiography/aortic surgery. Associated with thrombolytic and anticoagulant treatments.
- Cholesterol emboli (crystal emboli) that travel from the aorta or renal arteries → distal small renal vessels → inflammatory response and occlusion → ↓ O_2 → ischaemia and fibrosis
- Diagnosis is made using angiography and/or kidney biopsy.

Clinical features
- NAD urinalysis, ± heavy proteinuria
- ± fever, myalgia due to inflammatory response
- Eosinophilia and eosinophiluria
- ↓ C_3 C_4 complement levels
- Embolic infarcts of distal regions, e.g. retina and legs (livedo reticularis)
- ± AKI 2° multiple emboli or ↓ kidney function.

Management
Supportive with the aim to ↓ BP; (ACEI/ARB); ↓ cholesterol (statin).

Systemic disease

Multiple myeloma (MM)

In this cancer, affecting the plasma cells (a type of white blood cell (WBC)) responsible for the production of antibodies, an accumulation of abnormal plasma cells in the bone marrow form lesions ∴ affecting normal production of RBCs. There are Ig light chains produced by abnormal (neoplastic) plasma cells. Antibody light chains filtered through the glomerulus are reabsorbed in the proximal tubule.

- In MM there is a high concentration of light chains; not all reabsorbed → urinary excretion (Bence Jones proteinuria, see 📖 p. 56). Light chains are toxic, causing inflammation, blockage (light chain casts) and long-term damage → contrast–induced nephropathy and ↑ Ca^{2+} (↑ with dehydration)
- ↑ nephrotoxicity 2° to the use of NSAIDs, radiocontrast media, ACE or ARB to treat MM
- 3 stages: stage I—median survival 62 months; stage III—29 months.
  - More common in ♂; usually >60yrs; renal impairment in ~50%.

Clinical features

- Osteoporosis, bone pain or back pain, ± pathological fractures
- Weight loss, anaemia, ↓ WCC, ↑ risk of infection and pyelonephritis
- Proteinuria, ↑ Ca^{2+}, hyperuricaemia, amyloidosis
- Renal impairment with volume depletion or AKI.

Management

- Treat causes of AKI
- Dehydration: ↑ oral intake, IV fluids, may require large volume if ↑ Ca^{2+} (3–5L/24hrs)—high fluid input to minimize light chain precipitation in renal tubules
- Fluid balance, i.e. input and output, daily weight, lying and standing BP, closely monitor if history of heart failure (HF) and oliguric/anuric
- Refer to anaemia team—erythropoietin stimulating agent (ESA) may be required (blood transfusion associated with hyperviscosity with high paraprotein levels)
- IV bisphosphonate, e.g. zoledronic acid if still Ca^{2+} ↑ and euvolaemic, check Ca^{2+} daily to prevent hypocalcaemia
- Hyperuricaemia treated with allopurinol
- Avoid nephrotoxic drugs
- Observe for signs of infection and treat, e.g. fever, ± prophylactic antibiotics and influenza and pneumococcal vaccines
- Drugs: corticosteroids and alkylating agents, e.g. cyclophosphamide, melphalan, biological therapies, e.g. thalidomide or proteasome inhibitors (e.g. bortezomib) and dexamethasone to ↓ light chain production
- Stem cell Tx in those <70yrs of age and deemed clinically fit to withstand the treatment
- Administration of analgesia for bone pain, radiotherapy for bone pain

- Plasma exchange to ↓ light chain concentration in renal tubules (see 📖 p. 416)
- Acute HD for AKI (see pp. 116–18).
▶Tx is not contraindicated if the patient makes a good recovery and is stabilized. Implications of long-term prognosis need to be considered regarding choice about Tx options.

Common urinary conditions

Urinary tract infection (UTI)

- Lower UTIs involve the superficial mucosa of the bladder and urethra
- Upper UTIs involve the kidneys, ureters, and deep medullary tissue.

Risk factors for lower infections

- Uncommon in children or ♂, usually associated with urinary tract abnormality
- ♀ 50% likely to have one UTI in lifetime and 3–5% risk of recurrence due to pregnancy, recent or frequent sexual intercourse, use of spermicides that ↓ normal flora in the vagina, poor post-voiding hygiene
- Presence of an indwelling urinary catheter (IDC)
- Stagnant urine due to obstruction/incomplete bladder emptying
- Highly concentrated urine or non-acidic urine
- Prostatitis
- Bladder, ureteric, or kidney calculi
- Diabetics and those on IS.

- 70–90% are *Escherichia coli*; other organisms include *Klebsiella*, *Enterococcus faecalis*, and *Proteus*
- Diagnosis: urine dipstick +ve for nitrites and/or WBCs, ± mild haematuria or proteinuria, midstream urine (MSU) (see 📖 pp. 52–6):
  - rule out a sexually transmitted disease
  - presence of WBC casts are more indicative of pyelonephritis.

Clinical features

- Lower UTI: urinary, e.g. frequency, urgency, nocturia, offensive urine, ± haematuria. suprapubic pain, new episode of confusion, and/or incontinence in the elderly
- Upper UTI/pyelonephritis: loin pain, fever, ± rigors, night sweats, ± nausea/vomiting. ± signs of shock.

Management

- Treat causative organism with antibiotics, e.g. trimethoprim, co-trimoxazole, ciprofloxacin, or oral cephalosporin
- ↑ fluid intake
- Remove indwelling urinary catheter (IDC) if possible
- Educate the patient; hygiene post voiding; voiding post intercourse
- Avoid spermicides
- Hormone replacement therapy in postmenopausal women
- Recurrent UTIs are diagnosed if >4 culture +ve results/yr:
  - require further investigation
  - ± prophylactic antibiotics
- Interstitial cystitis is common in ♀ who have had recurrent UTIs and may present with UTI symptoms and sterile pyuria.

Reflux nephropathy

Accounts for 5–10% of ESKD in the developed world; occurs in infancy.

- Associated with vesico-ureteric reflux, inadequate bladder emptying or outflow obstruction:
  - progressive lesions and chronic tubulo-interstitial scarring due to repeated chronic infections in one or both kidneys
- Diagnosis is made by performing a ^{99m}Tc-dimercaptosuccinic acid (DMSA scan)/intravenous urogram (IVU) and biopsy.

Clinical features

- Haematuria and proteinuria (<1g/24hrs), heavy proteinuria if FSGS
- Renal colic ± passing a stone
- ± ↑BP
- Sterile pyuria with WBC casts on microscopy.

Vesico-ureteric reflux

Occurs in 0.1–1% of newborn babies; commonly diagnosed in infancy.

- The formation of scar tissue in the kidney slows at around 6yrs of age and completely stops at puberty.
  - In adults with no new scar formation, management is aimed at the prevention of CKD progression.

Management

- Management of BP and proteinuria—aim for BP <130/80mmHg with ACEI or ARB as first-line treatment (see 📖 p. 92)
- Immediate treatment of new infections
- More prone to UTIs, hypertension, and pre-eclampsia during pregnancy, refer for specialist care.

Nephrolithiasis

Kidney stones form due to concentrated or static urine, excess stone-forming substances, e.g. calcium oxalate (most common), cystine, phosphate or uric acid.

- It affects ~8–15% of the population most commonly between the ages of 20–60yrs with ♂ twice as prone to kidney stones.

Management

- Aimed at the stone-causing substance (e.g. dietary, ↑ oral fluids)
- Staghorn calculi are made of magnesium ammonium phosphate and may require nephrolithotomy or lithotripsy.

Urinary tract obstruction

Obstruction of urine causes increased pressure in the urinary tract causing kidney damage. In children, related to anatomical abnormalities; in older age, especially ♂, prostate disease, tumours, stones (see Table 1.1 for clinical features of acute and chronic obstruction).

Acute obstruction

Kidney damage is reversible, recovering in a few days, if obstruction relieved. Causes include prostatic disease, retroperitoneal fibrosis, calculi, tumours (rare), papillary necrosis, or blood clots.

Chronic obstruction

Slow to progress and may not be evident until patient presents with CKD. Obstruction can be corrected; kidney damage is irreversible.

Types of obstruction

- Upper tract:
  - involves a ureteric or higher obstruction
  - affects one or both kidneys
- Lower tract:
  - involves the bladder/prostate/urethra
  - affects both kidneys
- Bilateral obstruction or obstruction of one single functioning kidney causes renal impairment
- Obstruction can either be complete or partial.

Table 1.1 Clinical features of acute and chronic obstruction

Acute	Chronic
Anuria and progressive AKI—only when both kidneys obstructed/single functioning kidney	↑ BP
Localized pain or signs of sepsis (e.g. fever)	Nocturia, frequency, prostatic symptoms, e.g. hesitancy, urgency
± asymptomatic	± pain and feeling of fullness

Management

Acute obstruction

- Urgent decompression: ↑ risk of irreversible kidney damage if delay in treating obstruction
- IDC *in situ*:
  - check for any mechanical blockage, e.g. clamped or kinked tubing
  - check for blockage caused by blood clots and liaise with medical staff as the catheter may require a manual flush
- Bladder outflow—insert IDC/suprapubic if unable to insert IDC
- Ureteric—nephrostomy tube or retrograde ureteric stenting
- Urinary stone screen to identify cause of the stone.

Chronic obstruction

- Relieving the obstruction as for acute obstruction
- Management of CKD (see pp. 126–9).

Further reading

Chalmers, C. Applied anatomy and physiology and the renal disease process. In Thomas N (ed) *Renal Nursing*, 3rd edn, pp. 27–74. Edinburgh: Elsevier; 2008.

Daugirdas JT. *Handbook of Chronic Kidney Disease*. Philadelphia, PA: Lippincott Williams & Wilkins; 2011.

Davison A, Cameron S, Grünfeld JP. *Oxford Textbook of Clinical Nephrology*, 3rd edn, vol 1. Oxford: Oxford University Press; 2005

Steddon S, Ashman N, Chesser A, et al. (eds). *Oxford Handbook of Nephrology and Hypertension*. Oxford: Oxford University Press; 2006.

Warrell A, Cox T, Firth D (eds). *Oxford Textbook of Medicine*, 5th edn. Oxford: Oxford University Press; 2010.

References

1. NHS Kidney Care. *Kidney Disease: Key Facts and Figures*, September 2010. Available from: <http://www.kidneycare.nhs.uk/our_work_programmes/prevention/key_facts_kidney_disease>

2. The Renal Association and UK Renal Registry. *The Twelfth Annual Report*, December 2010. Available at: <http://www.renalreg.com/reports/2010.html>

Useful patient websites

EdRenInfo. Available at: <http://renux.dmed.ed.ac.uk/edren/edreninfohome.html>

NHS Choices. Available at: <http://www.nhs.uk/Conditions/Kidney-disease-chronic/Pages/Causes.aspx>

PKD charity. Available at: <http://pkdcharity.org.uk/>

Clinical assessment of the chronic kidney disease patient

Undertaking a clinical assessment

Many patients with kidney disease will be asymptomatic and may have been referred solely on account of a decreased estimated GFR (eGFR), proteinuria, haematuria, or uncontrolled hypertension. Those patients with an AKI or late stage 4/5 CKD will be referred as urgent cases. CKD and AKI require a thorough clinical evaluation in order to assess, diagnose, and treat the underlying condition effectively. It is important to have a good knowledge and understanding of the relevant available investigations in order to provide effective support and patient education and to be able to effectively manage the kidney patient.

The role of the nurse is to undertake a comprehensive clinical assessment including:
- Taking thorough histories:
  - medical, surgical, and drug
  - social and family
- Undertaking:
  - baseline observations and a physical examination
  - requesting preliminary investigations.

History
History taking from the patient and/or significant other is invaluable in completing an accurate assessment. If the patient is under the care of other physician/s, contact them or their GP for recent reports if required.

Presenting complaint
Current symptoms and signs in particular looking for:
- Urinary:
  - haematuria—microscopic or frank
  - proteinuria/microalbuminuria
  - pain, e.g. loin pain, burning on micturition, or suprapubic pain
  - alteration in urinary pattern, e.g. anuria/oliguria/polyuria, nocturia, new onset of incontinence, frequency, dysuria, frothy urine
  - urethral discharge, e.g. pus, blood
  - urinary tract symptoms, e.g. acute or chronic retention of urine, poor and/or interrupted flow, hesitancy, urgency, frequency, nocturia or urinary retention
- Abnormal BP, postural hypotension
- Peripheral oedema (pitting oedema to extremities), genital/sacral/periorbital oedema
- Dyspnoea on exertion/talking/at rest
- Lethargy/fatigue
- Abnormal bruising or bleeding
- Pruritus, rash
- Fever, night sweats, insomnia
- Seizures, cognitive impairment
- Altered bowel habit, e.g. constipation/diarrhoea
- Loss of appetite, nausea, vomiting, dyspepsia, weight loss

- Hiccups
- Painful/aching joints, restless legs
- Raynaud's phenomenon
- Myalgia
- Mouth ulcers
- Hair loss
- Pregnancy, history of pre-eclampsia, sexual dysfunction
- Psychological issues, e.g. depression/anxiety.

Past medical history

- Chronic conditions, e.g. cancer, diabetes, ischaemic heart disease (IHD), chronic HF, peripheral vascular disease (PVD), cerebral vascular disease, hypertension, SLE, respiratory disease, e.g. asthma or chronic obstructive pulmonary disease (COPD)
- Known kidney disease, e.g. polycystic kidney disease, renal calculi
- Recent illness/infections
- Surgical procedures/other procedures
- Childhood renal-specific problems, e.g. enuresis, vesicoureteric reflux, recurrent UTIs
- Pregnancy, e.g. number of live births, pre-eclampsia.

Family history

- Kidney disease
- Genetic diseases
- Cancers
- Primary hypertension
- Diabetes mellitus.

Current medications and allergies

- Potentially nephrotoxic drugs, e.g. NSAIDs, aminoglycosides, ciclosporin (see 🕮 p. 569)
- Antihypertensive medications, e.g. ACEI or ARBs
- Diabetes medications, e.g. insulin, oral hypoglycaemic agents
- Antibiotics either current or recent
- Analgesics, e.g. NSAIDs
- Oral contraception
- Steroids and immunosuppressants
- Recreational, e.g. alcohol, cocaine, heroin
- Herbal medicines, e.g. St John's wort, ginseng
- Over-the-counter (OTC) vitamins and supplements, cod liver oil.

Ethnicity

- Diseases such as diabetic nephropathy, SLE, IgA nephropathy, hypertensive nephropathy—more common in Afro-Caribbeans and Asians.

Psychosocial history

- Job/financial situation—prior and present occupational history, e.g. exposure to nephrotoxins
- Home/social, e.g. lives alone/family support
- Mobility and activity level
- Future plans for a family in case cytotoxic medications are considered

- Adherence with medications
- Smoking/recreational drugs/alcohol (quantity and duration)
- Risk of hepatitis B/C and HIV
- Previous resident/recent visitor to overseas country and/or history of illness, e.g. TB, malaria.

Assessment

▶ Many patients with CKD are asymptomatic and an examination may be normal—diagnosis will be by investigation only (see 📖 p. 171 for pain assessment and 📖 p. 587 for fluid assessment).

General

General observation and condition at rest:

- Colour of skin, is it pale or flushed, assess skin turgor and integrity
- Presence of scars, a fistula, and/or long-term HD or PD catheter
- Fistula—check thrill and bruit
- Check height and weight to calculate body mass index (BMI)
- Temperature (normal 35.5–37.2°C)
- Assess mucous membranes, observe for any signs of ulceration, excoriations, or oral thrush
- Peripheral or central oedema, e.g. pitting oedema to ankles.
  Respiratory (normal rate 12–20 breaths/min)
- Assess for dyspnoea, tachypnoea, or orthopnoea
- Observe the movement of their chest; is there chest symmetry, use of accessory muscles?
- Presence of cough; dry or productive (frothy, haemoptysis)?
- ± pulse oximetry (normal 95–100%), ABGs, CXR.

Cardiovascular (normal pulse 60–100bpm, systolic BP (SBP) 90–140mmHg, diastolic BP (DBP) 60–90mmHg)
- Check for sinus rhythm
- Perform both lying and standing BP if possible
- ± electrocardiogram (ECG)/echocardiogram (ECHO).

Neurological

- Conscious level—neurological observations
- Evidence of motor or sensory deficit.

Gastrointestinal

- Fluid allowance
- Loss of appetite, dietary restrictions.

Urine output

- Check output, if they have a catheter is urine output >0.5ml/kg/hr?
- Dipstick urine if not anuric ± MSU, early morning urine (EMU) for ACR/PCR, AFBs or 24hr urine collection to assess total urine output.

Diabetes

- Check blood glucose level (BGL) and prior glycosylated haemoglobin (HbA1c) results, patient's own blood glucose readings.

Neurovascular observations
- Assess feet for colour, warmth, movement, sensation, ulcers
- Check for presence of peripheral pulses in both legs. e.g. posterior tibialis (PT), dorsalis pedis (DP) and popliteal pulses
- Check for groin bruit (RAS).

Dressings
- Check dressings, e.g. exit site, temporary HD catheter, wound or ulcer signs of infection.

Investigations

The most common diagnostic investigations include haematology, biochemistry, serology, nephritic screen, urinary tests and radiological imaging.

Measuring kidney function

Serum creatinine

Cr is the product of the metabolism of creatinine phosphate in the muscles excreted by the kidney and is proportional to muscle mass. Ur is not used as a marker of kidney function as it is synthesized by the liver and is not produced at a constant rate like Cr.

- ↑ serum Cr levels only seen when there is a 50% decline in kidney function, so is not a good marker of early loss of kidney function
- Replaced by calculating eGFR for the early detection of CKD
- Monitoring Cr levels is useful in CKD stages 4 and 5 and Tx recipients as relatively constant over a 24hr period:
  - ↑ seen in progressive kidney disease and plot graphing Cr is used to monitor progress and predict timing of the commencement of RRT as there is a linear decline in kidney function (available online[1]).

Inaccurate assessment of kidney function can occur as Cr secretion is affected by:
- Ethnicity (↑ in Afro-Caribbeans)
- Gender
- Large muscle mass
- ↓ muscle mass (amputees, elderly)
- Malnutrition (↓ protein intake)
- Medications (trimethoprim, spironolactone, amiloride)
- Ketoacidosis.

Measuring creatinine clearance (CrCl)

- As kidney function declines, the proportion of Cr cleared by secretion increases relative to that cleared by glomerular filtration ∴ CrCl measurements will overestimate the GFR
- Not routinely used within clinical practice as:
  - inaccurate 24hr urine collection, i.e. poor collection technique
  - inter-laboratory variation in serum creatinine levels
  - altered Cr secretion
- Normal range is 70–125ml/min.

Estimated glomerular filtration rate (eGFR)

- GFR is the filtration rate of the functioning nephrons in the kidney
- Normal GFR >100ml/min/1.73m^2, GFR equates roughly to the % kidney function, e.g. GFR 60ml/min/1.73m^2 is ~60% kidney function
- eGFR is the recommended method for measuring kidney function and automatically reported by all laboratories, though online calculators available[3,4]
- The normal ageing process causes a decline in kidney function by 8–10ml/min per decade from the age of 40yrs in normal healthy adults:
  - eGFR <60ml/min may be normal in a 70yr-old with no other clinical indicators of kidney disease.

Advantages of using eGFR

- Effective method of early detection and monitoring of CKD and response to therapies, e.g. medications, management of BP
- Reliable tool which can be used to predict and plan the need for RRT.

Disadvantage of using eGFR

- Not very accurate when kidney function is very low or close to normal
- Inaccurate results when used in the very obese (BMI >30kg/m^2) or cachectic patients, multiple amputees (BMI <18.5kg/m^2) as overestimates eGFR.

▶ *eGFR should not be used in the following situations:*

- AKI—Cr levels may appear normal due to the delay between ↓ in eGFR and a steady state of Cr being achieved, i.e. needs stable kidney function
- Measurement of kidney function post living donor nephrectomy
- <18yrs of age
- Pregnancy
- ♀ >90yrs of age.

Normal variation in eGFR

↓ eGFR	↑ eGFR
• Low-protein diet (malnourished)	• Pregnancy
• Liver disease	• Diurnal variation
• Ageing	• High-protein diet
• Ethnicity (Afro-Caribbean)	

---

eGFR formulae

Two mathematical formulas are recommended for use:[2,3]

- Modification of diet in renal disease (MDRD):
  - requires gender, age, ethnicity, and serum Cr
- Cockcroft–Gault formulae:
  - requires age, weight, and serum Cr
- If a highly accurate GFR is required then the gold standard tools such as inulin, ^{51}Cr-EDTA or 125I-iothalamate or iohexol should be used (e.g. monitoring chemotherapy or evaluation of kidney function in potential live related donors)
- Ideally the patient should not eat any meat for 12hrs prior to the test:
  - the specimen is processed within 12hrs for most accurate results
  - although this is a NICE recommendation it is difficult to implement.

Other methods of measuring kidney function

Chronic kidney disease epidemiology collaboration (CKD-EPI) equation[4] requires further validation prior to implementation in the clinical setting but appears to be more accurate.

- Initial studies have found it to be better than MDRD when GFR is >60ml/min/1.73m^2, as MDRD tends to overestimate the prevalence of CKD stages 1 and 2

- When GFR <50ml/min/1.73m^2 MDRD and CKD-EPI have been found to give similar results
- NB It is likely that this calculation will be recommended as the preferred formula for clinical practice in the near future.

Inulin is a polysaccharide that is injected into the bloodstream.
- Not absorbed, secreted, or metabolized by the kidneys making it easy to measure the amount filtered by the kidneys by testing both urine and serum levels
- Remains the gold standard for measuring GFR, though not commonly used as it is a costly procedure.

Isotopic measurement of GFR involves the injection of a radioisotope such as ^{51}Cr-EDTA or ^{99}Tc-DPTA, and a series of blood samples over a 4hr period to measure renal elimination of the isotope.
- Normal range is the same as CrCl 70–125ml/min
- DPTA can also be measured using a gamma camera over the kidney. These techniques are expensive therefore not routinely used in the clinical setting. ⚠ Pregnancy.

Cystatin C is another method although not commonly used and is a low-molecular-weight protein and freely filtered by the kidneys.
- ↓ kidney function, cystatin C accumulates in the bloodstream and can be used to reflect GFR
- Unlike using MDRD or Cockcroft–Gault calculations, cystatin C is not affected by age, sex, diet, muscle mass, or the effects of inflammation
- Not currently available within the clinical setting.

Haematology

The main aim is to identify the presence of anaemia, malignancy, clotting disorders, infections, or inflammatory diseases. Table 2.1 provides an outline of the most common investigations, with a more comprehensive overview provided on anaemia management, see 📖 pp. 224–5.

Table 2.1 Common haematology investigations used in the assessment of CKD

Full blood count (FBC)	Interpretation
Hb	↓ anaemia
RCC—number of red cells/L of blood Show damage to RBC	↑ polycythaemia, dehydration ↓ anaemia, over-hydration
Mean cell volume (MCV)/mean cell haemoglobin (MCH)/mean corpuscular haemoglobin conc (MCHC)	Hypochromic/microcytic—iron deficiency anaemia or thalassaemia Macrocytic anaemia—B12 or folate deficiency
Haematocrit (HCT)—indicates % of RBC in whole blood volume	↓ anaemia, blood loss, myeloma ↑ dehydration, polycythaemia
Platelet count	Uraemia affects platelet function in later stages of CKD
WCC Differential—% of the 5 different WBCs	↑ inflammation, infection, leukaemia ↓ SLE, bone marrow/liver and spleen disorders E.g. ↑ eosinophils often indicative of an allergic process
Other tests	
Clotting profile	Activated partial thromboplastin time (APPT), DIC, prolonged in liver cirrhosis, ↑ with anticoagulant medications
Bleeding time	Prolonged in thrombocytopenia and vascular disorders
Ferritin	↓ iron deficiency anaemia
Vitamin B12 Folic acid	↓ macrocytic anaemia
% Transferrin saturation (% TSAT)	Diagnosis of anaemia ↑ thalassaemia, ingestion of iron, haemochromatosis ↓ iron deficiency anaemia
% hypochromic RBCs	>10% iron deficiency anaemia

Biochemistry

Urea and electrolytes (see electrolyte table, 📖 p. 593–601)
- Ur – ± ↑ in CKD stages 4 and 5
- ↑ associated with high protein intake (e.g. body builders taking protein supplements), medications (e.g. steroids, tetracycline), GI bleeding and haemorrhage
- ↓ associated with low protein intake (e.g. severe malnutrition), liver damage and pregnancy

Cr—↑ in CKD stage 4 and 5 (see 📖 p. 42).

Liver function tests (LFTs)
Alb is only produced by the liver
- ↑ in hypovolaemia
- ↓ in malnutrition, protein loss in PD, nephrotic syndrome and malignancy

Total plasma proteins
- ↓ associated with ↓ Alb in nephrotic syndrome, liver disease, haemorrhage, burns
- ↑ with normal albumin-globulin ratio seen in dehydration
- ↓ with ↓ albumin globulin ratio e.g. autoimmune diseases, SLE, myeloma, shock and chronic infections

ALP—↑ MBD, pregnancy, liver disease

Other tests
HbA1c – reflects mean blood glucose control over a 12 wk period
- Underestimates glycaemic control in stage 4 and 5 (false high –uraemia), low results in conditions with ↓ RBC lifespan e.g. sickle cell, use of ESAs (see 📖 p. 134)

Fasting BGL—to assess for diabetes

PTH
- ↑ stages CKD 4 and 5 (see 📖 p. 191)

Uric acid
- ↑ stages 4 and 5 CKD → gout due to the excess uric acid crystallizing in the joints, also seen in pre-eclampsia, MM and acute shock

Lipid and triglycerides
- ± ↑ CKD, nephrotic syndrome and kidney Tx patients
- ↓ HDL, ↑ LDL associated with CVD

± **PSA** (protein produced by the prostate) for ♂ over 50 yrs of age
- ↑ prostate cancer or prostatic hyperplasia

Pre-Tx workup—blood group, HLA tissue typing, virology status (include CMV, EBV) (see 📖 p. 456)

Serology

Investigations include inflammatory markers, viral serology and nephritic screen (see Table 2.2).

Inflammatory markers

ESR—↑ infection and inflammation

C-reactive protein (CRP)—↑ in inflammatory disease/infections, malignancy, later stages of pregnancy, use of oral contraceptives

Viral serology—hepatitis A/B/C and HIV
• Some kidney diseases are associated with hepatitis, HIV, polyarteritis nodosa (PAN), cryoglobulinaemia
• Screen at risk groups and patients requiring RRT.

Table 2.2 Nephritic screen for CKD assessment

Complements C3 and C4	↓ in inflammatory conditions e.g. SLE, infective endocarditis
Immunoglobulins e.g. IgG, IgA, IgM	↑ in autoimmune diseases and allergies e.g. IgA nephropathy, MM
Autoantibodies	
Anti-nuclear antibodies (ANA)	SLE, with anti-dsDNA antibodies more specific for SLE
Anti-neutrophil cytoplasmic antibodies (ANCA)	Systemic and renal vasculitis
cANCA + Antiprotenase 3 (anti-PR3) antibodies	Wegener's granulomatosis
Anti-glomerular basement membrane (Anti-GBM)	Goodpasture's syndrome
Creatine kinase (enzyme)	Rhabdomyolysis
Serum protein electrophoresis	Measures abnormal globulins in the blood e.g. to diagnose MM
Rheumatoid (Rh) factor	Autoimmune diseases particularly rheumatoid arthritis
Antiphospholipid antibodies	Cause coagulation disorders seen in pre-eclampsia, autoimmune diseases such as SLE
Cryoglobulins	Abnormal immunoglobulins found in diseases e.g. MM, autoimmune disease (e.g. SLE), infection (e.g. hepatitis)
Anti-streptolysin O titre (ASOT) or anti-DNase B titre	Assists in the diagnosis of past or present streptococcal infections i.e. post infectious GN

Urinary investigations

Proteinuria

Measuring proteinuria is useful for the early detection of kidney disease. Prolonged proteinuria left untreated will lead to loss of kidney function and is also a strong predictor of the increased risk of CVD and death. Those with diabetes, hypertension, and the elderly are more at risk.

- In healthy adults it is normal to have a small amount of protein present in the urine (tubular casts composed of Tamm–Horsfall protein) and a small amount of albumin.

Causes of proteinuria

- Glomerular (most common):
  - 1° GN
  - 2° GN, e.g. diabetes, SLE, amyloidosis
- Tubular:
  - tubulointerstitial nephritis (TIN), e.g. nephrotoxic drugs, toxins, e.g. tetracycline, lead
- Overflow:
  - MM, myoglobinuria, haemoglobinuria
- Tissue/secretory:
  - inflammation, e.g. UTI
  - urinary tract tumours
- Short-lived or transient episodes:
  - fever, excessive exercise
  - seizures
  - congestive cardiac failure (CCF) and in acutely unwell patients
- Orthostatic or postural.

Quantification of proteinuria

- Currently the NICE CKD guidelines (2008) recommend using (see 🕮 p. 130 for CKD for referral guidelines):
- *Albumin: creatinine ratio (ACR)*—measure the conc of albumin and creatinine
  - >sensitivity detecting lower levels of protein, especially in individuals with diabetes compared to PCR
- *Protein: creatinine ratio (PCR)*—measures the conc of protein and creatinine
  - it does not detect microalbuminuria
  - PCR is an accepted method in non-diabetes.

▶ Both tests require an EMU or MSU to avoid circadian changes. 24hr urine collections are not necessary for quantification purposes.

Table 2.3 provides an approximate correlation between dipstick readings, 24hr protein excretion, urinary protein or albumin to creatinine ratios.

- Normal protein excretion rate is <150mg/24hrs (<20 mg of albumin)
- ∴ persistent >150mg/24hrs requires further investigation as it may indicate kidney or systemic disease
- Investigate a +ve urine dipstick of ≥+1 with either an ACR or PCR
- Persistent proteinuria is only diagnosed when there have been 2 or more +ve tests repeated after 1–2wks as 5% of the healthy population may have a trace to +1 present in their urine
- Exclude UTI and orthostatic hypotension
- Preferable to use a EMU sample, 24hr protein urine collection may be requested
- Abnormal = PCR >50mg/mmol/L.

Table 2.3 Approximate correlation between dipstick readings, 24hr protein excretion, urinary protein or albumin to creatinine ratios

	Dipstick	Urine total protein excretion mg/24hrs (g/24hrs)	Urine PCR mg/mmol (urine prot mg/L)	Urine ACR microalbum-ininuria mg/mmol
Normal	−ve	<150 (<0.15)	<15 (<100)	<2.5 (♂) <3.5 (♀)
Microalbuminuria	−ve	<150 (<0.15)	<15 (<100)	2.5–30 (♂) 3.5–30 (♀)
'Trace' protein	Trace	150–449 (0.15–0.449)	15–44 (100–299)	
Clinical proteinuria	1+	450–1499 (0.45–1.499)	45–149 (300–999)	>30
	2+	1500–4499 (1.5–4.499)	150–449 (1000–2999)	100–299
Nephrotic range	3+	>4500 (>4.5)	>450 (>3000)	>300

Microalbuminuria

Abnormal amount of albumin excreted in the urine below the level detected using standard urinary protein dipsticks.

- 2 or more +ve results are required preferably within 1 month prior to the diagnosis of microalbuminuria
- Exclude acute metabolic crisis, intercurrent illness, and UTI prior to diagnosing the presence of microalbuminuria
- Optimize diabetes control prior to testing
- Exclude other causes of ↑ Alb excretion which include:
  - menstrual contamination, vaginal discharge, uncontrolled hypertension, HF, strenuous exercise and type 1 diabetes <5yrs
- Strongly associated with CVD
- Preferable to use an EMU sample
- Abnormal = ACR >30mg/mmol—indicative of either systemic or kidney dysfunction.

Haematuria

There are 2 types of haematuria; macroscopic (blood is visible in the urine) and microscopic (not visible but shows up positive on dipstick and on microscopy).
- Microscopic haematuria is often an incidental finding, asymptomatic, and may be of no clinical significance (5% of normal population):
  - further investigate to rule out kidney disease or urological malignancy (see 📖 p. 130, CKD for referral guidelines)
  - urinary dipstick is the recommended screening test and not urine microscopy.

Causes of haematuria
- Urinary tract—renal stones, polycystic kidneys, trauma, cancer, cystitis, prostatitis, urethritis, bladder and prostate cancer
- Glomerular—IgA nephropathy, Alport's syndrome
- Transient—menstruation, sexual activity, trauma, exercise, and viral infections
- Other—over-anticoagulation.

- Haematuria should be further investigated if >+1 when tested on 2–3 separate occasions a few wks apart
- MSU should be sent to exclude UTI
- Considered significant if >2 per hpf on microscopy
- Dysmorphic shaped RBCs are usually glomerular in origin
- Occur in UTIs, kidney injury/infarct, renal calculi, acute tubular necrosis, renal tumour, nephrotoxicity, e.g. medications and glomerular disease (usually dysmorphic cells)
- Exclude menstruation, excessive exercise, sexual intercourse, and recent trauma to the urinary tract, e.g. urinary catheter
- Ensure fresh sample as false +ve can occur with lysis of RBCs.

Urine tests

There are various types of urine tests which will be outlined in this chapter; however the initial nursing assessment should be observation of the urine sample for appearance, odour, presence of sediment, and volume.

Appearance/odour
- Normal urine—straw to dark yellow in colour and translucent with no distinct odour
- Ammonia smell usually indicates the presence of an infection
- Sweet smelling urine is more likely to be due to ketosis:
  - some foods can affect the odour of urine, e.g. asparagus.

Abnormal appearance of urine
- *Dark/red to bright red*—haematuria as a result of kidney injury or has a smoky appearance as a result of bleeding from the kidney itself or certain foods, e.g. beetroot or blackberries, menstruation, medications, e.g. phenytoin, and porphyria
- *Pink through to black/brown in colour*—(usually described as 'coca cola') due to myoglobinuria, e.g. rhabdomyolysis
- *Orange*—medications, e.g. rifampicin, senna
- *Dark yellow/brown*—hyperbilirubinuria, drugs, e.g. nitrofurantoin
- *Cloudy/turbid*—presence of UTI/pus and bacteria (can appear milky)
- *Milky*—lymphatic leakage into urinary system (chyluria). Other causes include the presence of crystals, e.g. oxalate/urate and Ca^{2+} or storage of the sample in the fridge
- *Frothy*—due to an excess of protein present in the urine and can be seen if you shake the sample as it will appear 'foamy'

▶ Old urine samples can also appear frothy so it is important to check the date of the sample. Keep sample refrigerated ($2–8°C$) to aid preservation, discard >24hrs.

Volume
Normal urine output is between 500–1500ml/24hrs with a minimum of 400ml/24hrs to maintain normal bodily function.
- Anuria <100ml/24hrs
- Oliguria <400ml/24hrs
- Polyuria >3000ml/24hrs.

Osmolality
The concentrating ability of the renal tubules can be assessed by measuring osmolality (more accurate than specific gravity (SG)).
- An EMU sample is required for an accurate result (normal range is 500–800mosmol/kg[1])

Dipstick urinalysis
A cheap and useful near patient test that can assist in the diagnosis and monitoring of CKD and can also be used for screening asymptomatic

patients, e.g. for the presence of proteinuria and haematuria (see Table 2.4 for the interpretation of the most common parameters on dipstick).

▶ Microalbuminuria dipsticks should only be used as a screening, not as a diagnostic tool

▶ False positive readings may be due to menstruation (blood present), medications, e.g. diuretics, ascorbic acid, antibiotics (erythromycin, trimethoprim) and some contrast media.

Table 2.4 Common urinary dipstick parameters and interpretation (see 📖 p. 48 for haematuria and proteinuria)

Parameter	Interpretation
Glucose	Hyperglycaemia or low renal glucose threshold, sepsis, pregnancy, renal tubular damage, Fanconi's syndrome
Ketones	Diabetes, alcoholic ketoacidosis, starvation, severe hypervolaemia
Bilirubin	Liver disease or bile duct obstruction
SG	>1.020 seen in hypovolaemia
Normal range 1.003–1.035	SG 1.000–1.005 in diabetes insipidus. ▶ Results may be affected by low protein diets, in chronic liver disease, pregnancy and fluid and electrolyte imbalance
pH Normal range 4.5–8	Useful in assessing the efficacy of treatment, e.g. uric stone disease and metabolic alkalosis <5 ↑ risk of uric stones >8 indicates renal tubular acidosis or UTI ▶ pH can be affected by dehydration, fever, heat stress, inflammation, excessive exercise, acute illness
Urobilinogen	Pre-hepatic jaundice
Nitrite	Indicates UTI with a urease producing organism −ve result does not rule out a UTI
Leucocytes	Usually indicative of inflammation/infection May also be +ve with a contaminated sample

Microscopy, culture, and sensitivity (MC&S)

Microscopy will assist in the identification of bacteria, casts, crystals, or blood cells.

- Advise laboratory if the patient is receiving antibiotics (take sample prior to commencing treatment where possible)
- MSU sample
- The presence of multiple organisms can indicate contamination and the specimen should be re-collected.

Bacteria

The risk of a bacterial UTI is greater in diabetes, ♀ (shorter urethra), pregnancy, urinary retention, vesicoureteric reflux and immunocompromised patients, e.g. Tx recipients.
- Bacterial infection present if >10^5cfu/ml and/or organisms 1–10hpf.

Fungi

- Risk factors include indwelling urethral catheters, ureteric stents, immunocompromised patients, antibiotic use and diabetes mellitus

Cells

- Assessment of urine for the type of cells is important as it can be indicative of damage to the kidney or urinary tract. See Table 2.5 for commonly found urinary cells and their interpretation in CKD.

Table 2.5 Clinical interpretation of urinary cells

Type of cells	Interpretation
WBC >5/hpf provides diagnostic disease/condition:*	
Neutrophils	UTIs/inflammation of urinary tract, GN, TIN
Lymphocytes	Chronic interstitial disease
Sterile pyuria >10 WBC/hpf with −ve culture	Chlamydia, partial treatment of a UTI, calculi, prostatitis, bladder tumours, TIN, appendicitis, TB
Eosinophils	Allergic interstitial nephritis, TIN, prostatitis, RPGN
Renal tubular cells	Normal finding ↑ tubular damage, ATN, TIN
Squamous and transitional epithelial cells	Normal finding
Renal epithelial	ATN, GN, rejection, viral infections

* ⚠ Possible contamination from vaginal or urethra.

Casts

Casts are made up of proteins from the kidney. There are various types of casts associated with different kidney diseases as outlined in Table 2.6.

Table 2.6 Types and causes of urinary casts

Type	Cause
RBCs	GN
WBCs	Interstitial nephritis
	Acute pyelonephritis
	TIN
Granular or cellular (quantified and follow for progression)	Renal parenchymal disease
Tubular	ATN
Epithelial	ATN, GN
Fatty	Nephrotic syndrome
Hyaline/Tamm–Horsfall proteins	Excessive exercise
	Fever
	Diuretic use
	CKD/pyelonephritis (large numbers)

Crystals

There are various factors that affect the formation of urinary crystals, e.g. urinary pH, solute concentration, and presence of crystallizing inhibitors.
- Cholesterol crystals may be seen in cases of heavy proteinuria and some drugs, such as antibiotics (e.g. amoxicillin), antiviral therapy (e.g. aciclovir), methotrexate, and vitamin C
  - may cause crystal precipitation with serious consequences as they precipitate in the renal tubules and can cause AKI.

Acidic pH urine
- Uric acid—acute urate nephropathy
- Calcium oxalate—hypercalciuria, hyperoxaluria
- Cystine—cystinuria.

Alkaline pH urine
- Calcium phosphate—risk factor for the formation of calcium stones
- Magnesium ammonia phosphate—*Proteus* UTIs.

Other urinary investigations

- Urinary cytology or more specialized tests, e.g. flow cytometry and immunochemistry—investigating cancer and inflammatory diseases of the urinary tract (MSU is required)
- Bence Jones protein—involves heating the urine which causes the protein to precipitate out, dissolve at 100°C, and precipitate again on cooling used in the diagnosis of MM, amyloidosis, Waldenström's macroglobuminaemia and cryoglobulinaemia (EMU required)
- Myoglobin level—myoglobin is found in muscles and is released into the bloodstream when there is injury to the muscle—myoglobin causes renal tubular blockage and subsequently ATN. The condition known as rhabdomyolysis (see 📖 p. 102) is seen in trauma cases such as crush injuries, excessive exercise, and status epilepticus (EMU sample preferable).

Diagnostic imaging

Plain x-ray

Kidneys, ureter, and bladder (KUB) x-ray is commonly performed to show the size, shape, position, and number of kidneys present.

- Quick, cheap, and easy to perform and useful in detecting radio-opaque renal calculi and calcifications of the renal tract. ▶Check if pregnant.

Renal ultrasound

One of the most common renal investigations as it is cheap, safe, and easy to perform.

- Provides an estimate of the size of the kidneys, echogenicity, any hydronephrosis, and differentiates between solid lesions and cysts
- Detect structural abnormalities and can be used to exclude urinary obstruction, e.g. cysts, reflux, and assess bladder emptying
- Guidance tool for kidney biopsies or insertion of nephrostomy tubes.

Renal Doppler studies

Used to evaluate renal vascular flow, e.g. renal thrombosis/infarction, ATN, RAS, assess transplanted kidneys for ATN, obstruction to urine out-flow and acute rejection.

- Normal resistive index (<0.7); a high reading may indicate intrarenal vascular disease, arteriosclerosis, ATN, obstruction to urine outflow, and acute rejection.

CT scan

Provides in-depth pictures of renal anatomy, surrounding structures and for identifying abnormal structures, e.g. mass/tumour/haematoma in kid-ney injury, retroperitoneal disease, abscess, pyelonephritis, renovascular disease, renal and ureteric calculi, and tumour staging.

- Useful in distinguishing cysts from tumours
- Contrast media may be used for improved visibility of the renal cortex. ▶Check if allergic to contrast media/iodine/shellfish, has asthma or any allergies.

Magnetic resonance imaging

Provides better visibility than a CT scan of renal anatomy, visualizing and evaluating lesions and masses, renal vein thrombosis and staging of tumours.

- May use contrast agent non-nephrotoxic agent, gadolinium. ⚠ Caution with ↓ kidney function as it has been associated with the development of nephrogenic systemic fibrosis (NSF)
- The European Medicines Agency risk categories for this agent:
  - high risk—should not be used in severe kidney disease, restricted dose in moderate kidney disease
  - medium/low risk—should be given in the lowest possible dose for severe kidney disease
- ↑ risk in older person as kidneys are less able to remove gadolinium.

Intravenous pyelogram (IVP) or intravenous urogram (IVU)

Contrast media is injected via a vein followed by x-rays to follow progress of the media which is excreted via the kidneys.

- An IVP or IVU is useful in detecting renal calculi, medullary sponge disease and papillary necrosis
- A post voiding x-ray may also be performed to assess bladder outflow
- Furosemide may be used to aid in the differential diagnosis of pelvic ureteric junction obstruction.

Pre-procedure nursing considerations

▶ Check for allergies to contrast media/iodine/shellfish and asthma/allergies
- Ensure written informed consent form signed and educate patient on pre and post-procedure care
- NBM 4–6hrs before procedure
- Bowel preparation 2 days prior to procedure (check with local radiology unit for policy)
- Prophylactic antibiotics may be required
- The medical staff may request a fluid restriction (~500ml) 24hrs prior to the procedure but only if GFR is normal (assists with concentrating the contrast media)
▶ Check metformin stopped 24hrs pre-procedure—↑ risk of lactic acidosis
- ± corticosteroids if there is a history of atopy or asthma

Post-procedure nursing considerations

- Check kidney function in patients with known renal impairment
- Check urinalysis for haematuria
- Observe for signs of bleeding and infection, e.g. fever
- Observe for signs of allergy to contrast medium, e.g. pruritus, nausea/vomiting, sneezing. Antihistamines may be prescribed by the medical staff and note in medical file. Severe anaphylaxis, e.g. ↓ BP, shock, bronchospasm is a medical emergency
- ↑ fluid intake unless on a fluid restriction to flush through contrast media
- Check Cr at 48hrs organized prior to re-starting metformin.

Retrograde pyelogram

- Involves the insertion of a catheter and an injection of contrast media into the pelvis of the kidney and ureter via cystoscopy, followed by a series of x-rays.
- This test detects calyceal defects, tumours of the ureter and pelvis, hydronephrosis, and calculi
- Pre-procedure and post-procedure as for IVU.

Renogram

- Involves the injection of an IV radioisotope which is excreted by the kidneys, then followed immediately by a series of x-rays usually over a 2–4hr period

- Used to assess tubular secretion and kidney function, e.g. ↓ blood supply to the kidney the radioisotope will not be visible:
  - assess the area of obstruction, e.g. renovascular disease
  - provides a complete image of renal cortical lesions e.g. identify tumours and renal contusions.

Types of radioisotopes
- DMSA (^{99m}Tc-dimercaptosuccinic acid)—retained by the proximal tubule cells and functioning parenchyma:
  - detection of congenital abnormalities, e.g. vesicoureteric reflux and scarring
- DPTA (^{99m}Tc-diethylenenetriamine pentaacetic acid)—rapidly excreted and provides details of blood supply, overall kidney function, identifying the percentage function for each kidney and urinary excretion:
  - not as effective when Cr >200mmol/L.
- MAG 3 (^{99m}Tc-benzoylcaptoacetyltriglycerine)—quantifies renal blood flow, kidney function and excretion, and visualizes aorta and renal perfusion:
  - diagnose renal artery thrombosis/emboli and stenosis
  - IV furosemide may be given which provides quantification of kidney function.

Captopril (ACEI) test dose may be used with either DPTA or MAG3 renograms to assess kidney perfusion and identify RAS. The patient is given a dose of captopril and if occlusion is present, it will cause a reduction in blood flow.

Pre-procedure nursing considerations
- Ensure patient is well hydrated if possible
- ▶ Check if patient is pregnant as contraindicated. Breastfeeding mothers will require advice on contact with baby and discarding breast milk post procedure
- Check with medical staff if taking antihypertensive medication as they may be required to stop a few days prior to the test.

Post-procedure nursing considerations
- BP should be monitored post procedure for 2hrs if given a test dose of captopril.

Voiding cysterourethrogram
A non-invasive investigation using radionuclide to detect vesicoureteric reflux.

Renal angiogram/angiography
This involves an injection of radiopaque contrast media into the blood vessels, usually the femoral, but occasionally the brachial, artery. It is then followed by a series of fluoroscopic x-rays used to identify any blockages. Used for the diagnosis of renovascular disease (e.g. RAS), acute renal ischaemia, emboli/thrombosis, tumours, polyarteritis nodosa, Tx donor assessment, and identify area of bleeding post kidney biopsy.

Complications post procedure
- Bruising, haematoma, false aneurysm (1:1000)
- Infection
- Allergic reaction to the contrast

- Embolism or dissection of a vessel
- Failure of the procedure.

Pre-procedure nursing considerations

- Patient education and preparation, check consent form signed:
  - notify staff of any altered sensations to insertion area such as warm or wet. Advise patient they may feel a 'hot flush' sensation when the contrast media is being injected
- Complete pre-procedure checklist and record if allergic to contrast medium/iodine/shellfish, asthma or any known allergies
- Baseline haemodynamic and neurovascular observations (feet colour, warmth, movement, sensation and pedal pulses (PT and DP)
- Ensure adequately hydrated pre-procedure:
  - ± IV 0.9% n/saline or sodium bicarbonate 1.26%, usually given at 125ml/hr over 4hrs prior to the procedure
- Other agents which may be used: antioxidant N-acetylcysteine (NAC), nephroprotective drug for ↓ kidney function and low urine output
- ± FBC, U&Es, clotting profile
- ► Check anticoagulant therapy stopped pre-procedure as per medical orders as there is a risk of bleeding (e.g. usually stop warfarin 3 days prior so INR <1.7:
  - ± IV heparinization pre-procedure
- ► Check metformin stopped 24hrs pre-procedure—↑ risk of lactic acidosis
- Fast from food <4hrs prior and clear fluids 2hrs prior as contrast media can cause nausea and vomiting.

Post-procedure nursing considerations

- Observations according to local policy to detect any signs of bleeding, e.g. pulse, BP 30 min for 2hrs, 1hrly for 2hrs until not lying flat
- Observe for signs of haemorrhage ↓ BP ↑ pulse (thready), pallor sweating or the patient may become agitated
- Check puncture site for signs of bleeding/haemorrhage/haematoma
- Neurovascular observations, check colour, warmth, movement and sensation of both feet and for the presence of pedal pulses, e.g. DP, PT
- Bed rest, usually flat or at 45° for the first 1–2hrs, then bed rest 3–24hrs depending on local policy
- Check kidney function in known renal impairment
- Check Cr at 48hrs has been organized prior to re-starting metformin
- Recommence anticoagulants the evening post procedure as per medical orders
- ↑ oral fluid intake if not on fluid restriction to flush through contrast media which is nephrotoxic and monitor urine output (check voided 6–8hrs post procedure)
- Educate patient on to avoid strenuous exercise for 48–72hrs and a bath or shower for 24hrs. Post washing, pat dry the puncture site.

Kidney biopsy

A kidney biopsy is undertaken to provide a diagnosis or to guide treatment. It is performed percutaneously with the patient lying prone for native kidneys and in a supine position for transplanted kidneys. In native biopsies the left kidney is usually chosen for ease of access. Rarely Tx biopsies are performed as an 'open' procedure if clinical circumstances dictate, e.g. high risk of bleeding.

- Percutaneous biopsy is performed by introducing a Tru-Cut® needle or a spring-loaded biopsy gun into the lower pole of the kidney to obtain a sample of kidney tissue, which must include the cortex:
  - LA is used for this procedure
  - The patient is asked to hold their breath when the needle is inserted into the kidney
- US is used to assist in the location of the kidney and identify any cysts
- CT guidance can be used where identification of renal cortex is impossible, e.g. in gross obesity.

Contraindications

- Uncontrolled hypertension
- Diagnosed kidney disease
- Uncooperative patient
- Profound psychological problems (e.g. needle phobia)
- UTI
- Uncontrolled coagulopathy
- Hydronephrosis or cystic kidneys
- Gross obesity
- Severe anaemia
- Small kidneys
- Acute pyelonephritis/abscess
- Solitary kidney
- Possible renal tumour.

Complications

- Pain
- Other organs biopsied, e.g. bowel, spleen, or liver
- 0.1% arteriovenous fistula
- Most patients will have transient microscopic haematuria which will resolve itself
- <5% prolonged bleeding/haemorrhage/haematoma as the risk of bleeding increases 2–3-fold with renal impairment and may require transfusing in 1% of cases
- 1:1500 irreversible kidney damage with subsequent nephrectomy required <0.1%
- 0.01% risk of death.

Pre-procedure nursing considerations

- Check consent form signed as per unit policy and educate patient on the pre- and post-procedure care:
  - patient may have anxiety about kidney biopsy, particularly if they have undergone a previous biopsy of their native or transplanted kidneys
- Check if the patient is allergic to iodine if used as antiseptic solution
- Baseline urinalysis, haemodynamic observations, check no current UTI:
  - if BP >140/90mmHg inform medical staff for review
- Check FBC, group and save taken, check Hb >10g/dl
- Check clotting profile, platelet count taken and within normal limits:
  - contact medical staff if INR >1.2, bleeding time >10mins, platelets <100 × 10⁹/L
- Check anticoagulants have been stopped 5 days prior, e.g. warfarin, heparin, clopidogrel as ordered by the medical staff
- Check the patient has not been taking NSAIDs or aspirin
- ± infusion of desmopressin or a blood transfusion if abnormal bleeding times and/or Ur ≥20mmol/L or Cr ≥300mmol/L.

Post-procedure nursing considerations

- Haemodynamic observations according to local policy:
  - signs of haemorrhage ↓ BP, ↑ pulse (thready), pallor sweating, aching pain to shoulder/back or abdomen and become agitated
- Check puncture site according to local policy for signs of bleeding/haemorrhage/haematoma
- Check urinalysis for the presence of haematuria prior to discharge
- Bed rest dependent on local policy, many units now discharge within the same day:
  - lie flat for the first 2–6hrs
  - transplanted kidney biopsy will not require as long on bed rest, usually 6hrs
  - overnight stay usually recommended in the presence of persistent frank haematuria
- Pain assessment (flank) and provide analgesics as required
- Follow up anticoagulation therapy if stopped pre-biopsy and discuss with medical staff recommencement
- Patient education on discharge:
  - no strenuous lifting for 4wks post procedure
  - check puncture site for signs of redness, swelling, and bleeding
  - notify unit if evidence of back pain, fever, dizziness, or haematuria.

Further reading

Daugirdas, J. *Handbook of Chronic Kidney Disease Management*. Philadelphia, PA: Wolters Kluwer/ Lippincott Williams & Wilkins; 2011.

NICE. *Chronic Kidney Disease: Early identification and management of chronic kidney disease in adults in primary and secondary care*. Clinical Guideline 73. London: National Institute for Health and Clinical Excellence; 2008.

Steddon S, Ashman N, Chesser A, et al. *Oxford Handbook of Nephrology and Hypertension*. Oxford: Oxford University Press; 2006.

Warrell A, Cox T, Firth D (eds). *Oxford Textbook of Medicine*, 5th edn. Oxford: Oxford University Press; 2010.

References

1. National Kidney Disease Education Program. GFR calculators. Available at: ℅ <www.nkdep.nih. gov/healthprofessionals/tools/Reciprocal>

2. EdREN. *Reciprocal creatinine plots*. Available at: ℅ <http://renux.dmed.ed.ac.uk/edren/ Handbookbits/HDBKgfrest.html> (accessed 6 May 2012).

3. CKD-EPI calculator. Available at: ℅ http://mdrd.com/>

4. The UK Renal Association. *About eGFR*. Available at: ℅ <http://www.renal.org/whatwedo/ InformationResources/CKDeGUIDE/AbouteGFR.aspx> (accessed 6 May 2012).

Useful patient websites

European Medicines Agency. Available at: ℅ <http://www.ema.europa.eu/ema/>

UK Renal Association. Patient information leaflets for kidney biopsy (native and transplanted), angioplasty and stent insertion. Available at: ℅ <http://www.renal.org/whatwedo/information-resources/patients.aspx>

Patient information leaflets

EdRenINFO. Available at: ℅ <http://www.edren.org/pages/edreninfo/ckd-chronic-renal-failure-an d-its-progression.php>

The Royal College of Radiologists. Available at: ℅ <http://www.rcr.ac.uk>

UK NKF. Available at: ℅ <http://www.kidney.org.uk>

Chapter 3

Management of hypertension

Introduction

Hypertension is a largely preventable and is the most commonly treated chronic condition in primary care. It is associated with increased morbidity and mortality and management strategies are aimed at preventing associated complications, e.g. cerebrovascular disease, CVD, and CKD. Untreated hypertension will often lead to a progressive rise in BP which may be increasingly resistant to treatment as a result of vascular and kidney damage.

The publication and implementation of the National Service Framework for CVD prevention and the British Hypertension Society (BHS) and NICE guidance for the management of hypertension (updated in 2011)[1] have had a major impact by improving:

- Routine BP surveillance
- Strategies aimed at targeting high-risk groups and those with non-modifiable risk factors
- Early detection and management of hypertension:
  - modifiable risk factors, e.g. lifestyle modification
  - pharmacological interventions.

The current guidelines are based on many recent, large, randomized controlled hypertension drug trials assessing not only the efficacy of agents in reducing BP, but also whether they reduce cardiovascular events over and above their ability to reduce BP. There is evidence of the importance of lifestyle measures in the prevention and treatment of hypertension, efficacy of different drug groups, and the importance of assessing absolute risk of CVD.

Blood pressure facts

- BP is measured as systolic and diastolic pressure:
  - Systolic blood pressure (SBP) indicates the pressure during ventricular contraction
  - Diastolic blood pressure (DBP) indicates the pressure during ventricular relaxation
- BP varies between individuals, between ethnic groups, and also at different times of the day:
  - SBP continues to rise until the 8th decade of life
  - DBP rises until about the 5th decade of life and after this remains about the same or declines slightly
  - DBP is the best predictor of risk for patients aged <50yrs; SBP is the best predictor for patients aged >50yrs
- BP within the general population has a normal distribution, with no clear cut-off between hypertensive and normotensive subjects
- Long-term health benefits have been documented when BP is maintained at <140/90mmHg in those without diabetes and <130/80mmHg in those with diabetes:
  - ↑ risk of complications with higher values
- For every increase of 20/10mmHg in BP there is a doubling of the risk of CVD.

Definition of hypertension

Hypertension is diagnosed in the clinic (which should be confirmed by ambulatory BP monitoring (ABPM)) when:
- BP >140/90mmHg in those without diabetes
- BP >130/80mmHg in those with diabetes.

NICE guidance[1] for the definition of hypertension
- Stage 1: clinic BP >140/90mmHg and ABPM daytime average BP or home BP monitoring (HBPM) average is >135/85mmHg
- Stage 2: clinic BP is >160/100mmHg and subsequent ABPM daytime average or HBPM average BP is >150/95mmHg
- Severe: clinic SBP is >180mmHg or clinic DBP is >110mmHg.

- All adults should have their BP checked every 5yrs until the age of 80yrs
- Those with high-normal SBP (130–139mmHg) should have their BP checked annually
- NICE guidance[1] recommends the use of ABPM to confirm a diagnosis of hypertension in all people with a clinic BP >140/90mmHg. Whilst waiting for the ABPM, evidence of target organ damage (TOD) should be investigated
- Referral to a specialist with an interest in hypertension is recommended if BP is uncontrolled on 4 antihypertensive agents.

Types of hypertension

Types of hypertension

Primary hypertension

The term primary hypertension is now preferred and has superseded the term 'essential' hypertension.

- Accounts for approximately 90% of people with hypertension where there is no identifiable cause for the raised BP
- It is estimated that 25% of the UK population suffer from hypertension (BP ≥140/90mmHg)
- Prevalence is influenced by advancing age, modifiable risk factors, e.g. obesity, dietary factors, lack of exercise, alcohol consumption (see 🕮 pp. 84–5)
- Isolated ↑ SBP is more common in the elderly and ↑ DBP in <50yrs.

Secondary hypertension

About 5–10% of people will have secondary hypertension where the rise in BP is due to an identifiable cause. Treating the cause can help to treat the hypertension.

Causes of secondary hypertension

- Obesity
- Drugs, e.g. NSAIDs, corticosteroids, erythropoietin, calcineurin inhibitor (CNIs), combined oral contraceptive pill, nasal decongestants, cocaine and amphetamines
- CKD
- Renovascular disease e.g. renal artery stenosis (RAS)
- Hormonal disturbances e.g. phaeochromocytoma
- Endocrine tumours e.g. Conn's adenoma
- Other causes: obstructive sleep apnoea, hyper/hypothyroidism, coarctation of the aorta.

White coat hypertension

15–30% of the population suffer from white coat hypertension which is more common in pregnancy and advancing age. There is a risk of commencing treatment for hypertension in normotensive people, e.g. causing orthostatic hypotension and risk of falls in the elderly. Features of white coat hypertension include:

- The clinic BP is raised and soon returns to normal once the person has left the clinic. The HBPM and/or ABPM are normal
- The person may be tachycardic (common), sweaty, and experience palpitations (rarely) when in the clinic which they would not usually exhibit as a result of anxiety associated with attending the clinic
- This phenomenon can also occur in known treated hypertensive persons, so requires review of HBPM or ABPM to prevent over-medicating
- If white coat hypertension is suspected, then arrange HBPM or ABPM.

Accelerated phase hypertension

This condition requires immediate treatment and is defined as a DBP >120mmHg with grade 3 or 4 hypertensive retinopathy (grade 3 = exudates AND haemorrhages; grade 4 = papilloedema). The BP needs to be lowered in a controlled way, as lowering it too fast may cause further TOD, e.g. stroke, renal infarction.

A hypertensive emergency requires immediate BP lowering due to acute TOD.

A hypertensive urgency may have similar BP readings but without severe symptoms or signs of TOD and BP can be lowered in hrs to days usually with oral medication.

Clinical features
- Headache, visual disturbance—hypertensive retinopathy
- Confusion—hypertensive encephalopathy (cerebral oedema)
- SOB—LVF
- Chest pain—angina, MI
- Proteinuria, haematuria, and AKI—nephrosclerosis
- Microangiopathic haemolytic anaemia
- CVA—intracerebral haemorrhage.

Causes
- Primary hypertension
- Renal, e.g. glomerulonephritis, renovascular disease
- Systemic, e.g. SLE, scleroderma
- Pre-eclampsia/eclampsia
- Endocrine—phaeochromocytoma
- Drugs, e.g. ecstasy, ciclosporin, ESAs, MAOIs.

Investigations
- Check patient's current medications and adherence to regimen
- Any use of recreational drugs, e.g. amphetamines, ecstasy
- Assessment for underlying cause
- Urine—proteinuria, haematuria and casts
- U&Es
- FBC
- ECG
- CT head if neurological changes
- Kidney biopsy—but only once BP stabilized for 2wks.

Management
- Treatment is dependent on whether the patient is symptomatic and there is any TOD i.e., whether a *hypertensive urgency* or *emergency*
- Where possible, gradual ↓ of BP will minimize any adverse effects, e.g. CVA, kidney damage or coronary event.

Hypertensive urgency
- Admit—renal/medical/CCU/obstetric HDU
- Oral nifedipine retard 10mg—other CCBs onset too slow
  - if BP still ↑ further dose at 2hrs. Titrate up to 30mg tds over 24–48hrs
- Convert to longer-acting CCB once stable (e.g. amlodipine)
- β blockers and α blockers can be added in as needed
- ACEI/ARB should only be used once fluid levels stable—danger of precipitant ↓ in BP
- Discharge for follow-up within 3 days when BP <180/110mmHg
- Further agents added to ↓ BP to target levels

Hypertensive emergency
- Admit—HDU/ICU
- Check fluid status:
  - IV fluids if hypovolaemic
- Speed and extent of initial reduction dependent on associated complications:
  - e.g. acute aortic dissection requires immediate ↓ of SBP <110mmHg conversely in an acute ischaemic stroke necessitating thrombolysis the BP should be ↓ by only 15% over 1hr
  - with AKI the BP should be ↓ by 20–25% over several hrs
- Choice of agent also varies with complications:
  - IV nitroprusside has historical value in cases of aortic dissection and pulmonary oedema at immediate onset. ⚠May result in cyanide poisoning in CKD and not commonly used due to potential toxicity
- Labetalol (oral or IV)—onset in 5–10mins:
  - commonly used in AKI, CVA, encephalopathy, eclampsia. May precipitate severe drop in BP, heart block/bradycardia, HF
- Glyceryl trinitrate or isosorbide dinitrate infusion—onset 1–5mins:
  - used if angina/MI especially if LVF
- α-blockers (phenoxybenzamine)—onset 1–2mins:
  - used in phaeochromocytoma may precipitate angina
- BP will require close monitoring as per unit policy
- Patient education on the importance of taking prescribed antihypertensive medications.

Resistant hypertension
- NICE[1] have defined resistant hypertension as uncontrolled BP >140/90mmHg despite optimal or best tolerated 3rd line treatment
- Most common cause is poor medication adherence
- Leads to stiffening and calcification of arteries, LVH, and further resistance to treatment.

Predisposing factors
- Non-adherence
- Obesity
- Alcohol

- Ethnicity
- CKD
- Diabetes mellitus.

Management
- Assess and treat predisposing factors or underlying causes, e.g. drugs, alcohol, adherence
- Assess for white coat hypertension by either ABPM or HBPM
- Provide advice and educational information on ↓ salt diet ± refer to dietitian if required
- May require the use of diuretic therapy with low-dose spironolactone if K^+ ≤4.5mmol/L:
  - ⚠️↑ risk of ↑ K^+ with ↓ eGFR., if K^+ >4.5mmol/L, consider a ↑ dose of a thiazide-like diuretic
- May require the addition of another agent e.g. β or α blocker.

Orthostatic hypotension
- Defined as a fall of >20/10mmHg in SBP/DBP within 2–5mins of standing still
- Caused by reduced venous filling and pre-load leading to ↓ cardiac output and ↓ BP
- More common in the elderly due to ↓ baroreceptor sensitivity
- Anaemia can exacerbate symptoms.

Clinical features
- Dizziness, falls
- Pre-syncope
- Weakness and visual disturbances.

Causes
- Drugs, e.g. antihypertensives (CCB, vasodilators, and nitrates), opiates, alcohol, antidepressants (tricyclic and phenothiazines)
- Dehydration
- Parkinson's disease
- Diabetes mellitus
- Amyloidosis
- Endocrine—hypoaldosteronism,
- Advanced age.

Management
- No treatment is required if asymptomatic.
Symptomatic
- Investigate and treat underlying cause, e.g. drugs, dehydration
- Treat anaemia (see 📖 pp. 226–7)
- Conservative options:
  - ↑ Na^+ intake /fluid intake
  - advise patient to get out of bed slowly in the morning in stages or when lying down

(Continued)

(Continued)
- postural counter manoeuvers, e.g. leg crossing, muscle tensing,
- ↑ physical activity levels
- advise patient to avoid the hot weather, straining, early morning activity and exercise especially after a meal, avoid caffeinated drinks
- compression aids, e.g. support stockings
- pharmacological options may include mineralocorticoids, e.g. fludrocortisone.

Role of the kidney in blood pressure control

The kidney plays a major role in BP control by causing the constriction of arteries and veins and increasing the extracellular fluid volume via the renin–angiotensin pathway (see Figure 3.1).

The mechanisms include:
- In kidney failure, the kidneys produce more renin as a result of ↓ perfusion, which further ↑ BP and kidney damage:
  - even in ESKD the kidney continues to produce renin. This explains why CKD and kidney damage can cause hypertension and why hypertension can also be the cause of kidney damage
- The ↓ in the number of nephrons → inability to excrete an adequate Na^+ –H_2O load → ↑ BP to compensate for this.

Hypertensive nephropathy/nephrosclerosis

Damage to blood vessels is caused by persistently elevated BP and occurs in all blood vessels throughout the body, in particular the cerebral, coronary, and kidney. Kidney involvement is due to sclerosis (narrowing) of the renal arterioles → ↓ blood supply to the glomeruli, tubules, and interstitium → scarring to the renal tissue.
- Associated with chronic hypertension
- Risk factors include black ethnicity and uncontrolled hypertension with underlying CKD.

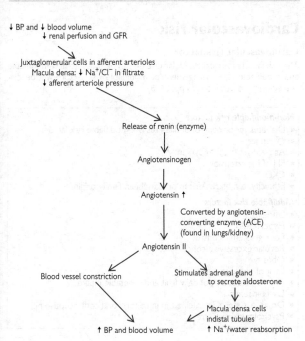

↓ BP and ↓ blood volume
↓ renal perfusion and GFR

Juxtaglomerular cells in afferent arterioles
Macula densa: ↓ Na$^+$/Cl$^-$ in filtrate
↓ afferent arteriole pressure

Release of renin (enzyme)

Angiotensinogen

Angiotensin ↑

Converted by angiotensin-
converting enzyme (ACE)
(found in lungs/kidney)

Angiotensin II

Blood vessel constriction

Stimulates adrenal gland
to secrete aldosterone

Macula densa cells
indistal tubules
↑ Na$^+$/water reabsorption

↑ BP and blood volume

Fig. 3.1 Renin–angiotensin pathway.

Cardiovascular risk

Cardiovascular risk factors

The risk factors for cardiovascular disease can be split into non-modifiable and modifiable (the management of modifiable risk factors will be discussed in more detail on 📖 pp. 84–5).

Non-modifiable risk factors
- Diabetes (poor control of diabetes is a modifiable risk factor)
- ♂ gender
- Age >55yrs in ♂ >65yrs in ♀
- FH of hypertension
- CKD
- Ethnicity, e.g. black African or Caribbean family origin.

Modifiable risk factors
- Smoking
- Hypertension
- Poor glycaemic control
- Regular excessive alcohol
- Obesity
- Lack of exercise
- Poor diet, e.g. lack of daily fruit and vegetable intake
- Dyslipidaemia
- Drugs, e.g. steroids, calcineurin inhibitors, oral contraceptive pill
- Psychological, e.g. stress.

Cardiovascular risk (CVR) assessment tools
- CVR equations[2] provide a score which is an approximation and should be used in conjunction with clinical assessment and judgement:
  - CVR may be underestimated if already taking an antihypertensive or lipid lowering drug, or has stopped smoking recently
  - CVR tools should be used in partnership with the person to discuss risk factors and treatment options
  - severe obesity (BMI >40kg/m²) and socio-economic status will affect CVD risk and should be taken into consideration when using risk calculators
- Those >75yrs are considered already at an ↑ risk of CVD, in particular if they smoke or have hypertension
- Previously the Framingham risk equation was used, however NICE lipid modification guidance[3] advises adjustment for the presence of any FH of premature coronary heart disease (CHD), or South Asian ethnicity due to its limitations:
  - tends to overestimate risk in low/medium-risk groups
  - underestimates risk for certain groups, e.g. South Asians, diabetics, familial hypercholesterolaemia, strong FH of premature CVD, LVF on echo, CKD and ♂ in lower socio-economic groups

- Many CV risk equations are not suitable for use in people with pre-existing CHD-angina, stroke/TIA, PVD, high risk of CVD, e.g. familial hypercholesterolaemia, diabetes, HIV, autoimmune disorders (SLE, rheumatoid arthritis), CKD
- An alternative is the QRISK®2 online calculator[4] which adjusts for ethnicity, social deprivation, and co-morbidities such as CKD and diabetes.

Cardiovascular disease and CKD

The majority of people with CKD die from CV-related complications, so reducing the risk of these is extremely important. However, reducing cholesterol levels in people with CKD does not reduce CV deaths as significantly as in the general population. All people with CKD should be considered to be in the highest risk group for CVD irrespective of levels of traditional CVD risk factors.

The causes of CVD in CKD include:

- Atherosclerosis—fatty material collects along the walls of the arteries. As these deposits thicken and harden they can cause a blockage in the vessel wall or result in the formation of emboli
- Arterial calcification—hardening or stiffening of the blood vessels due to a variety of uraemic toxins and calcium deposition in the blood vessels
  - arterial pressure depends in part on the stiffness of the arteries and SBP tends to be higher
  - vascular calcification, particularly coronary calcification and arterial stiffness, occurs in CKD as a result of hyperparathyroidism, inflammation, hyperphosphataemia, Ca^{2+} loading from phosphate binders and vitamin D metabolites
  - anaemia (see 📖 pp. 226–7).

Management of cardiovascular risk

NICE guidance[3] for the management of CV risk includes:

- 1° prevention (no previous cardiovascular event):
  - statins recommended for 1° prevention of CVD in adults who are 20% or have a >10yr risk of developing CVD (i.e. includes CKD)
  - use of a CV risk assessment calculator and/or clinical assessment, e.g. in older people, high-risk ethnic groups, diabetes
  - patient education on lifestyle modification (see 📖 pp. 84–5)
- 2° prevention (previous cardiovascular event):
  - statins should be used in conjunction with lifestyle modification
  - assessment should include: smoking, alcohol intake, BP, BMI or other measure of obesity, fasting lipids and BGL, LFTs, TSH if dyslipidaemic
  - aim for cholesterol <4mmol/L or LDL <2mmol/L.

Treatment in CKD

- Provide education and support on lifestyle modifications (see 📖 pp. 84–5)
- Promote a healthy diet:

- liaise with dietitian and educate person about a low-fat diet to
  ↓ cholesterol levels if required
- The Renal Association, 2010[5] recommend:
  - CKD 1–4 and transplant patients with 10yr risk of CVD calculated
    >20% should be commenced on a statin
  - aim for a total cholesterol <4mmol/L or 25% ↓ from baseline, or
    fasting LDL cholesterol <2mmol/L or a 30% ↓ from baseline
  - use of antiplatelet drugs for 2° prevention, e.g. low-dose aspirin.
    ⚠ ↑ risk of minor bleeding in CKD patients who are given multiple
    antiplatelet drugs
- Good glycaemic control, HbA1c to be maintained between
  48–58mmol/mol/HbAo or 6.5–7.5%.

Use of statins
- A baseline LFT should be taken prior to commencing statin treatment,
  re-checked at 3 months, and then annually
- ⚠There is an ↑ risk of statin-induced myositis with CKD and fibrates
  are contraindicated in advanced kidney disease.

Complications of hypertension

There are often no symptoms of hypertension and it is only diagnosed at a routine health check-up, as part of ongoing management of other chronic conditions (e.g. diabetes) or after one of the complications has arisen, e.g. CVA.

Complications include:
- CVA or TIA
- MI, LVF, IHD
- Atherosclerotic disease, PVD
- HF
- Multi-infarct dementia
- Retinopathy
- Hypertensive nephropathy/nephrosclerosis → CKD:
  - a ↑ 5mmHg in DBP results in a 35–40% ↑ in the risk of a stroke
  - a ↓ 5mmHg in SBP is associated with a 25% ↓ in the risk of CKD.

Measurement of blood pressure

Accurate measurement of BP is an extremely important clinical skill and requires regular training, use of validated equipment and implementation of recommendations on procedure.

Factors that can influence BP readings as much as 20mmHg:

- Time of day
- Emotional state, anxiety
- Exercise
- Caffeine
- Smoking—BP is elevated for 15–30mins after smoking a cigarette
- Drugs
- Bladder fullness
- Pain/shock
- Acute changes in temperature.

Blood pressure monitoring devices

The BHS website provides detailed guidance on the use of validated automated and manual BP devices, including a list of suitable machines, in various price brackets, to recommend to people. The manual sphygmomanometer remains the gold standard for measuring BP.

Automated

- Automated devices can give inaccurate results with an irregular pulse, e.g. atrial fibrillation:
  - check radial or brachial for rhythm of pulse and use a manual device if irregular
  - may underestimate SBP and overestimate DBP
- Automated devices can be used for measuring BP at home. These can be bought relatively cheaply from pharmacies
- Wrist BP monitors are not recommended due to their inaccuracy
- BP should be checked manually if there is concern about the results

Home blood pressure monitoring (HBPM)

Encouraging people to measure their own BP can motivate them to act on the other lifestyle measures to help reduce BP. For those unable or unwilling to monitor BP at home, BP can be checked between visits, e.g. at the GP surgery or by a community nurse to assess efficacy of drug therapy and a history of BP.

- Home measurements should be taken by the person in a sitting position:
  - twice, 1min apart, twice a day, e.g. am and evening for a minimum of 4 days, preferably 7 days
  - the 1st day's readings should not be included and an average taken of all of the other readings
- Comparing clinic readings with measurements made at home can identify white coat hypertension (see 📖 p. 70).

Ambulatory blood pressure monitoring (ABPM)

ABPM is recommended if the clinic reading is ≥140/90mmHg prior to commencing treatment, excluding severe hypertension.

- ≥2 measurements/hr as a minimum taken during the person's normal 'wake' time (e.g. 7a.m. to 9p.m.).
- The daytime average BP should be based on a minimum of 14 measurements
- A diary is kept by the person of their activities during the 24hrs
- Useful as an assessment for:
  - inconsistent BP readings
  - evaluation of nocturnal hypertension
  - efficacy of drug treatment over 24hrs
  - diagnose possible white coat hypertension.

Assessment of postural hypotension

The correct measurement of BP is required in people with suspected postural hypotension, e.g. symptoms such as falls and dizziness. Autonomic neuropathy in diabetes is a common cause of postural hypotension. Possible causes in CKD include hypovolaemia and hyponatraemia.

- BP should be measured with the person in either the supine or sitting position
- Measure BP again when the person has been standing for at least 1 min
- Management includes review of medications, assess for underlying cause, e.g. nausea/vomiting, volume depletion post HD.

Manual procedure for measuring BP

- Promote a quiet and relaxed atmosphere
- Sitting for at least 5mins, relaxed, and not moving or speaking
- Check the person does not need to void, has recently had any caffeine or food, undertaken exercise, or smoked
- Remove restrictive clothing from the arm—measurement should not be performed through clothes as it requires direct skin contact
- The arm must be outstretched and be supported with the cuff at the level of the heart (in line with the mid-sternum)
- Use an appropriate sized cuff for the upper arm.
  - a standard adult cuff is for an arm circumference of <33cm
  - a cuff of the wrong size will give an incorrect reading. See the BHS website for correct sizing chart[6]
  - as a guide the cuff should encircle ≥80% and not more than 100% of the upper arm
- Palpate brachial pulse in the antecubital fossa
- Quickly inflate the cuff to above the point where the brachial pulse disappears. Deflate the cuff and palpate until the pulse re-appears
- Quickly inflate the cuff to 30mmHg above the estimated systolic level needed to occlude the pulse identified above
- Place the stethoscope diaphragm over the brachial artery and deflate the cuff by 2–3mmHg/sec until Korotkoff sounds can be heard, this is the SBP
- Continue to deflate the cuff until the tapping sound disappears. This is DBP
- This process should be repeated 3 times for greatest accuracy and the mean level recorded

(Continued)

(Continued)

- If possible BP should be taken at the beginning and end of consultation
- Inaccurate readings can occur as a result of:
  - practitioners rounding off to the nearest zero
  - inability to identify Korotkoff sounds
  - practitioner bias, e.g. assuming same as last BP reading.

For automated machines, place the correct sized cuff around the arm with the indicator mark on the cuff over the brachial artery. The monitor will then inflate and deflate to give a BP reading. Again, take 2 readings and record the mean value.

Assessment and diagnosis of hypertension

- An initial BP should be measured in both arms
- Normal to have a difference of <10mmHg between the arms:
  - if the difference between the 2 arms is >20mmHg—repeat
  - if on the next measurement the difference remains >20mmHg—measure all further BP on the arm with the higher reading
  - >20mmHg may indicate underlying vascular disease and the practitioner should notify the medical staff
- If BP in clinic ≥140/90mmHg:
  - take a further measurement during the clinic visit
  - if this 2nd measurement is significantly different from the 1st, then take a 3rd measurement and record the lower of the last 2 measurements
- For clinic BP ≥140/90mmHg, offer ABPM to confirm diagnosis of hypertension prior to treatment, excluding accelerated hypertension
  - if the person is unable to have ABPM, then HBPM should be used to confirm the diagnosis
- Investigate for TOD which includes:
  - examining the fundi for retinal damage
  - ECG to check for LVH
  - ECHO to confirm LVH if indicated on ECG
  - U&E, eGFR to check for kidney damage
  - urine dipstick to test for the presence of blood
  - ACR to test for the presence of protein
  - blood glucose level
  - fasting blood lipid profile
- Other features on clinical assessment or investigations that might be sought or indicated in selected patients include:
  - peripheral vascular disease, e.g. absent peripheral pulses, ankle-brachial pressure index
  - cerebral complications, e.g. cognitive function, carotid bruits
- CV risk assessment (see 📖 p. 76)
- PMH, including FH of hypertension, diabetes, CVA, risk factors, kidney disease or any prior history or treatment of hypertension.
- Assessment for recent events, e.g. bereavement, loss of job
- Assess for white coat hypertension with ABPM
- Current medications and any allergies or contraindications to drugs, e.g. pregnancy, HF.

Management of hypertension

All people should be offered education and support on non-pharmacological treatment, e.g. lifestyle modification (see 📖 pp. 84–5).

- Stage 1, <40yrs and no evidence of TOD, CVD, CKD or diabetes—do not require antihypertensive treatment and should have an annual review
- However, current risk prediction charts will often underestimate lifetime risk in this age group and treatment or more specialist assessment for TOD may well be appropriate.

Commencement of antihypertensive treatment

- Stage 1 hypertension <80yrs with 1 or more of the following:
  - TOD
  - CVD
  - CKD
  - Diabetes
  - 10yr cardiovascular risk ≥20%
- Stage 2 hypertension of any age.

Non-pharmacological treatment

Advice on lifestyle modification can help to reduce BP and lower overall CV risk. This should be provided to all people with high and borderline BP on a regular basis. Encourage people to discuss the following with a healthcare professional for individualized advice and provide educational resources, e.g. leaflets, websites, audiovisual aids.

Dietary/salt management

- There is good evidence to suggest that a diet high in salt ↑ BP, causes fluid retention and is associated with CVD:
  - restrict salt intake <100mmol/day (6g/day)
  - avoid adding salt in cooking or at the table, e.g. 5g sodium chloride (NaCl) ≈to 1 teaspoon of salt, give advice on the use of seasoning as an alternative
  - avoid processed foods as high in salt
  - check packaging and labels for salt content, e.g. some breakfast cereals have a high salt content. Choose foods that contain ≤0.1g Na^+ per 100g
  - ⚠ CKD patients should not use salt substitutes e.g. 'Lo Salt' as NaCl is often replaced with potassium chloride (KCl)— ↑ risk of hyperkalaemia
- Low-fat, high-fibre diet with 5 portions of fruit and vegetables per day and to maintain an ideal body weight (IBW)
  - it is recommended that people at risk of CVD should eat 2 portions of fish per week and one of these should be oily fish
- There is a strong link between being overweight and hypertension:
  - provide advice and support to achieve IBW
  - losing 10kg can ↓ SBP by 5–10mmHg

Exercise

- A good stress reliever and can also help people to lose weight, maintain IBW, and ↓ BP
- Aim to for 20–30mins of brisk exercise, i.e. that gets them out of breath, at least 3 times a week:
  - advise patients who are less physically able that 10min of physical activity in episodes during the day is just as effective
- Regular aerobic exercise can ↓ SBP by 4–9mmHg
- A brisk walk for 1/2hr per day ↓ relative risk by 20% (see 📖 pp. 558–61)

Alcohol

- Excessive alcohol intake can lead to ↑ BP and reduce efficacy of antihypertensive medication
  - ↓ alcohol intake can ↓ SBP by 2–4mmHg
- Drinking a moderate amount may be beneficial for coronary heart disease and is not harmful. People should be advised to stick to national levels for alcohol intake:
  - 21 units/week in ♂ and 14 units/week in ♀, and not more than 3 units for ♂ and 2 units for ♀ on any day
  - excessive alcohol intake, i.e. binge drinking is associated with hypertension.

Smoking

- Smoking has not been directly linked to ↑ BP; however it does reduce life expectancy as a result of CVD and pulmonary disease
- Smoking cessation lowers the risk of blood vessel damage that can lead to an MI or CVA.
  - if this is achieved before middle age, it returns life expectancy to near that of a life-long non-smoker
- Smoking cessation reduces cardiac events by 50% in the first 2yrs.

Weight

- ↓ weight to a BMI of 20–25 is recommended
- ↓ 5–10% of initial body weight can ↓ BP and improve BGLs.

Relaxation therapy

- Associated with a beneficial effect on lowering BP in those with stress and anxiety.

Support groups/organization

- Referral to organizations and local support groups can be beneficial for advice and support on making lifestyle modifications.

General information

- Provide information, websites, and leaflets on hypertension and CVR
- Patient education on medicines to be taken and promote adherence, e.g. simple dosage regimen, multicompartmental medicine box (see 📖 p. 572)
- Encourage patient to monitor their condition, e.g. HBPM.

Pharmacological treatment

Choice of antihypertensive

There are many groups of antihypertensive agents available, each with different licensed indications, contraindications, cautions, and side effects. (See individual summary of product characteristics for full detailed information.)

- When treating an individual, the relevant contraindications and other indications for the drugs also need to be considered, see 📖 Table 3.1, p. 87. If a person is on one of the drugs for another reason it can be used out of place in the antihypertensive drug recommendation algorithm
- The order of use and titration of antihypertensive drugs to attain BP targets should follow the NICE guidance,[1] see Figure 3.2, 📖 p. 90.

The main groups

- Angiotensin converting enzyme inhibitors (ACEIs), e.g. ramipril
- Angiotensin receptor blockers (ARB), e.g. candesartan, losartan
- Calcium channel blockers (CCBs), e.g. amlodipine
- Thiazide and thiazide-like diuretics, e.g. bendroflumethiazide, indapamide
- Centrally acting, e.g. moxonidine
- Vascular smooth muscle relaxants, e.g. minoxidil
- β blockers, e.g. atenolol
- α blockers, e.g. doxazosin.

Specific points

- Treatment is split into RAS-blocking drugs, e.g. ACEI and β blockers
- Younger (<55yrs), non-black patients tend to have a greater RAS activation so may respond better to a RAS-blocking drug
- CCBs should be considered as 1st-line drug treatment
- ACEI and ARB should not be used in combination
- Ideally, the dosage should be simplified to promote adherence, however many people are likely to require >1 drug
- Treatment of BP in isolation will leave many patients at high risk of cardiovascular complications
  - absolute CVD risk should be assessed and interventions including statins and aspirin should be used where appropriate (see 📖 pp. 76–7).

Table 3.1 Antihypertensive agent summary[7]

Drug	Action	Additional indications	Side effects	Caution	Contraindications
βblockers e.g. atenolol, metoprolol, sotalol, bisoprolol	Block β adrenoreceptors and sympathetic response Block renin release from juxta-glomerular apparatus	Post MI or for angina, HF Consider: resistant hypertension, ♀ of childbearing age	Fatigue, ED, depression, nightmares, tingling, numbness or coldness in the extremities, ↑ risk of diabetes (esp. if used with thiazide or thiazide-like diuretics) and bronchospasm	PVD, HF, and diabetes	Asthma, COPD, heart block when used with a rate-limiting CCB Some drugs, e.g. NSAIDs, antidepressants (MAOIs), rifampicin
Angiotensin-converting enzyme inhibitors (ACEIs), e.g. captopril, ramipril, perindopril	Inhibit ACE—stops conversion of angiotensin I to angiotensin II conversion—vasodilation, natriuresis, and ↓ fluid volume and BP	Diabetic nephropathy, LVD post MI or established CHD, and proteinuric kidney disease, 2° stroke prevention	Angioedema, postural hypotension and dizziness with the 1st dose Rash, dry cough, renal impairment, and altered taste	Renal impairment (see 🔲 p. 92 for monitoring management)	Pregnancy, renovascular disease
Angiotensin receptor blockers (ARBs), e.g. candesartan, irbesartan	Selective inhibition of the angiotensin AT-1 receptor *Different drugs within the class have different licensed indications	ACEI intolerance, diabetic nephropathy, HF, hypertension with LVH, proteinuric kidney disease and post MI	Renal impairment, rash, headache, altered taste	Renal impairment (see 🔲 p. 92 for monitoring management). Interactions with some drugs e.g. NSAIDs, lithium, antifungals	Pregnancy, renovascular disease

(Continued)

Table 3.1 (Continued)

Drug	Action	Additional indications	Side effects	Caution	Contraindications
Thiazide diuretic e.g. bendroflumethiazide hydrochlorthiazide Thiazide-like diueretic e.g.chlortalidone, indapamide	Vasodilation Moderate diuresis ↑excretion Na⁺, K⁺, H₂O	HF Hypertension and oedema 2° stroke prevention	Diabetes, ED, hypokalaemia, ↓ efficacy of NSAIDs, ↑ LDL, cholesterol and triglyceride, impaired glucose tolerance (esp if taken with β blocker) Gout	Thiazides are less effective as kidney function declines Monitor serum K⁺ levels	Gout, lithium
K⁺-sparing diuretics, e.g. spironolactone, amiloride	Moderate diuresis	Resistant hypertension	Gynaecomastia in ♂ (spironolactone only) Hyperkalaemia in kidney failure	Not used with K⁺supplements, renal impairment	Avoid if baseline K⁺ >4.5mmol/L
Calcium channel blockers (CCBs), e.g. amlodipine, felodipine, nifedipine Two groups dihydropyridines, e.g. amlodipine and non-dihydropyridines, e.g. diltiazem.	Vasodilation	Angina Hypertension	Ankle swelling, headaches, palpitations, facial flushing Constipation associated with verapamil	Rate limiting CCBs when used in combination with β blockers Grapefruit juice inhibits the metabolism of some CCBs, e.g. nifedipine so co-administration should be avoided	Heart block, HF (non-DHP CCBs only)

					Q stress incontinence / Vary with drug
α receptor blockers, e.g. doxazosin, prazosin	Antagonists of α-1 receptor	Benign prostatic hypertrophy / Resistant hypertension	Initial dizziness and fluid retention / Postural hypotension, headache, flushing, ankle swelling and tachycardia	HF	
Vascular smooth muscle relaxants, e.g. minoxidil, hydralazine	Vasodilator	Severe hypertension	Tachycardia, fluid retention, headache. Minoxidil can cause hirsuitism	Minoxidil should be given with diuretic to control salt and water retention and β blocker to control reflex tachycardia—unless on dialysis. Dose adjustment in CKD due to poor clearance	

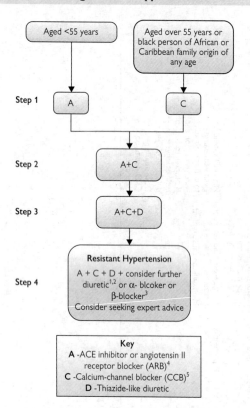

Antihypertensive agent use in CKD

Hypertension can increase the rate of progression to ESKD and ∴ controlling the BP can delay the time to ESKD. Uncontrolled hypertension can be a reason for commencing RRT.

In CKD, expect to administer ≥3 antihypertensive drugs to control BP. A suggested order for Caucasian patients is:

- Limit salt intake and employ non-pharmacological measures for modifiable risk factors, see 📖 pp. 84–5
- ACEI especially if proteinuria is present
- CCB
- Thiazide ± loop diuretic
- β blocker
- Vascular smooth muscle relaxant
- α blocker
- Centrally acting agents.

As discussed previously the exact order depends upon the patient's co-morbidities. Consider following the order given but change to suit the patient. Strategies should also be implemented to reduce CV risk.

ACEI and ARB monitoring

ACEI and ARB can cause kidney dysfunction so close monitoring is required after the commencement, or increased dosing, of the drug.

Monitoring of kidney function (e.g. GFR)

- Baseline result prior to commencement
- Within 2wks of commencement
- 2wks after a dose increase
- If patient has intercurrent illness; particularly if risk of hypovolaemia
- Ongoing regular monitoring to check for any ↓ in kidney function
- More frequent monitoring if taking other medications that promote hyperkalaemia
- If a ↓ in eGFR ≥25% or ↑ plasma creatinine ≥30% is seen following ACEI or ARB introduction or dose ↑, check kidney function again in 1–2wks
- If ↓ in kidney function is confirmed whilst still taking ACEI or ARB discuss with medical staff as to whether to stop or investigate for RAS (see 📖 p. 28)
- Investigate other causes of ↓ in kidney function, e.g. volume depletion or NSAIDs
- If no cause found, stop ACEI or ARB or ↓ dose to previously tolerated dose, add alternative medication if required (if taking for diabetes or proteinuric kidney disease a slow ↓ of kidney function is likely to be attributed to the disease itself)
- Educate patient on the importance of reaching optimal BP
- Advise patients to take the 1st dose at bedtime to allow for any ↓ in BP.

NB Although contraindicated in RAS, nephrologists may prescribe ACEIs or ARBs under controlled circumstances if they are unable to control hypertension with any other drugs and losing kidney function is the only way of doing this.

Management of hyperkalaemia and the use of ACEI and/or ARB

- If K$^+$ >5.0mmol/L do not start ACEI or ARBs, exclude and treat other factors that promote hyperkalaemia and recheck K$^+$
- If K$^+$ >6.0mmol/L, stop K$^+$-sparing drugs, e.g. K$^+$-sparing diuretic, NSAIDs
- Stop ACEI or ARB if K$^+$ ≥6.0mmol/L and not on the drugs that could elevate K$^+$
- Check diet, e.g. low salt substitutes should be stopped. If K$^+$ remains elevated then need to discuss with medical staff stopping ACEI or ARB.

Diuretics

- Thiazide diuretics may be ineffective once the GFR <25ml/min
- Metolazone can be added daily or on alternate days to the diuretic regimen:
  - patients will often weigh themselves at home daily and add metolazone once their weight reaches a predetermined level to increase diuresis and remove excess fluid to avoid accumulation
  - kidney function needs to be monitored carefully as it can deteriorate with metolazone-induced fluid loss
- Loop diuretics are often used in high doses to obtain sufficient diuresis:
  - doses of furosemide of 250mg or 500mg daily are not unusual
  - in those with normal kidney function the usual dose would be 40–80mg daily
- K$^+$ sparing diuretics, e.g. amiloride are not recommended due to the risk of hyperkalaemia
- Spironolactone for heart failure is used with caution when the GFR <10ml/min:
  - in CKD, spironolactone is more likely to cause hyperkalaemia so K$^+$ levels should be monitored closely.

Haemodialysis patients

When a patient requires RRT, antihypertensive medications should be reviewed. For patients undertaking HD, there are 3 potential issues:

- Timing of doses needs to be considered, since some drugs are removed by dialysis and therefore may benefit from being taken after dialysis
- The BP that a patient presents with at the start of the dialysis session may be high partly due to the extra fluid the patient has accumulated and they may have rushed for dialysis, whereas the BP they have at home may be lower:
  - measuring BP at home between dialysis sessions can help to assess this but can be difficult to achieve

- If a patient's BP is brought down too low by an antihypertensive medication they may not be able to tolerate HD and their BP may ↓ further
- Refer to a renal drug reference sources for guidance on whether a drug should be given after HD.[6]

Management of BP in HD patients

- Control of BP in the HD patient needs a multifactorial approach looking at the patients: IBW, salt and fluid intake, length and quality of HD, and their antihypertensive medications
- Antihypertensive medication dosage should be kept low to avoid hypotension during HD:
  - some patients will miss out their drugs on dialysis days to avoid this. There is limited evidence to support this, but anecdotally it may help
- ⚠ Anaphylactic reactions can occur in patients on an ACEI dialysing on polyacrylonitrile membranes so this combination should be avoided.

Transplant recipients

Hypertension occurs in up to 80% of kidney transplant recipients and is a risk factor for faster progression to CKD and development of CVD. Many transplant recipients will have serum Cr levels within the CKD range, i.e. they rarely return to normal baseline even if they have stable kidney function post transplantation. The risks are increased by IS agents which either have a direct hypertensive effect, e.g. CNIs or those that increase risk factors for hypertension such as BMI and hyperlipidaemia, e.g. steroids.

Promotion of healthy living and self-management is an important aspect of long-term, post-Tx follow-up care and in many units is nurse-led through initiatives such as annual review clinics (see 📖 pp. 472–3).

Monitoring and management

- The target BP <130/80mmHg but can be challenging to achieve
- Diurnal variation in BP—24hr ABPM may be useful as clinic BP reading may be misleading
- All antihypertensive drugs are effective in kidney Tx recipients but special considerations apply:
  - dihydropyridine CCBs are the treatment of choice for recipients who take CNIs (ciclosporin and tacrolimus) because CCBs dilate the afferent arterioles, ∴ reversing the vasoconstriction of the afferent arteriole induced by the CNIs
  - non-dihydropyridine CCBs can ↑ blood levels of ciclosporin, tacrolimus, and sirolimus so should be used with extreme caution.

- ACEI and ARB ↑ the risk of hyperkalaemia so although they are widely used, the patients should have their K^+ levels closely monitored
- β blockers are often used since the patients have a high incidence of IHD
- diuretics are useful since hypertension in ciclosporin treated patients may be Na^+ dependent.

Further reading

van den Born BJH, Beutler JJ, Gaillard CA, *et al.* Dutch guideline for the management of hypertensive crisis—2010 revision. Neth J Med 2011; **69**:248–55.

Williams B, Poulter NR, Brown MJ, *et al.* The BHS Guidelines Working Party. British Hypertension Society Guidelines for Hypertension Management, IV: Summary. *BMJ* 2004; **328**:634–40.

References

1. NICE. *Hypertension: Clinical Management of Primary Hypertension in Adults.* Clinical Guideline 127. London: National Institute for Health and Clinical Excellence; 2011. Available at: ℳ <http://www.nice.org.uk> (accessed 1 May 2012).
2. ℳ http://www.bhsoc.org/Cardiovascular_Risk_Charts_and_Calculators.stm
3. NICE. *Lipid Modification: Cardiovascular Risk Assessment and the Modification of Blood Lipids for Primary and Secondary Prevention of Cardiovascular Disease.* Clinical Guideline 67. London: National Institute of Health and Clinical Excellence; 2010.
4. ℳ <http://qrisk.org/>
5. Holt S, Goldsmith D. *The Renal Association Guideline: Cardiovascular Disease and CKD,* 5th edn. London: Renal Association; 2008. Available at: ℳ <http://www.renal.org/Libraries/Guidelines/Cardiovascular_Disease_in_CKD_-_FINAL_DRAFT_26_May_2010.sflb.ashx>
6. British Heart Society. *Measuring blood pressure.* Available at: ℳ <http://www.bhf.org.uk/heart-health/conditions/high-blood-pressure.aspx>
7. Ashley C, Currie A. *Renal Drug Handbook,* 3rd edn. Oxford: Radcliffe Medical Press; 2009. Available at: ℳ <http://www.kidneycare.org.uk/upoloaded/renaldrughandbook.pdf>

Patient information websites

EdRenINFO. *Blood pressure and kidneys.* Available at: ℳ <http://www.edren.org/pages/edreninfo/blood-pressure-and-kidney-disease.php>

NHS Choices. *Eatwell plate.* Available at: ℳ <http://www.nhs.uk/Livewell/Goodfood/Pages/eatwell-plate.aspx>

NICE. *High blood pressure,* 2011. Available at: ℳ <http://www.nice.org.uk/nicemedia/live/13561/56013/56013.pdf>

Patient.co.uk. *Medication for high blood pressure.* Available at: ℳ <http://www.patient.co.uk/health/Medication-for-High-Blood-Pressure.html>

Chapter 4

Acute kidney injury

AKI epidemiology and prognosis

AKI, previously known as acute renal failure (ARF), is defined by a fall in eGFR, a rise in serum Cr and/or oliguria, resulting in a reduction in excretory function and accumulation of waste products from metabolism. It is now recognized that even minor increases in serum Cr are associated with poorer patient outcomes.

Onset of AKI can occur over a matter of hrs or days and is seen in ~20% of all hospital admissions, 7% of inpatients, and up to 25% critical care patients. AKI is often seen in critically ill patients due to reduced renal perfusion secondary to reduced cardiac output, sepsis, or surgery. 5–6% of ITU patients require RRT. AKI accounts for >60% of patient admissions to ITU. The mortality rate for those who do not respond to treatment varies from 15–60%. Mortality is mainly due to infection.

▶ The worst indicator for survival is AKI associated with multiple organ failure.

Definition

The Renal Association (2011) Guideline 1.1 AKI: Definition, Epidemiology and Outcomes recommends using the international Kidney Disease: Improving Global Outcomes (2012) (KDIGO) to define AKI.

Defining AKI
- Serum Cr rises by ≥26.5µmol/L within 48hrs *or*
- Serum Cr rises ≥1.5 times baseline, which is known *or*
- Presumed to have occurred within 7days *or*
- Urine output is <0.5ml/kg/hr for 6hrs
- The reference serum Cr should be the lowest Cr value recorded within the past 3 months
- If a reference serum Cr value is not available within 3 months and AKI is suspected, repeat serum Cr must be taken within 24hrs.

Risk factors for developing AKI
- Advanced age >75yrs
- Underlying chronic kidney disease (eGFR <60ml/min/1.73m^2)
- Sepsis
- Hypovolaemia
- ↓ cardiac output
- Nephrotoxic drug administration
- Atherosclerotic peripheral vascular disease
- Diabetes mellitus
- Multiple myeloma
- Liver failure
- ♂/ethnicity/genetics.

Causes of AKI

Pre-renal failure

GFR decreases, which → ↓ urine output <400ml/day. This can be caused by:

- Intravascular depletion (severe vomiting/diarrhoea, haemorrhage burns, dehydration)
- Hypotension (sepsis, trauma)
- Anaphylaxis
- Impaired cardiac output (myocardial infarction, arrhythmias, cardiomyopathy)
- Medications (NSAIDs, contrast medium, ACEIs, ciclosporin).

The kidneys are structurally normal, but due to ineffective nephron perfusion AKI occurs. Pre-renal failure causes are linked to hypoperfusion of the kidneys. If this is noted quickly and perfusion is restored to the kidney, normal kidney function rapidly returns. If delayed and renal hypoperfusion continues, ischaemic damage to the kidneys will occur.

Intrinsic renal failure

Intrinsic renal failure is caused by damage to the kidney or its surrounding vasculature. There are 4 possible categories of damage:

- Vascular
- Tubular
- Glomerular
- Interstitial.

Intrinsic renal failure is responsible for 10–40% of cases of AKI.

Acute tubular necrosis (ATN) is the most common cause of intrinsic renal failure with a mortality rate of ~50%. It is predictable in high-risk clinical settings ∴ preventable.

See Figure 4.1 for classification and major causes of AKI.

Correction of AKI at this stage does not guarantee return to normal kidney function as it does with pre-renal failure. This is due to the damage that occurs to the nephron, the functional unit of the kidney, which cannot be reversed.

Post-renal failure

This is caused by an obstruction which can occur in the ureters, bladder neck, or urethra. The obstruction can be unilateral or bilateral.

The most common causes are:

- Renal calculi
- Ureteric obstruction
- Bladder cancer
- Blood clot
- Debris
- Benign prostatic hypertrophy
- Prostate cancer
- Medications (anticholinergics, acyclovir, sulfonamides).

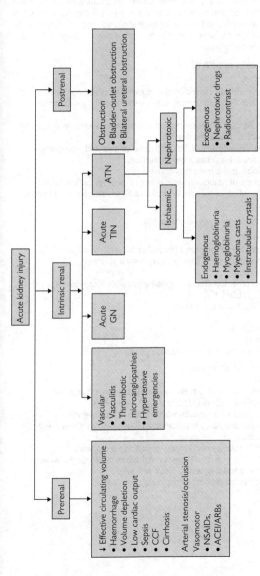

Fig. 4.1 Classification and major causes of acute kidney injury. Reproduced from Steddon S, Ashman N, Chesser A, et al. *Oxford Handbook of Nephrology and Hypertension*, Oxford: Oxford University Press; 2006, with permission from Oxford University Press.

As with pre-renal failure, post-renal failure can be fully reversible if the cause is identified and treated early. An urgent US can be undertaken to determine obstruction and/or hydronephrosis in the kidneys. A nephrostomy may be performed initially to allow urine drainage before the obstruction is corrected.

Complex causes of AKI

Rhabdomyolysis

- A clinical syndrome caused by the release of cellular contents following significant striated muscle injury. Also known as 'crush injury'
- Injury can be caused at reperfusion in ischaemic skeletal muscle or by energy depletion and cell death
- If cell death is widespread, intracellular elements and membrane products are released into the circulation:
  - myoglobin is the main nephrotoxin
- A key feature of rhabdomyolysis is large quantities of fluid being retained in inflamed muscle, → profound hypovolaemia in addition to toxic kidney injury.

▶ Not all rhabdomyolysis results in AKI.

Clinical features

- Urine dipstick +ve for blood (no red cells on microscopy)
- Urinary myoglobin +ve (not present in normal urine)
- ↑ Cr:urea ratio
- ↑ Alb if volume depleted or hypoalbuminaemia if capillary leak
- ↑ AST, ALT, LDH, CK
- ↑ K^+, ↑ PO_4, ↑ urate, ↑ lactate
- ↓ Ca^{2+}
- Myalgia/weakness (rare)
- ↓ urine output.
  See Table 4.2 for causes of rhabdomyolysis.

Management of rhabdomyolysis

Prevent AKI:

- Aim to resuscitate the patient; up to 12L/day may be required
- Aim for CVP 8–12mmHg (normal CVP 2–6mmHg)
- IV 0.9% normal saline and bicarbonate are normally given
- Urine output should be maintained ≥150ml/hr or ≥300ml/hr with traumatic injury
- Continue IV therapy until urinary myoglobin disappears
- Dialysis may be required if overt renal failure develops. However prognosis is good if causative insult removed
- Physiotherapy to debilitated muscle is required.

Table 4.2 Causes of rhabdomyolysis

Physical causes	Trauma and disasters (crush injury)
	Prolonged immobility
	Compartment syndrome
	Muscle vessel occlusion
	Sickle cell disease
	Shock and sepsis
	Excessive exertion
	Delirium tremens
	Electric shock
	Status epilepticus or asthmaticus
	Neuroleptic malignant syndrome
	Malignant hyperthermia
Myopathies	Polymyositis/dermatomyositis
	McArdle's disease and other inherited myopathies
Drugs and toxins	Alcohol, heroin, amphetamines, cocaine and ecstasy
	Statins & fibrates
	Antimalarials
	Zidovudine
	Snake and insect venoms
	Infections
	Pyomyositis and gas gangrene
	Tetanus, legionella, salmonella
	Malaria
	HIV, influenza and coxsackie
Electrolyte abnormalities	$\downarrow K^+, \downarrow Ca^{2+}, \downarrow PO_4, \downarrow Na^+, \uparrow Na^+$
Endocrine disorders	Hypothyroidism
	Hyperglycaemic emergencies

Acute glomerular nephritis (AGN)

AGN encompasses diseases such as crescentic glomerulonephritis, Wegener's granulomatosis, Goodpasture's syndrome, and lupus glomerulonephritis. AGN should be suspected if a patient is admitted with:

- Haematuria
- Rising urea and Cr
- Proteinuria
- Hypertension
- Fluid overload/oedema
- Arteritis of skin and retina
- Haemoptysis
- Rashes.

To accurately determine the cause a kidney biopsy needs to be performed, as laboratory results can suggest more than one cause of intrinsic renal failure. See 📖 p. 9 for more detail.

With AGN the patient may require immunosuppressive medication to reduce antibody production and plasmapheresis to remove any antibodies already made.

Nephrotoxic medications

There are a range of nephrotoxic medications that can cause damage to the renal tubules so it is imperative to be aware which medications are nephrotoxic or require dose adjustments in AKI. Examples include:

- NSAIDs
- Aminoglycosides (gentamicin)
- Amphotericin
- ACEIS and ARBs
- Contrast dye.

Contrast-induced AKI (CI-AKI)

Contrast medium can be nephrotoxic and patients who develop CI-AKI have a greater risk of death or prolonged hospitalization.

Pre-existing renal impairment is the most important risk factor for developing CI-AKI. Screening for both AKD and CKD is recommended for all patients at risk, i.e. the elderly, those with diabetes who are to have contrast medium investigations. See 📖 p. 60.

Classification of AKI

AKI is divided into 3 stages, pre-renal, intrinsic renal, and post-renal, each with its own impact on the kidney.

▶ Patients with CKD can have an episode of AKI that may cause their renal impairment to progress more rapidly.

▶ Conditions affecting kidney structure and function can be considered acute or chronic, depending on their duration.

> **AKI stages**
> - Pre-renal: ↓ renal blood flow
> - Intrinsic: structure within the kidney(s) is damaged
> - Post-renal: obstruction within the urine collection system.

- RIFLE (Risk, Injury, Failure, Loss, End-stage) classification defines severity of AKI based on changes to serum Cr and urine output (Table 4.3)
- AKIN (Acute Kidney Injury Network) modified criteria to include the entire spectrum of AKI which reviews serum Cr, urine output, and time (Table 4.4):
  - AKIN advocates a uniform standard for diagnosis and classification of AKI in order to optimize the treatment of patients with kidney disease
- KDIGO (Kidney Disease: Improving Global Outcomes) staging classification based serum Cr changes from baseline, urine output and time (Table 4.5).

All 3 systems are current clinical guidance recommendations for AKI and use of one of these classification systems should promote earlier detection of AKI, → appropriate and timely treatment prior to kidney injury.

▶ The Renal Association (2011) recommends using the KDIGO classification.

Table 4.3 RIFLE classification of AKI

Category	GFR criteria	Urine output	
Risk	↑ Cr × 1.5 eGFR ↓ >25%	<0.5ml/kg/h × 6hrs	High sensitivity
Injury	↑ Cr × 2 eGFR ↓ >50%	<0.5ml/kg/h × 2hrs	
Failure	↑ Cr × 3 eGFR ↓ >75%	<0.3ml/kg/h × 2hrs Anuria × 12hrs	High specificity
Loss	Complete loss of kidney function >4 wks		
ESKD	End stage kidney disease (>3 months)		

Table 4.4 AKIN classification of AKI

Category	Serum Cr	Urine output
Stage 1	↑ serum Cr ≥150–200% from baseline	<0.5ml/kg/h for ≥6hrs
Stage 2	↑ serum Cr >200–300% from baseline	<0.5ml/kg/h for ≥12hrs
Stage 3	↑ serum Cr >300% from baseline or serum Cr >54mmol/L with an acute rise of at least 44mmol/L or commencement of RRT	<0.3ml/kg/h for ≥24hrs or anuria for ≥12hrs

Table 4.5 KDIGO classification of AKI

Category	Serum Cr	Urine output
Stage 1	↑ ≥1.5 to 1.9 × baseline ≥0.3mg/dl (≥26.5μmol/L)	<0.5mL/kg/hr for 6–12hrs
Stage 2	≥ 2–2.9 × baseline	<0.5ml/kg/h for ≥12hrs
Stage 3	3 × baseline or ↑ in serum Cr ≥4mg/dl ≥353.6μmol/L or initiation of RRT	<0.3ml/kg/h for ≥24hrs or anuria for ≥12hrs

Prevention

Prevention during admission to hospital

The National Confidential Enquiry into Patient Outcome and Death (NCEPOD 2009) report reviewed the care of patients who died in hospital where their 1° diagnosis was AKI. Its recommendations include:

- All patients admitted as an emergency must have Cr and electrolytes taken on admission and routinely during admission
- Acute admissions must have a senior medical review within 12hrs
- Acute hospitals must have access to a nephrologist, 24hr US, and surgery
- Patients should have physiological observations undertaken and monitoring plans made which take into consideration their illness and risk of deterioration.

> *Prevention of AKI for people admitted to hospital*
> - Adequate hydration:
>   - Daily weight/fluid assessment
>   - Daily BP
>   - Fluid balance chart
> - Stop nephrotoxic drugs
> - Daily observation of indwelling catheter (if present) to detect possible post-renal obstruction.

A simple and effective way to monitor a patient's condition in hospital is to use a Modified Early Warning Score (MEWS) (Table 4.6). Each observation is given a score and a score of 2 in any area means the patient requires frequent observation. A score of 4 or an increase by 2 from the previous score requires urgent medical attention.

Table 4.6 MEWS scoring system

Score	3	2	1	0	1	2	3
Respiratory rate (min⁻¹)		≤8		9–14	15–20	21–29	>29
Heart rate (min⁻¹)		≤40	41–50	51–100	101–110	111–129	>129
SBP (mmHg)	≤ 70	71–80	81–100	101–199			
Urine output (ml/kg/hr)	Nil	<0.5					
Temperature (°C)		≤35	35.1–36.0	36.1–38.0	38.1–38.5	≥38.6	
Neurological				Alert	Reacting to voice	Reacting to pain	Unresponsive

Clinical features

It is important to differentiate between AKI and CKD. A history of these chronic clinical features implies CKD:
• Lethargy
• Weight loss
• Anorexia
• Nocturia
• Unexplained anaemia.

▶ AKI clinical features can include these, with additional features arising over a period of hrs or days.

Genitourinary
• Oliguria/anuria/polyuria:
  • urine may be coloured or foamy
• Enlarged bladder:
  • suggestive of chronic urinary retention (post-renal failure).

Neurological
• Headache
• Drowsiness
• Confusion
• Seizures
• Coma
• Neuropathy.

Mouth
• Metallic taste in mouth
• Distinctive breath odour (due to uraemia).

Cardiorespiratory
• Fluid overload
  • Often prevalent with ↑ JVP, peripheral and pulmonary oedema
  • Sudden weight gain.

Gastrointestinal
• Nausea, vomiting
• Persistent hiccups.

Skin
• Pallor.

Bloods
• Electrolyte imbalances
• Clotting abnormalities.

Understanding urine output
• Oliguria usually indicates AKI (or risk of if patient dehydrated)
• Abrupt anuria implies acute urinary obstruction, acute and severe glomerulonephritis, or renal artery occlusion
• Slowly decreasing urine output can signify a stricture outlet obstruction due to prostate enlargement.

Assessment

Accurate and effective assessment of the patient ensures treatment occurs in a timely manner.

Recent clinical events
• Renal angiogram with or without contrast medium (contrast medium is nephrotoxic). Any other contrast studies.

Clinical features
• Recent changes in physical condition
• Urinary or gynaecological symptoms that may identify an obstruction.

Previous medical history
• Underlying chronic kidney disease (eGFR <60ml/min/1.73m²)
• Sepsis
• Hypovolaemia
• ↓ cardiac output
• Nephrotoxic drug administration
• Atherosclerotic peripheral vascular disease
• Diabetes mellitus
• Multiple myeloma
• Liver failure.

Family history
• Is there a family history of CKD or ESKD?

Medication review
• Are they taking any non-prescribed OTC/herbal/Chinese medication?
• Have they recently commenced any nephrotoxic medication?

Observations
• What are their recent clinical observations?
  • baseline temperature, pulse, BP measurements, MEWS score
• Fluid assessment 📖 p. 587, commence fluid chart.

Investigations
Urinalysis
• Urinalysis should be done on admission as a baseline test and daily thereafter. Various urinary findings can assist with diagnosis
• After collecting a urine sample for dipstick analysis send an MSU for microscopy and culture
• Consider urine electrolytes, ACR or PCR (avoid PCR in DM).

Urinalysis assisting diagnosis
- Nitrites indicative of pyelonephritis/UTIs
- Protein indicative of tubular damage, glomerulonephritis, pyelonephritis
- Haematuria indicative of glomerulonephritis, pyelonephritis, renal infarction, kidney stones, tubular necrosis, rhabdomyolysis
- ↑ specific gravity indicative of pre renal
- ↑ specific gravity indicative of tubular necrosis
- Urobilinogen indicative of haemolysis associated-induced necrosis.

Blood testing
- FBC
- Group and save—in case blood transfusion required
- Serum Cr, U&Es
- Renal bone profile
- CRP
- Clotting times
- Glucose levels
- Arterial blood gas
- Immunological blood tests
- Virology:
  - Hep B/C, HIV, MRSA swabs

Daily blood sampling for urea, Cr electrolytes and FBC, should continue (coagulation studies if deranged). Virology screening of hepatitis B/C and HIV are mandatory in the context of infection control, and to exclude AKI causes.

Diagnostic imaging
- Renal US (size, number, position of kidneys, obstruction, hydronephrosis). See 📖 p. 58
- Chest x-ray
- Abdominal x-ray if renal calculi suspected.

Other investigations
- *ECG:* ECG can be used routinely or continual cardiac monitoring may be required if the patient is in ITU, IHDU, CCU, or MAU to assess cardiac rate and rhythm
- *Kidney biopsy:* occasionally this may be requested, but this should only be performed once all outstanding pre- and post-renal factors have been addressed. A biopsy in AKI is looking for intrinsic causes. Kidney biopsy is an invasive procedure which carries a risk of bleeding and/or further damage to the kidney/death. For further details see 📖 p. 62.

▶Contrast medium studies should be avoided because of the risk of contrast nephropathy unless benefit outweighs risk, e.g. renal infarction suspected.

Management of AKI

Assessment

Management depends on the cause of AKI. Obtain baseline information in all cases:

- Underlying cause of the kidney injury
- Assess the clinical course, including co-morbidities—obtain a full patient history
- Volume status (dehydration/overload)
- BP
- Anaemia
- Clotting screen
- Correction of electrolyte abnormalities
- Nutritional support if catabolic
- Medication adjustment—reduce dose discuss with pharmacist
- ▶ Avoid nephrotoxic drugs
- RRT if required.

Fluid balance

- Daily weight
- Accurate fluid balance monitoring and recording
- Fluid intake may be limited to previous day's urine output + GI loss + 500ml insensible loss
- ▶ Fluid allocation may need to be substantially ↑ if patient has a fever or in a warm environment where insensible loss is more
- Observe daily for signs of fluid overload or dehydration, oedema, SOB, thirst, ↓ skin turgor
- Diuretics may be required to treat fluid overload
- ▶ Diuretics can ↓ the circulating volume excessively and worsen AKI, evaluate usefulness of diuretics.

Pulmonary oedema

Pulmonary oedema is the most serious complication caused by salt and water overload. It is often due to the misuse of IV fluids given to patients who are anuric or oliguric.

Managing pulmonary oedema

- Sit patient in a comfortable position that assists them to breath
- The patient will be restless, confused, and frightened—reassure them
- Give O_2 via a facemask with a reservoir bag if sats <90% on air.
  ▶ Caution in known COPD patients:
  - regular monitoring of O_2 sats, arterial blood gases, BP, pulse
- Morphine 2.5–5mg, can be given to relieve symptoms rapidly.
  ▶ Observe for signs of respiratory depression, have naloxone available
- Maintain accurate fluid balance chart/daily weight
- Give IV diuretics to assist with fluid removal if oliguric
- May require RRT
- Communication/psychological support, patient, and family.

Anaemia

Blood transfusions should be avoided where possible, but may be required in AKI, hence FBC and group and save are required upon admission. Check FBC daily.

▶ ESA therapy is not usually given to treat anaemia in AKI.

Clotting

Clotting levels need to be taken daily if deranged. Visual inspection for bruising and extended bleeding times need to be documented and appropriate staff informed. Exclude use of heparin being a possible cause.

Nutrition

Malnutrition is noted as a predictor of mortality during hospitalization for patients with AKI, regardless of complications or co-morbidities. Hypercatabolism occurs with AKI patients and so dietetic input is necessary. The Renal Association (2010) recommends AKI patients receive 25–35kcal/kg/day, with a maximum of 1.7g/kg/day amino acids for those patients who are catabolic and receiving RRT. Nutritional support can also include protein shakes and parenteral nutrition. For further information see 📖 pp. 213–14.

Daily requirements

- K^+ restriction is often required, mmol/kg/day is used as a guide
- Daily blood samples of U&Es, bone profile, FBC, CRP
- Na^+ intake should be matched to output—for those who are oliguric, it may be as little as 15–30mmol/day. For those who are polyuric, urine Na^+ concentrations are much higher (50–70mmol/L), resulting in an intake requirement of up to 200mmol/day if passing 3L urine.
  ▶ Remember Na^+ and fluid balance are inter-related
- Dietetic input and nutritional support are required due to their catabolic state.

Hyperkalaemia

Patients with AKI are at risk of hyperkalaemia. Hyperkalaemia can cause cardiac arrhythmias. An ECG may show peaked T waves, which is indicative of hyperkalaemia with a K^+ >6.0mmol/L. During the oliguric phase when passing <400ml/day, ↑ risk of hyperkalaemia. See 📖 pp. 593–601 for further information about electrolyte imbalance.

Neurological

The systemic retention of urea and other toxic waste products during AKI leads to neurological changes within the central and peripheral nervous system. Monitor for any changes in physical and mental condition, e.g. lethargy, confusion, lapses of consciousness or depression.

Blood analysis

- Daily serum urea, Cr, electrolytes (including PO_4, Ca^{2+}) CRP, FBC, HCO_3, glucose
- Arterial blood gases as required
- Identify and treat acute complications (e.g. hyperkalaemia, acidosis)
- Monitor Hb, blood transfusion may be required.

Management in the ward setting

Nurses on the ward should be aware of the causes of AKI the investigations and treatments required and the importance of timely intervention.

Role of the nurse caring for the acutely unwell patient

- Complete nursing admission record as per local procedure:
  - include all medications the patient normally takes (OTC and prescribed), note any nephrotoxic drugs
- Undertake baseline and then continue regular clinical observations of the patient, reporting any abnormalities to the medical staff
- Implement strategies to prevent infection, this is a leading cause of death in AKI, ensure blood cultures are taken if patient is pyrexial
- Observe the patient for signs of fluid overload, electrolyte imbalances, and changes in mental capacity and level of consciousness
- Ensure fluid balance chart is completed daily (daily volume status essential)
- Daily weight
- Daily urinalysis (with microscopy if required)
- If an in-dwelling catheter is present, ensure cleanliness of genital area:
  - observe for signs of infection
- Liaise with the dietitian regarding appropriate dietary management for each stage of their AKI
- ECG may be undertaken as a baseline and done regularly if patient has been hyperkalaemic
- Offer information about AKI to the patient and their family/carers to help understand their illness
- Offer psychological support and help alleviate their anxieties, this is an acute, unplanned admission and the patient is likely to be anxious and afraid
- Consider social circumstances, dependents, effect admission has had on home circumstances
- Refer to counsellor/social worker for added support
- Care for the patient post kidney biopsy as per unit policy (for further information see 📖 Clinical assessment, p. 63)
- Ensure reviewed by medical staff daily
- Review care plan daily, adjust as condition improves
- Liaise with other members of the multiprofessional team in a timely manner
- If the patient is on RRT, provide handover to the RRT staff
- Each patient will have differing individual requirements depending upon the cause and prognosis of AKI and any additional co-morbidities.

Follow-up care

When the patient is ready for discharge it is important that they are followed up by the nephrologist. Some patients may continue to require dialysis and will attend as an outpatient until such a time their kidney function recovers. Some will not regain adequate function to manage without dialysis and will enter the chronic dialysis programme.

Patients will need assistance with fluid balance, nutritional support, and lifestyle management.

Renal replacement therapy

RRT is required to treat:
- Refractory hyperkalaemia
- Intractable fluid overload
- Metabolic acidosis (when causing circulatory compromise)
- Overt uraemia (encephalopathy, pericarditis, uraemic bleeding).

▶ Initiation of RRT may be deferred if the underlying clinical condition is improving and there are early signs of renal recovery.

RRT for AKI can be undertaken in the main ward setting, acute IHD unit, or ITU and there are 3 options:
- Continuous RRT (CRRT)
- Sustained low efficiency daily dialysis (SLEDD)
- Intermittent HD (IHD)
- Acute PD (see 📖 p. 120).

Whilst RRT is often provided under the support of a nephrologist, CRRT is mostly provided in the ITU or HDU by intensivists. It is the responsibility of the intensivist to make the referral to nephrology services, if the patient is likely to be transferred to the renal unit once stable.

The decision to commence RRT depends upon biochemical or clinical indicators including:
- Fluid overload (may include pulmonary oedema)
- Hyperkalaemia (resistant to medical therapy)
- Serum urea >27mmol/L or symptomatic prior to this level
- pH <7.15 (metabolic acidosis)
- AKI with multiple organ failure
- Urine output <0.3ml/kg for 24hrs or anuria for 12hrs
- Drug toxicity, which can be removed via IHD.

Preparation of patient for dialysis
- Inform patient/family/carer of need for dialysis—why/how/type/frequency
- Describe and explain vascular access
- Prepare patient for line insertion, explain procedure, consent, clotting screen
- Describe and explain dialysis
- Carry out pre-dialysis nursing assessment as per HD (📖 pp. 384–6)
- Reassure patient.

Vascular access

The patient will require insertion of a temporary vascular double lumen catheter preferably into the right internal jugular vein or right or left femoral vein.

Subclavian access should be avoided in patients at risk of progressing to CKD stage 4 or 5 due to the risks of compromising future, permanent vascular access. For further information see 📖 pp. 380–1.

Dialysis will be performed on the ward either by an Acute Dialysis team who visit the ward or by the ward nurses who have HD skills and competencies.

Intermittent HD

The prescription of IHD will be based on the fluid, metabolic, and electrolyte status of the patient.

Suggested IHD prescription
- 1–2hrs HD
- Low blood flow rate (150–250ml/min)
- Small surface dialyser
- Repeat daily for 3–4 days
- If no signs of DDS increase blood flow rate and duration of dialysis
- Marked fluid overload—consider ultrafiltration.

▶ Each patient must have an individualized IHD prescription.

Complications of IHD include dialysis disequilibrium syndrome and dialyser reactions.

For further information on complications, causes, clinical features, nursing considerations and prevention see 📖 pp. 402–5.

Nursing considerations
- Accurate fluid management
- Patient assessment: weight/ fluid/bloods medication review/clinical condition (1st IHD and subsequent sessions as required)
- Dialysis prescription: fluid/dialysate/hrs/anticoagulation
- Access, check for patency/signs of infection
- Clinical observations as per patient clinical condition
- Continuous ECG monitoring if indicated
- Regular monitoring of the extracorporeal circuit to ensure appropriate anticoagulation:
  - anticoagulation is required to prevent clotting in the extracorporeal circuit and heparin is most commonly used
  - heparin adds to the risk of bleeding and heparin-induced thrombocytopaenia (HIT)
- Provide effective, ongoing communication with both patient/carer/family
- Manage other co-morbidities, e.g. diabetes mellitus, hypertension, COPD and include these in the nursing assessment.

Dialysis disequilibrium syndrome (DDS)

The symptoms of DDS are caused by water movement into the brain, leading to cerebral oedema. There are 2 possible theories: reverse osmotic shift induced by urea; and a fall in cerebral intracellular pH. HD rapidly removes small solutes such as urea, particularly in patients who have raised nitrogen levels. The reduction in BUN (blood urea nitrogen) and plasma osmolality creates a transient osmotic gradient, which promotes water movement into the cells. The loss of extracellular water can also cause extracellular volume depletion, which can contribute to the development of hypotension.

New HD patients are at greatest risk, particularly if the BUN is markedly elevated (>175mg/dl). Normal BUN ~6–20mg/dl.

Other predisposing factors include severe metabolic acidosis, older age, paediatric patients, and the presence of other CNS disease. Preventative methods include initiating dialysis slowly and gently to ensure that urea is removed slowly and fluid removal is carefully controlled.

DDS symptoms

Acute symptoms developing during or immediately after HD:
- Headache
- Nausea
- Disorientation
- Restlessness,
- Blurred vision
- Cramps
- Hypertension.

More severely affected patients progress to confusion, seizures, coma, and even death. It is now recognized, however, that many milder signs and symptoms associated with dialysis, such as muscle cramps, anorexia, and dizziness developing near the end of a dialysis treatment, are also part of this syndrome.

Other disorders should be considered and excluded including uraemia itself, subdural haematoma, metabolic disturbances (hyponatraemia, hypoglycaemia), and drug-induced encephalopathy. Drug accumulation is a particular problem in AKI with drugs that are normally excreted by the kidney.

Preventing DDS
- Gentle frequent dialysis
- Gradual reduction in BUN
- Slow urea removal
- Ultrafiltration
- Consider peritoneal dialysis.

Severe DDS is now rare in adults because of the standard use of preventive recommendations.

Nursing management
- The major focus is on prevention and, as the clinical features can be non-specific, diagnosis is difficult
- Regular monitoring and close clinical observation of the patient are essential at each dialysis
- If mild symptoms are present consider reducing blood flow, duration of treatment or using co-current flow
- If severe (e.g. seizure) discontinue dialysis. Call doctor, observe patient
- Medication, which reduces intracranial pressure, e.g. 50% glucose, mannitol, or hypertonic saline may be prescribed
- Medical review of patient before subsequent HD sessions.

Continuous RRT

This follows the same principles as IHD, and is undertaken as a continuous process over a 24hr period as the patient is often haemodynamically unstable. As it is a continuous process, fluid and waste removal occur at much slower rates. Blood flow and dialysate flow rates (if dialysate is being used) are lower which reduces risk of dialysis disequilibrium syndrome. Fluid and toxin clearance per 24hr period is greater than IHD.

As with IHD there are several options for CRRT
- Continuous venovenous HD (CVVHD)
- Continuous venovenous haemofiltration (CVVHF)
- Continuous venovenous haemodiafiltration (CVVHDF)
- Slow continuous ultrafiltration (SCUF).

Sustained low efficiency daily dialysis

SLEDD has the benefits of both intermittent and continuous therapies, in that it can be slow and gentle and easily tolerated by the patient. As it occurs daily and the duration of therapy is longer, it allows for gradual fluid and toxin removal. Treatment hrs can be reduced as time goes on, so that the patient could be attached to the machine for 12hrs a day, with 12hrs of respite to allow for physiotherapy and other necessary investigations without interruption to the HD regimen.

Anticoagulation

Anticoagulation should be tailored according to individual patient needs and the RRT modality undertaken. CRRT require continuous anticoagulation at a higher dosage than required for SLEDD and this needs to be taken into consideration when choosing which form of therapy is appropriate. Alternatives to systemic anticoagulation in AKI include heparin free dialysis where regular saline flushes into the extracorporeal circuit are performed. Epoprostenol is a suitable alternative to unfractionated heparin in those at ↑ risk of bleeding. For further information see 📖 pp. 364–6.

Plasmapheresis

Plasmapheresis may be used to treat the underlying cause of AKI, e.g. AGN, SLE, Goodpasture's, syndrome, ANCA-associated vasculitis (see 📖 p. 416).

Acute peritoneal dialysis

Acute PD is an effective alternative to HD for treating AKI although its use is limited for rapid fluid removal and treatment of hyperkalaemia. It tends not used routinely in all UK hospitals and is more common in the developing world, where it may be the only method of RRT available. Acute PD can be commenced immediately once the PD catheter has been inserted if the percutaneous method is used.

Advantages
- PD is widely available in UK units as a form of RRT for ESKD patients and is technically easy to perform
- PD access placement is simple to carry out with percutaneous insertion which can be performed under a local anaesthetic
- ↓ risk of systemic infections as the alternative form of access is usually temporary vascular access which can be prone to infection
- Minimal bleeding risk
- Minimal risk of disequilibrium syndrome
- Electrolyte and acid–base imbalances are effectively corrected
- ↑ amounts of fluid can be slowly removed, which enables more flexible administration of TPN
- ↓ hypotension as fluid removal less aggressive
- PD saves precious vascular access and preserves residual renal function
- If the patient requires long-term RRT, PD can be continued as the access placed is suitable for permanent use. This causes less disruption for the patient and promotes the use of home-based therapies.

Disadvantages
- Less rapid electrolyte/acid–base and fluid correction is a possibility
- Difficult if the patient has had previous abdominal surgery, particularly if adhesions are present
- Surgical PD catheter insertion using laparoscopy may be required if percutaneous insertion is not possible. If neither of these options work then laparotomy would be required
- Risk of peritoneal infection
- Protein losses.

- Automated PD machine to perform the dialysis exchanges would be the preferred method of treatment
- The patient should be in the supine position and small fill volumes used to minimize the risk of leakage of PD fluid at the exit site
- Patients should be instructed to remain in bed during the treatment, usually 12hrs overnight, but can be allowed to walk around during the daytime as long as the fluid has been drained out of the peritoneal cavity.

Contraindications include:
- Severe hyperkalaemia
- Uraemic pericarditis
- Severe fluid overload with pulmonary oedema
- Uraemic encephalopathy.

Further reading

Bagshaw S, George C, Bellomo R. A comparison of the RIFLE and AKIN criteria for acute kidney injury in critically ill patients. *Nephrol Dial Transplant* 2008; **23**:1569–74.

Himmelfarb J, Joannidis M, Molitoris B, et al. Evaluation and initial management of acute kidney injury. *Clin J Am Soc Nephrol* 2008; **3**:962–7.

Mehta RL, Kellum JA, Shah SV, et al. Acute Kidney Injury Network: report of an initiative to improve outcomes in acute kidney injury. *Crit Care*. 2007; **11**(2):R31.

Steddon S, Ashman N, Cunningham J, et al. *Oxford Handbook of Nephrology and Hypertension*. Oxford: Oxford University Press, 2006.

Uchino, S, Kellum JA, Bellomo R, et al. Acute renal failure in critically ill patients. A multinational, multicenter study. *JAMA* 2005; **294**(7): 813–18.

Warrell DL, Cox TM, Firth JD (eds). *Oxford Textbook of Medicine*, 5th edn, chapter 21.5. Oxford: Oxford University Press; 2010.

Useful websites

Kidney Disease: Improving Global Outcomes (KDIGO). Available at: ℘ <http://www.kdigo.org/clinical_practice_guidelines_3.php>

NCEPOD Report. Available at: ℘ <http://www.ncepod.org.uk/>

Renal Association website. Available at: ℘ <http://www.renal.org/Clinical/GuidelinesSection/AcuteKidneyInjury.aspx>

Chronic kidney disease stages 1–3

Identification and prevalence of CKD

CKD affects ~10% of the adult population worldwide. Stage 3–5 CKD is present in 6–7% of the adult UK population. More people are now aware of having reduced kidney function or proteinuria as a result of the consensus and subsequent publication of various CKD guidelines, such as NICE, KDOQI, and the UK Renal Association. These guidelines provide recommendations for clinical practice and include regular measurement and reporting of kidney function. Registers such as the quality outcomes framework (QOF) used in general practice, records the prevalence of CKD. The CKD register ensures an annual assessment of kidney function for people in high-risk groups.

CKD strategies are aimed at the early identification, prevention where possible, and the effective management to delay progression of CKD to ESKD.

Risk factors for CKD include:

- Diabetes
- Hypertension
- Cardiovascular disease (IHD, CHF, PVD, cerebral vascular disease)
- Structural renal tract disease
- Kidney stones
- Prostatic hypertrophy
- Multisystem diseases with potential kidney involvement, e.g. SLE
- FH of stage 5 CKD or hereditary kidney disease
- Opportunistic detection of haematuria or proteinuria.

People in these at-risk groups should be offered an eGFR and an ACR check at least once per yr (see 📖 p. 2 for causes of CKD).

Stages of CKD

CKD is divided into stages depending on the level of eGFR (Table 5.1).

Table 5.1 Stages of CKD

Stage	eGFR ml/min/1.73m²	Description
1	≥90	Normal or ↑ eGFR with other evidence of kidney damage
2	60–89	Slight ↓ in eGFR, with other evidence of kidney damage
3A	45–59	Moderate ↓ in eGFR with or without evidence of kidney damage
3B	30–44	
4	15–29	Severe ↓ in eGFR with or without evidence of kidney damage
5	<15	Established renal disease
5D		Dialysis
5T		Transplant

* Suffix P may be added to indicate proteinuria at any stage, suffix D = Dialysis (stage 5) Suffix T = Transplant (stage 4/5)

See 📖 p. 42 for measurement of kidney function.

Stages 1–3 CKD screening and monitoring

Screening, early recognition and monitoring of patients with stage 1–3 CKD can delay progression of the disease.

Stage 1 CKD is kidney disease with normal kidney function. Stage 2 is 60–89% function.

Stage 1–2

Almost all patients with stage 1–2 CKD can be managed in primary care with the aim being to:

- Identify people at risk of progressive kidney disease, e.g. those with normal or near normal eGFR but evidence of kidney disease:
  - haematuria, proteinuria
  - genetic diagnosis of kidney disease, e.g. reflux nephropathy
- Reduce the associated risks as the risk of a cardiovascular event and death is substantially ↑ by the presence of CKD 1–2, particularly when proteinuria is present.

⚠ Need to ensure the eGFR result has been corrected for ethnicity as it is an estimate of kidney function only. Repeat serum Cr level if elevated and no baseline comparisons within 14 days.

Further assessment

- Evidence of proteinuria i.e. ACR >70mg/mmol or PCR >100mg/mmol
- Presence of haematuria (non-kidney causes excluded)
- Significant decline in eGFR that indicates the presence of progressive disease.

Management includes annual:

- Serum Cr/eGFR—consider referral if short-term ↓ in eGFR >15% or ↑ Cr >20% or loss in GFR over 1yr of 5ml/min, or 10ml/min over 5yrs
- Urinary protein, e.g. ACR (in DM) or PCR
- BP: 140/90 max (130–139/90), or 130/80 max (120–129/80) for patients with proteinuria: (ACR>30 or PCR>50)
- Cardiovascular risk assessment (see 📖 p. 76).

Lifestyle considerations

- Avoid high fat, high salt, processed foods (see 📖 p. 84–5).
- Stop smoking
- Keep to an ideal body weight
- Regular exercise
- Diabetes—keep blood sugar within targets
- Hypertension—keep BP <140/90 and <130/80 in diabetes.

CKD stage 3A and 3B

Most stage 3A/B CKD can be managed in primary care but may require more frequent review to identify progression of kidney disease and reduce the associated risks, e.g. cardiovascular event.

Progression of kidney disease highlighted by

- Proteinuria
- Haematuria (renal)
- ↓ eGFR.

Further assessment required if:

- Proteinuria ACR ≥70mg/mmol or PCR ≥100mg/mmol
- Haematuria (non-renal causes excluded)
- ↓ eGFR of 5ml/min/1.73m² within 1yr or 10ml/min/1.73m² within 5yrs
- Young person.

Initial assessment

- May require referral from 1° care if:
  - unwell, history of significant disease, systemic disease involving kidneys with urinary abnormalities, or other indicators
- Repeat serum Cr level if elevated and there are no baseline comparisons within 14 days
- Clinical assessment, e.g. bladder enlargement (e.g. urinary obstruction), hypovolaemia, HF:
  - consider imaging (US) to exclude obstruction or if FH of polycystic kidney disease
- Urine test, e.g. dipstick for blood, ACR or PCR which may indicate progressive disease
- Medication review for potential nephrotoxic drugs or drugs which need dose alterations with a reduced GFR
- Patients with stage 3B CKD will require an Hb level as there is an ↑ risk of anaemia with an eGFR <45ml/min/1.73m².

The following can be used to help identify progressing CKD:

- Obtain a minimum of 3 eGFR results over a period of no less than 90 days
- If a new finding of ↓ eGFR:
  - repeat the eGFR within 2wks to exclude causes of acute deterioration of GFR, e.g. AKI or initiation of ACEI/ARB therapy
- Define progression as ↓ in eGFR of >5ml/min/1.73 m² within 1yr, or >10ml/min/1.73m² within 5yrs.

Management stage 3B: 6–12-monthly screening of:
- Serum Cr/eGFR and serum K^+ level:
  - consider referral if ↓ eGFR of 5ml/min/1.73m^2 within 1yr or 10ml/min/1.73m^2 within 5yrs
  - if an unexplained ↓ in eGFR, repeat within 2 wks to exclude acute causes of deterioration, i.e. AKI or initiation of ACEI or ARB therapy
  - Hb (exclude non-renal causes below normal parameters), in CKD <11g/L may require treatment
- Urinary protein, e.g. ACR or PCR:
  - tighter BP control if ACR ≥30mg/mmol or PCR ≥50mg/mmol
  - consider referral and/or discussion with nephrologist if ACR ≥70mg/mmol or PCR ≥100mg/mmol
- BP:
  - CKD without diabetes: keep SBP <140mmHg (target range 120–139) DBP <90mmHg
  - CKD, diabetes, and ACR ≥70mg/mmol: maintain SBP <130mmHg (range 120–129mmHg) DBP <80mmHg
- Cardiovascular risk review at each appointment
- Provide education as required on lifestyle modifications
- Aim for plasma cholesterol <5mmol/L:
  - ↓ total cholesterol by 25%; or LDL by 30% to reach <4.0mmol/L or <2.0mmol (whichever is greatest)
  - commence lipid lowering medication if required
  - liaise with dietitian if a low-fat diet is required
  - antiplatelet drugs for 2° prevention, e.g. low-dose aspirin
- Medication review for potential nephrotoxic drugs or drugs which need dose alterations with a ↓ eGFR
- Immunization for influenza and pneumococcal advised
- Patient information on CKD, preventing progressive kidney disease.

The older patient with CKD

- The prevalence of CKD is higher in the older population and correct identification and assessment of CKD in older people requires caution
- After the 4th decade, kidney function declines at a rate of 8–10ml/min/1.73m^2 per decade
- An eGFR in the range 45–59ml/min/1.73m^2, if stable over time and without any other evidence of kidney damage, in people aged >70yrs should be considered unlikely to be associated with CKD
- A ↓ eGFR is more likely to be the effect of normal decline of the kidneys with age
- Those who are referred to nephrology services may never progress to ESKD or require RRT; however, they will require some specific management of CKD-associated complications management and to prevent progression.

Nursing considerations

Medications

- Prescribing in the older person requires caution, e.g. dose adjustments are needed due to a ↓ eGFR and age (see 📖 Pharmacology, p. 568).
- Educate the patient on avoiding the use of nephrotoxic agents, e.g. NSAIDs
- It is important to remember to check patients' medications regularly as changes may have been made by other clinicians and not communicated to the renal team.

Hb

- Declines with age and the prevalence of anaemia ↑
- Nutritional inadequacies → serum iron, vitamin B_{12}, and folate deficiencies and along with low endogenous erythropoietin levels predispose the older person to anaemia
- Anaemia is an independent risk factor for mortality and hospitalization in the older population.

Malnutrition

- Is an independent risk factor for death. It is a multifactorial problem involving social, economic, and psychological factors (see 📖 p. 212).

Risk of AKI

- Older people are at risk of episodes of AKI whether they are known or not to renal services
- Prevention of AKI, avoid episodes of dehydration, e.g.↓ circulatory volume → ↓ renal blood flow and perfusion → AKI
- ▶ Seek medical advice if they have diarrhoea and vomiting and unable to take oral fluids.

Older people often have several co-morbidities and maybe under the care of more than one disease area/consultant, e.g. cardiac, diabetes, care of the older person. It is important to liaise with other teams for any changes in management, e.g. medications.

- Practitioners express concern about labelling older patients as having CKD when their condition can be a consequence of the normal ageing process
- An age-related decline in eGFR is common, e.g. expected eGFR in an 85yr-old would be <60ml/min (Stage 3A)
- ▶ A stable eGFR 45–59ml/min without evidence of kidney damage is unlikely to be associated with CKD-related complications
- Patients in this group should be informed that a slight reduction in kidney function is a normal part of the ageing process and if their kidney function remains stable it is unlikely to get much worse over time.

Referral criteria

People with CKD in the following groups should normally be referred for specialist assessment by a nephrologist:
- Higher levels of proteinuria (ACR >70mg/mmol) unless known to be due to diabetes and already appropriately treated
- Proteinuria (ACR >30mg/mmol) together with haematuria
- Rapidly declining eGFR (>5ml/min/1.73m^2 within 1yr, or >10ml/min/1.73m^2 within 5yrs)
- Poorly controlled hypertension despite the use of at least 4 antihypertensive drugs at therapeutic doses
- Suspected of having rare or genetic causes of CKD
- Suspected renal artery stenosis
- African-Caribbean ethnicity to ensure correct diagnosis and assessment.

▶ Renal outflow obstruction should be referred to urological services, unless urgent medical intervention is required.

Desired minimal referral information
- Previous eGFRs
- Past medical and drug history
- BP
- Urinalysis
- ACR/PCR if proteinuria present
- Renal US
- Electrolytes, HCO_3
- Ca^{2+}, PO_4, Alb
- Hb
- Cholesterol
- HbA1c if applicable.

Many people will remain stable at stage 3 or 4 and will not progress to stage 5 and require RRT. Unless management of complications of CKD such as anaemia, hyperparathyroidism, or metabolic bone disease is required, it is possible to continue monitoring patients in primary care and seek advice from nephrology services when needed.

Proteinuria management

See 📖 p. 48 for further information on the measurement of protein and microalbuminuria. The recommended interventions are shown in Table 5.2.

Table 5.2 Recommended interventions for proteinuria and microalbuminuria

ACR/PCR mg/mmol	eGFR ml/min1.72m²	Risk factors	Action
ACR <30 PCR <50	≥60	None	None
ACR <30 PCR <50	≥60	Yes	Repeat 12 months
ACR <30 PCR <50	≥30	Hypertension Diabetes	Offer ACEI or ARBs
ACR ≥70 PCR ≥100	Irrespective of eGFR		Refer to nephrologist

Microalbuminuria

- Screened for in diabetes, HF, and evidence of kidney damage
- Defined as ACR 20–200mcg/min or 30–300mg/24hrs
- ACEI or ARBs used in:
  - diabetes and ACR >2.5mg/mmol (♂) or >3.5mg/mmol (♀) irrespective of presence of CKD or hypertension
  - CKD and hypertension without diabetes and ACR <30mg/mmol
  - CKD, without diabetes and ACR ≥70mg/mmol, irrespective of presence of hypertension or cardiovascular disease
- The use of ACEI and ARBs reduce microalbuminuria in both diabetic and non-diabetic nephropathy
- ↓ in proteinuria of 0.5g/day is associated with a slower progression of both renal and cardiovascular disease
- ACR >2.5mg/mmol in ♂: ACR >3.5mg/mmol in ♀ with diabetes is clinically significant (see Table 5.3 for ACR interventions in people with diabetes).

Table 5.3 ACR interventions in diabetes

ACR measurement mg/mmol	eGFR ml/min/1.72m²	Action
≤2.5 ♂ ≤3.5 ♀	≥60	Check eGFR annually
≤2.5 ♂ ≤3.5 ♀	≥30–59	Check eGFR annually
≤2.5 ♂ ≤3.5 ♀	<30	Refer to nephrologist
>2.5 ♂ >3.5 ♀	≥30	Offer ACEI or ARB
>2.5 ♂ >3.5 ♀	<30	Refer to nephrologist

Management of co-morbidities

Diabetes and CKD
- Leading of cause of CKD in developed countries due to the ↑ prevalence of type 2 diabetes mellitus (DM)
- DM damages large and small blood vessels → damage to the kidneys, eyes and vascular system.
- Associated with persistent hyperglycaemia 2° to poor glycaemic control and ↑ risk of CVD.

Type 1 DM
- Usually occurs in children, young adults but can occur at any age
- Result of autoimmune destruction of pancreatic beta cells
- Destruction of cells that produce insulin
- Managed with diet and insulin injections.

Type 2 DM
- Result of insulin deficiency and insulin resistance
- Contributory factors: obesity, sedentary lifestyle, ethnicity (Asian/Afro-Caribbean) and genetic factors
- Present with ↑ BP and microalbuminuria
- Managed with combination of lifestyle changes and oral medication
- As disease progresses may require insulin.

▶ In both type 1 and 2 DM blood glucose concentration is related to the development of microalbuminuria and over time to overt proteinuria.

▶ Not all patients with DM will develop diabetic nephropathy.

- Advanced CKD is associated with ↑ insulin resistance, leading to ↑ insulin dosage or addition of insulin to oral agents for glycaemic control (i.e. metformin).

▶ Consider reducing metformin when eGFR <45ml/min.

- As CKD progresses towards stage 5 a ↓ in insulin degradation occurs and often results in ↓ insulin requirements
- ↑ urea levels may interfere with some methods used to measure HbA1c:
  - laboratory assays should be checked if unusual results occur
- 1° or 2° care diabetes teams should be consulted if dose adjustments are needed
- Good diabetes control and monitoring can ↓ the risk of developing microvascular complications:
  - 1% reduction in HbA1c is associated with 21% reduction in morbidity and death related to DM
  - a target HbA1c of <48mmol/mol (6.5%) is recommended.

▶ Changes in the reporting of HbA1c values were introduced in the UK in 2009 and from June 2011 HbA1c is reported in mmol/mol (Table 5.4).

Table 5.4 HbA1c conversion

%	mmol/mol
6.0	42
6.5	48
7.0	53
7.5	58
8.0	64
8.5	75

All people with diabetes should have annual:
- eGFR and cardiovascular assessment checks
- HbA1c
- Hb if stage 3B CKD
- Eye screening and assessment for retinopathy
- Foot assessments and referred to a chiropodist if required.

Hypertension
Current BP targets are:
- CKD without diabetes
  - maintain SBP <140mmHg (range 120–139mmHg), DBP<90mmHg
- CKD, with diabetes and ACR ≥70mg/mmol:
  - maintain SBP <130mmHg (range 120–129g), DBP<80mmHg.

Cardiovascular risk and CKD
Increased cardiovascular risk starts early in patients with CKD. As eGFR falls, the risk of death and cardiovascular events such as stroke and heart disease rises. All patients with CKD should be considered to be in the highest risk group for cardiovascular disease irrespective of levels of traditional CVD risk factors

See p. 76 for further information on hypertension, cardiovascular risk assessment, and management.

Interface with primary care

Quality Outcome Frameworks

The Quality Outcomes Framework (QOF) is part of the payment system for GPs based on achieving nationally agreed targets. Payments are adjusted depending on disease prevalence and performance in managing the disease. Income generated from the QOF contributes to the running costs of GPs' surgeries and staff. Chronic disease registers were developed as part of the QOF to assist with routine screening for and management of diseases such as hypertension, diabetes, and chronic heart failure. CKD was added in 2006.

> *QOF indicators for CKD*
> - CKD 1: register of patients age 18yrs and over with CKD stages 3–5
> - CKD 2: % with BP recording in past 15 months
> - CKD 3: % on register with last BP recording 140/85mmHg or less
> - CKD 5: % on register with hypertension and proteinuria who are treated with an ACEI or ARB (unless contraindicated or side effects recorded)
> - CKD 6: % on register with ACR (or PCR) value in last 15 months.*

▶ *Thresholds for definition of proteinuria for QOF are under discussion but evidence suggests ACR >30mg/mmol and PCR >50mg/mmol.

The CKD register

The CKD register captures assessment data for people in high-risk groups see Table 5.5.

Table 5.5 Risk categories requiring annual assessment

Co-morbidities	Drugs	Urinary
DM	ACEI	Recurrent UTIs
Hypertension	ARB	Bladder outflow obstruction
HF	Long-term NSAIDs (>12 months' duration)	Recurrent kidney stones (>1/yr)
Vascular disease: PVD, CHD, stroke	Diuretics	Neurogenic bladder
Multisystem disease involving the kidney, e.g. SLE, rheumatoid arthritis	Lithium carbonate	Polycystic kidney disease
	Mesalazine and other 5-aminosalycilic drugs	Reflux nephropathy
	Calcineurin inhibitors (ciclosporin, tacrolimus)	Persistent proteinuria
		Persistent haematuria (urological)

Register criteria
- There must be at least 2 results of eGFR <60ml/min at least 3 months apart before coding a patient as having CKD
- Patients with an eGFR >60ml/min/1.73m² should have other evidence of kidney damage before they can be coded as CKD
- If there are 2 eGFR readings in different stages, the patient should be coded as the higher stage (e.g. a result of 35ml/min and 29ml/min code as stage 3)
- ▶ Referral should be based on the progression of CKD not a one-off abnormal measurement of eGFR, e.g. ↓ eGFR>5ml/min/1.73m² within 1yr or >10ml/min/1.73m² within 5yrs
- CKD registers can be used in conjunction with national and local referral guidelines to assist with referral to nephrology services for advice and further management
- Running reports from a GP practice system to identify all those with an eGFR <60ml/min/1.73m² and cross referencing with a CKD register highlights patients who may have CKD stage 3–5 but not yet on the register
- 95% of patients with CKD 3–5 will already be on registers for hypertension, DM, or CHF.

Read codes
The following read codes are used to identify the different stages of CKD on the register:
- CKD stage 1 = 1Z10
- CKD stage 2 = 1Z11
- CKD stage 3 = 1Z12
- CKD stage 4 = 1Z13
- CKD stage 5 = 1Z14.

Data from CKD registers enables the prevalence of CKD to be identified by local practices.

Quality standards

CKD quality standards have been devised by NICE (2011) to assist health-care professionals to provide high-quality, cost-effective care. The aim being, when delivered collectively is to improve the care and experience of adults with CKD.

Aims of quality standards
- Prevent people from dying prematurely
- Enhance quality of life for people with long-term conditions
- Help people to recover from episodes of ill health or following injury
- Ensure that people have a positive experience of care
- Treat and care for people in a safe environment and protect them from avoidable harm.

NICE CKD quality standards for stages 1–3
- People with risk factors for CKD are offered testing, and people with CKD are correctly identified
- People with CKD who may benefit from specialist care are referred for specialist assessment in accordance with NICE guidance
- People with CKD have a current agreed care plan appropriate to the stage and rate of progression of CKD
- People with CKD are assessed for cardiovascular risk
- People with higher levels of proteinuria, and people with diabetes and microalbuminuria, are enabled to safely maintain SBP within a target range 120–129mmHg and DBP <80mmHg
- People with CKD are assessed for disease progression
- People with CKD who become acutely unwell have their medication reviewed, and receive an assessment of volume status and renal function
- People with anaemia of CKD have access to and receive anaemia treatment in accordance with NICE guidance.

To compliment national guidance for management of CKD and to assist with the implementation of quality standards NICE has produced a CKD pathway See Figure 5.1, which includes:
- Overview of CKD
- Risk factors, identification and testing for those with and without diabetes
- Recommendations of investigations for CKD
- Management of CKD
- CKD progression and complications.

These guidelines and standards enable the majority of patients with CKD stages 1–3A to be monitored and managed in 1° care with advice being sought from nephrologists if complications arise.

Patient education for CKD stages 1–3

Patients should be informed of their condition and given information and advice on strategies to prevent the progression of the disease.

Advice for patients
- Take moderate exercise
- Healthy eating
- Maintain ideal body weight
- Good blood sugar control in those with diabetes
- Moderate alcohol intake
- Smoking cessation
- Maintain good BP control
- Adherence to medications
- Inform pharmacist about having kidney disease when buying OTC medicines
- Importance of attending clinic appointments
- Maintain independence.

Those with stage 3A CKD should be informed that they have been put on the CKD register with a careful explanation as to what this means. Terminology such as reduced kidney function or damage to the kidneys rather than CKD reduces the anxiety of being 'labelled' with another chronic disease. Patients with early kidney disease may not experience any symptoms but need to be aware that they need regular monitoring.

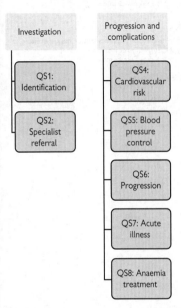

Fig. 5.1 Quality standards patient pathway stage 1–3 CKD. Adapted from 'QS 5 Chronic Kidney Disease quality standard'. London: NICE. Available from www.nice.org.uk/guidance/QS5. Reproduced with permission.

Further reading

Patient information websites

Blood tests and kidney function for patients. Available at: ◌ <http://www.edren.org>

Chronic kidney disease: Available at: ◌ <http://www.kidney.org.uk/Medical-Info/ckd-info/index.html>

Kidney damage and what it means to you. Available at: ◌ <http://www.bjpcn-cardiovascular.com/download/3337>

◌ <http://guidance.nice.org.uk/CG73>, update due for publication 2014

◌ <http://pathways.nice.org.uk/pathways/chronic-kidney-disease>

◌ <http://www.bnf.org>

◌ <http://www.diabetes.org.uk>

◌ <http://www.kidney.org.uk>

◌ <http://www.nice.org.uk/guidance/qualitystandards/chronickidneydisease/ckdqualitystandard.jsp>

◌ <http://www.nice.org.uk/nicemedia/pdf/CG67NICEguideline.pdf>

◌ <http://www.patient.co.uk/health/Chronic-Kidney-Disease.htm>

◌ <http://www.qof.ic.nhs.uk>

◌ <http://www.nice.org.uk/guidance/QS5>

Chronic kidney disease stages 4–5

Introduction

People with stage 4–5 CKD require specialist input to delay progression and manage associated complications.

- Stable stage 4 who do not progress may be transferred back to 1° care for monitoring, especially if they have no associated complications, e.g. anaemia, MBD
- People with progressive stage 4 should be regularly reviewed by nephrology services
- NICE quality standards have been developed to improve the care and experience of adults with stage 4–5 CKD.

NICE CKD quality standards for stages 4–5[1]

- People with progressive CKD whose eGFR is <20ml/min/1.73m^2, and/or who are likely to progress to established kidney failure within 12 months, receive unbiased personalized information on established kidney failure and renal replacement therapy options
- People with established renal failure have access to psychosocial support (which may include support with personal, family, financial, employment and/or social needs) appropriate to their circumstances
- People with CKD are supported to receive a pre-emptive kidney transplant before they need dialysis, if they are medically suitable
- People with CKD on dialysis are supported to receive a kidney transplant, if they are medically suitable
- People with established kidney failure start dialysis with a functioning arteriovenous fistula or PD catheter *in situ*
- People on long-term dialysis receive the best possible therapy, incorporating regular and frequent application of dialysis and ideally home-based or self-care dialysis
- People with CKD receiving haemodialysis or training for home therapies who are eligible for transport, have access to an effective and efficient transport service.

Advanced kidney care clinic

Patients may be transferred to the AKCC from the general nephrology clinic or may be referred directly by the GP or another specialist medical team, e.g. from the diabetes, cardiac, rheumatology, or immunology clinic (often as a result of an incidental finding). Figure 6.1 provides an example of a patient pathway for an AKCC.

AKCC referral criteria
- Advanced stages of kidney disease (stages 4–5)
- eGFR is declining at rate of >5ml/min/1.73 m² per year
- Current recommendation by both the NSF for Renal Services[2] and the UK Renal Association[3] 1yr prior to requiring RRT.

Purpose and structure of the AKCC
- Delay progression of kidney disease and prolong time to ESKD
- ↓ cardiovascular risk by good lipid, BP, and diabetes control
- Promote a healthy lifestyle
- ↓ risk of associated complications, e.g. anaemia, MBD, fluid overload, acidosis, malnutrition
- Access to a MPT, e.g. dietitian, social worker
- Timely preparation for RRT, planning and formation of access
- Support and management for those opting for conservative treatment
- Promote pre-emptive transplantation
- Tx work up and list for cadaveric transplantation where appropriate
- Maintain good QOL, continue with normal activities and employment
- Promote an integrated care approach to RRT; facilitate informed decision-making and choice of treatment to suit the patient both physically and psychologically
- Patient information and education on treatment options by the MPT renal team at least 6 months prior to reaching ESKD
- Psychological support to the patient, family, and carers
- Improve patient experience, satisfaction, and self-esteem
- Inform 1° care of any changes in medication and update with current treatment plan, e.g. RRT choice.

The AKCC requires an integrated approach with a dedicated renal MPT as follows:
- Medical staff: nephrologist, specialist renal registrar, vascular access and Tx surgeon
- Specialist nursing staff: advanced kidney care, anaemia, access, and Tx nurses, community nurses
- Other allied professionals: dietitian, pharmacist, social worker and counsellor/psychologist
- Liaison with external agencies: community nurses, GPs, other specialties (diabetes, HF, palliative care teams).

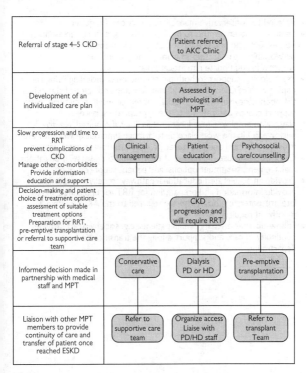

Fig. 6.1 Stage 4 and 5 CKD patient pathway.

Function and role of the nurse in the AKCC

Nurses working in the AKCC play a very important role in the ongoing management of patients with advanced kidney disease:

- In collaboration with the medical staff and MPT assess, monitor, and co-ordinate ongoing clinical management:
  - optimize BP control
  - liaise with the renal dietitian to ensure optimal nutritional state
  - anaemia management
  - hepatitis B vaccination
- Preparation, planning, and coordination of RRT, including dialysis access
- Home assessments working with the social worker, e.g. assess suitability for home-based treatments, re-housing, and adaptations
- Tx work-up, organize investigations, and collate results

- Referral to conservative management services if required
- Liaise with other healthcare professionals, e.g. district nurses, nursing homes, GPs and practice nurses, cardiac and diabetic teams who will be working in partnership to manage the patient:
  - provide and update patient care plan
- Psychological support to both patient and carer including living and coping with ESKD, support available, function and roles of staff within the nephrology service, e.g. social worker, counsellor, dietitian, patient support groups and referral to the appropriate service
- Liaise with employer or educational facilities if required, e.g. to perform PD in the workplace or to arrange time out of work for HD
- Provide individual and structured group educational programmes on
- CKD, discuss cause (if known) of their condition/disease, medications, management, treatment options, and patient support groups
- Provide an accelerated educational pathway to deliver education, provide information and preparation for RRT for unplanned starters/ late presenters or those who are referred to the AKCC within 3 months of requiring RRT
- Follow-up after discharge of all patients, e.g. social visit to provide continuity of care and support during the transition to new department.

Late presentation to nephrology services

Patients are classified as late presenters if they are first seen by a nephrologist <90 days prior to commencing RRT. Within the UK, as a result of the publication and implementation of CKD guidelines and inclusion of CKD in the quality outcomes framework (QOF) for primary care, the number of late presenters has declined from 27.1% in 2004 to 19% in 2009.[4] Late presentation also includes those patients who present for urgent treatment and are referred to as unplanned starters.

Reasons for late presentation/unplanned starters (excluding AKI) to nephrology services include:

- Previously undiagnosed CKD presenting once becoming symptomatic
- Denial or failure to cope with CKD diagnosis presenting only when symptomatic
- Diagnosed CKD patients who experience a sudden deterioration in kidney function 2° to:
  - episode of dehydration, e.g. in summer with excessive sweating, diarrhoea
  - cardiac event, e.g. MI, arrhythmia, HF
  - urinary obstruction, e.g. calculi, blood clot, or tumour
  - use of nephrotoxic agent, e.g. contrast media, medications such as NSAIDs, lithium, aminoglycosides, herbal remedies
- Late referral from 1° or 2° care
- Overseas residents who travel to the UK knowing that they require dialysis which is unavailable in their own country.

Consequences of late presentation

- ↑ risk of mortality and morbidity rates compared with patients who have been managed in a specialist renal clinic
- Development of associated complications of advanced kidney disease as a result of poorly controlled biochemical, metabolic, and fluid control, e.g. metabolic bone disease, anaemia
- Insufficient time to adequately prepare for RRT and plan permanent access. ↑ incidence of unplanned dialysis and use of temporary vascular access
- ↑ length of stay and healthcare costs
- Urgent discussion about choice of treatment may result in patients feeling rushed and ill-prepared for making life changing decisions
- Less likely to opt for self-care treatment
- Tendency to remain on their initial therapy choice which may not be the best option, e.g. a home-based treatment such as PD may suit their lifestyle better
- Lack of education and information may lead to adherence problems
- Inability to cope with the diagnosis of CKD can lead to depression, anxiety and stress
- Subsequent withdrawal of treatment by the patient following urgent commencement of dialysis instigated by family/medical staff.

Clinical management in AKCC

New patient assessment

- Assess urgency of referral; previous blood results, e.g. Cr, Ur and eGFR, e.g. rapid ↓ in GFR, are they a 'late presenter' likely to require RRT within 3 months?
- Late presenters—patient educator to provide an accelerated educational programme to support the patient/family/carer to make informed decisions about treatment options:
  - refer for counselling, social worker
  - access to peer support, patient organizations, expert patient groups
- Past medical and surgical history/co-morbidities, e.g. diabetes, cardiac, auto-immune disease, e.g. SLE:
  - specifically assess for any prior urinary/kidney problems, e.g. obstruction, enuresis as a child
  - significant renal FH, e.g. polycystic kidney disease
- Cardiovascular risk assessment (see 🕮 pp. 76–7)
- Haemodynamic observations, assess for presence of infection, ↑ BP
- Fluid assessment—see 🕮 p. 587
- Nursing assessment and commence patient care plan
- Assess cognition and language ability, e.g. carer, interpreter
- Nutritional assessment by renal dietitian
- Review current medications—check for:
  - nephrotoxic medications, e.g. NSAIDs, lithium
  - non-prescription medications, e.g. Chinese herbal remedies, St John's wort
  - need for dose alteration due to ↓ eGFR, e.g. statin, or consider stopping, e.g. metformin when eGFR <30 ml/min/1.73m²
  - use of antacids, effervescent tablets (may have high salt content)
  - spironolactone if GFR <30ml/min, discuss with medical staff if patients has diarrhoea/vomiting or HF and CKD as may cause hyperkalaemia and dehydration. Stop if K⁺ >6.0mmol/L
- Provide initial patient information and education
- Investigations will depend on level of patient assessment prior to review in the AKCC but will include up-to-date:
  - urinalysis for blood/protein, ACR, MSU if infection suspected
  - blood tests: U&E, Cr, eGFR, HCO_3, chloride, bone profile, lipid profile, Alb, glucose, LFTs, FBC (haematinics if Hb < 11g/dl), clotting profile, HbA1c (diabetes)
  - viral serology for HBsAg, anti-HBsAg antibodies, anti-HCV, HIV test if late presenter requiring RRT
  - blood group and tissue typing
  - ± serology for ANA, ANCA, anti-GBM, complements, and plasma and urine protein electrophoresis
  - ± ECG/CXR
  - renal US if not already undertaken or urinary obstruction suspected ± kidney biopsy which is usually performed prior to AKCC.

Follow-up

Review is usually 3-monthly for stage 4 CKD and will vary for stable 5, depending on clinical condition. Cardiovascular risk and BP management continues as for CKD stages 1–3. (For information on the assessment and management of anaemia see 📖 pp. 219–40, nutrition in CKD see 📖 pp. 199–217 and mineral bone disorders see 📖 pp. 185–97.)

- Clinical condition—assess for any change in the patient's condition
- Investigations: blood tests: Cr, eGFR, FBC (haematinics if Hb <11g/dl), Ca^{2+}, PO_4. PTH, K^+, HCO_3, HbA1c (diabetes), urinalysis, e.g. dipstick for protein and blood
- Check serology up to date, e.g. HBsAg, anti-HBsAg antibodies, anti-HCV, HIV test if preparing for RRT or Tx
- Monitor and manage electrolyte imbalance and acidosis, see 📖 pp. 593–601
- Assess fluid status, see 📖 p. 587
- Management of fluid overload:
  - salt restriction of <6g/24hr, fluid restriction, refer to renal dietitian for dietary advice if required (see 📖 p. 84)
  - ± use of a diuretic, e.g. a loop diuretic such as furosemide → Na^+ excretion ∴ ↓ Na^+ retention, possibly adding a thiazide-like diuretic to ↑ effect
  - monitor weight, lying and standing BP for postural hypotension, serum Na^+ and K^+ levels if diuretic effect causes excessive diuresis
  - patient to contact the clinic if they have any symptoms of hypotension, e.g. dizziness, light headiness
  - gradual weight loss over a period of days until euvolaemic
  - severe fluid overload—admission to manage fluid removal
  - ⚠ risk of ↓ kidney function in HF patients as they need to be in a state of physiological oedema to maintain kidney perfusion
- RRT if conservative measures cannot adequately control fluid overload to prevent long-term complications, e.g. LVH
- Management of dehydration: risk of further ↓ of kidney function → lack of kidney perfusion 2° ↓ extracellular fluid i.e. fluid deplete:
  - most common renal-related causes are inadequate fluid intake 2° to osmotic diuresis causing polyuria (up to 3L/24hr), diarrhoea, vomiting. anorexia
  - identify and treat underlying cause, e.g. diarrhoea/vomiting, anorexia, osmotic diuresis
  - ± $NaHCO_3$ and ↑ oral fluid intake
  - ↑ oral intake if appropriate
  - educate patient to avoid episodes of dehydration (especially in the older person), e.g. in hot weather, diarrhoea/vomiting—maintain fluid intake and seek medical advice
  - ± IV fluids if inadequate oral intake to prevent further ↓ kidney function

- Diabetes—management continues as for CKD stages 1–3, aim for tight glycaemic control—HbA1c <53mmol/mol (7.0%) (see 📖 p. 134, 135):
  - ↑ risk of hypoglycaemia 2° accumulation of some oral hypoglycaemic drugs or their metabolites, prolonged insulin half-life, ↓ or absent gluconeogenesis by the kidneys
  - consider stopping metformin when eGFR <30ml/min—risk of lactic acidosis
  - liaise with diabetic team if required for change of medication, e.g. commencement of insulin
- Recommend vaccination against influenza, pneumococcal infections, and hepatitis B—associated with ↑ response if immunized against HBV preferably 6 months prior to commencing RRT
- Bleeding times: prolonged → impaired platelet function:
  - usually no specific treatment required, unless undergoing a procedure or operation—may need clotting profile and prophylaxis, e.g. desmopressin
- Medications—review as per initial assessment
- Planning future care and ongoing education. Arrange for attendance at group education sessions
- Assessment, planning, and co-ordination of RRT or referral for conservative treatment (see 📖 pp. 160–1 and 📖 pp. 511–29)
- Tx work-up if pursuing pre-emptive living donor transplantation or suitable to be listed for cadaveric transplant when eGFR <20ml/min (see 📖 p. 456)
- Ongoing psychosocial support:
  - refer to MPT as required, e.g. dietitian, social worker, counsellor
  - refer to patient support groups
  - promote self-care and encourage patient involvement in treatment and decision-making
  - update patient's care plan, e.g. My Kidney Care Plan.[5]

Other information that should be provided in the AKCC

- Preservation of access, no venepuncture or cannulation of peripheral blood vessels
- Notify nephrology service if attending other clinics/hospitals for procedures in case any special preparation is required
- Attend appointments with other specialists and GP. Inform other hospital departments or specialists that they have advanced kidney disease, e.g. procedures such as angiograms using contrast media which is nephrotoxic
- Oral hygiene as more prone to gingivitis, dry mouth, halitosis/bad taste which includes:
  - regular dental/hygienist check-ups, check dentures are well fitted as may lead to ulceration
  - techniques to assist with dry mouth
  - notify nephrology service if having any dental procedures as may require prophylactic antibiotics

- Financial—refer to social worker for assistance with welfare benefits, prescription charges
- Sexual problems, pregnancy, and contraceptive advice (see 📖 pp. 180–1, 544–6)
- Importance of preventing any episode of dehydration (see 📖 p. 149)
- Travelling and vaccinations (see 📖 pp. 556–7)
- Requirement to notify the DVLA of a change in medical condition.

Patient education

The patient/family should be provided with access to a structured information and education programme covering all aspects of advanced kidney disease, treatment options, and associated complications. Specific information about RRT is usually commenced when eGFR <20ml/min and is dependent on clinical condition, speed of progression towards ESKD, and the individual patient.

Individual or group educational programmes should include:

- CKD—causes, symptoms, associated complications and long-term management of CKD with focus on delaying progression to ESKD and RRT, e.g. good BP, lipid and diabetes control
- Signs and symptoms of advanced kidney disease and action to take
- Medications and preservation of kidney function (see 📖 pp. 568–71):
  - review medications and discuss the side effects, dosage, and method of taking for efficacy, e.g. iron tablets, phosphate binders
  - advise patients not to take other drugs without consulting medical staff, e.g. OTC medicines, herbal remedies such as St John's wort, nephrotoxic medications, e.g. NSAIDs
  - not to accept changes to medications, e.g. generic medications on the advice of the pharmacist, they should only take what is written on their prescription
- Integrated approach when discussing treatment options providing:
  - advantages and disadvantages of each modality
  - efficacy, risks, potential benefits, adverse effects of dialysis, e.g. older person or those with co-morbid conditions may do worse on dialysis than conservative treatment
  - consequences of inadequate dialysis
  - life expectancy
  - all aspects of transplantation if appropriate (see 📖 pp. 446–7)
  - conservative treatment and end of life care (see 📖 p. 512) even if the patient opts for RRT, it is important to provide some information on end of life strategies
- Planning and preparation involved in dialysis:
  - vascular and PD access, home assessment, liaison with community teams if assisted dialysis for support requirements
  - concept of the MPT, their role, meeting the team
- Review cardiovascular risks and promote a healthy lifestyle, e.g. exercise, smoking cessation (see 📖 pp. 76–7, 84–5)
- Psychosocial aspects (see 📖 pp. 532–3)
- Education should be culturally sensitive taking into consideration the ethnic/religious background of the patient and family
- Encourage patients to self-manage and be aware of ideal blood results and know and record their own blood results:
  - suggest accessing programmes such as Renal PatientView[6]
  - encourage the use of a care plan, e.g. My Kidney Care Plan[5]
- Patient support groups, expert patients, i.e. attendance at educational events, patient evenings, one-to-one meetings.

Treatment options for stage 5 CKD

- Peritoneal dialysis (PD):
  - continuous ambulatory PD (CAPD)
  - automated PD (APD)
  - assisted PD, either aCAPD or aAPD
- Haemodialysis (HD):
  - home-based HD
  - hospital-based HD
  - satellite HD
- Transplantation:
  - pre-emptive
  - cadaveric
  - living related
  - living unrelated
- Conservative management:
  - supportive care.

Choice and suitability for RRT

Age is not a contraindication to RRT: many older people have a good QOL and do well on RRT. The effects of multiple co-morbidities, poor physical or mental functioning, and a life expectancy of <1yr on RRT need to be considered. Commencing RRT may cause a significant decline in functional ability and QOL whilst only providing a few extra months of life. Conservative interventions may be more appropriate providing a longer life expectancy and the best possible QOL. in the following situations:

- Significant physical or mental impairment, e.g. severe dementia or older person with disabilities who have no family/carer support.
  - ▶ Mental competence will need to be assessed in line with Mental Capacity Act[7]
- Multiple co-morbidities, e.g. severe cardiac disease, diabetes
- Terminal disease, e.g. metastatic cancer with a poor prognosis (see pp. 511–29).

Choice of dialysis modality

The decision and choice of treatment should be made by the patient/family/carer in partnership with the nephrologist and in collaboration with the MPT. Table 6.1 provides a comparison between HD and PD as a treatment option. See 📖 pp. 446–7, Transplantation for choice and suitability.

- An integrated approach to RRT should provide balanced and accurate information about both modalities, and discuss with the patient and family that at some point they may need to switch from between modalities, e.g. PD to HD, with loss of UF capacity or RRF
- Encourage and facilitate self-efficacy and to self–manage treatment:
  - patient/family to participate in their care as much as possible in those not suitable for a home-based treatment
- Access to support groups, e.g. expert patient, local, and national kidney patient organizations
- Psychological assessment:
  - person's ability to adjust to proposed routine, how it will fit in to their normal day-to-day living with work, social activities, and household routine
  - identify attitude and health beliefs—how a person views illness and healthcare professionals together with their ability to cope with living with a chronic condition.

NICE guidance on choice of dialysis8

- Offer all people with stage 5 CKD a choice of PD or HD, if appropriate, but consider PD as the 1st choice of treatment modality for:
  - children 2yrs old or younger
  - people with RRF
  - adults without significant comorbidities
- When discussing choice of treatment modalities, healthcare professionals should take into account that people's priorities are not necessarily the same as their own clinical priorities
- Before starting PD, offer all patients a choice, if appropriate, between CAPD and APD (or aAPD if necessary)
- For children for whom PD is appropriate, offer APD in preference to CAPD if they are on a liquid diet, especially if they have low RRF.

PD versus HD

- Comparisons of PD and HD survival rates are similar, younger patients without diabetes have a slightly better survival rate on PD
- The RR of death varies and is dependent on the length of time on PD with PD having ↓ mortality rates during the first 1–2yrs
- After this time mortality risk is influenced by age, diabetes and the presence of co-morbidities, e.g. in those people >50yrs of age with diabetes, survival rates decline after 2yrs on PD which may suggest a timely transfer to HD
- Overall mortality rates for the first 2yrs are similar between PD and HD, with ↑ RR of death in PD older population >2yrs.

Barriers to self-care treatment

There are potential barriers that may significantly impact whether a home-based treatment is chosen by both the patient and healthcare staff.

- Physical:
  - poor upper body strength, e.g. to lift dialysate bags
  - impaired manual dexterity, e.g. unable to open equipment
  - impaired vision, e.g. difficulty with connection
- Cognitive/psychological:
  - non-adherence
  - psychiatric condition
  - dementia, impaired memory/cognition
  - barriers to communication i.e. language, literacy, sensory loss.

Table 6.1 Comparison between HD and PD

	Peritoneal dialysis	Haemodialysis
Frequency	Continuous dialysis: 4 exchanges/day or APD machine overnight (possibly additional day exchanges)	Intermittent, 3 times per wk, daily or nocturnal may be available
Access surgery	Rest for 2wks post insertion, if used immediately (supine position with smaller volumes)	Fistula—few months to mature prior to use
	Drainage problems common post insertion	Difficult to form access in diabetes, severe vascular disease
	May require surgical/laparoscopic insertion	May be performed under LA or regional anaesthetic—GA less common
	No vascular access required	VA can be problematic—↑ use of temporary access → ↑ risk multiple complications
Adequacy	Determined by membrane permeability i.e. ↑ adequacy → ↑ volume, number of exchanges, time	Determined by blood flow, dialysate flow rate, and dialysis membrane characteristics
	Difficult to maintain with RRF loss	↑ adequacy ↑ number of hrs or size of dialysis membrane
	↑ muscle mass ± switch to HD	
	Removal of β_2-microglobulins and other middle molecules	

(Continued)

Table 6.1 (Continued)

	Peritoneal dialysis	Haemodialysis
Fluid balance/UF	Determined by peritoneal membrane permeability ± ↓ fluid restriction Maintain RRF for longer ↓ UF with time on PD Not as effective as HD ↑ reliance on hypertonic dialysate with loss of RRF and UF	Programme UF volume required in to HD machine at beginning of session—more certain of UF volume UF can be difficult—intradialytic ↓ BP, e.g. HF
Haemodynamic	More steady state blood figures and continuous fluid removal Better haemodynamic stability, e.g. HF, angina ↓ haemodynamic changes ∴ ↓ episodes of ↓BP Improved BP control ↓ incidence of arrhythmias	Risk of ↓ BP associated with poor cardiac function—may require longer slower dialysis
Flexibility	Some flexibility with times Could be undertaken at work/educational institution	Fixed sessions either in the unit, satellite unit so may be difficult to fit in around work/university Flexibility with home HD as self-caring
Self-care/home	Self-care or assisted by a family member or carer Independence—maintain normal social routine Easy to learn, requires motivation Need suitable housing, e.g. space to store fluids/clean	Not a pre-requisite as nursing staff undertake HD, patient encouraged to participate unless on home HD which is a self-care treatment Does not require specific home environment
Travelling (see 📖 pp. 556–7)	PD fluid can be delivered to most places around the world APD machine is transportable, can switch to CAPD for convenience if needed Does not require any arrangements with a renal unit for HD session	More involvement to arrange a space in another renal unit and transfer, i.e. medical letters Risk of contracting hepatitis B and C if travelling to high-risk countries May not be accepted to other units if hepatitis B, C or HIV +ve

Table 6.1 (Continued)

	Peritoneal dialysis	Haemodialysis
Transport	↓ travel and appointments to tertiary hospital Community team visit at home if required Home-based treatment: no travelling, missed meals	Need to travel to either main unit or satellite unit 3 times/wk Use of hospital transport → large amount of time away from home 3 times per wk—causing fatigue, missed meals Home HD requires clinic appointments only and community visits
Psychosocial	May become isolated → depression Altered body image, i.e. PD catheter or weight gain May experience 'burn-out' after long time on PD	Good social structure and support Altered body image, e.g. fistula in young patient Needle phobia
Other	Fewer dietary restrictions Worsen pre-existing malnourished state—protein loss ↑ weight gain, ↑ lipids, ↑ glucose load, difficult to control diabetes May exacerbate back pain ↓ anaemia ∴ ↓ ESA use Cheaper	↑ blood loss → ↑ use of ESAs
Infection	Risk of peritonitis and exit site infections—need good technique	Risk of temporary VA infection

Dialysis and the older person

- The median age for commencement of RRT in the UK at the end of 2009 was 64.8yrs (19.4% aged 65–74 and 14.6% >75yrs)
- 9% of prevalent RRT ≥65yrs of age are on PD compared to 68% on HD
- In the NECOSAD study those >70yrs of age were found to be 6 times more likely to choose HD than those aged 18–40yrs
- UK BOLDE (Broadening Options for Long-term Dialysis in the Elderly) study, of >65yrs of age on HD and PD. Found QOL similar in PD and HD but possibly ↑ slightly in PD.

Factors which can impact on the choice of treatment

- The effect on QOL
- Impaired cognitive ability necessitating support from family/carer in making decisions on treatment options
- Anxiety and fear of not being able to learn a new skill and undertaking the treatment themselves at home, e.g. due to impaired physical functioning (poor eyesight or manual dexterity) or cognitive impairment if no family/carer support available
- The personal and family burden of dialysis
- Feeling of isolation if on a home-based treatment
- Presence of other co-morbid conditions, e.g. diabetes and vascular disease, e.g. poor vascular access
- Location of dialysis and the distance to travel:
  - may take too much time away from home, cause pain as a result of long travelling times to hospital, e.g. osteoarthritis
- Family circumstances:
  - patient may also be a carer themselves and have additional responsibilities at home, e.g. a home-based treatment may be socially unsuitable
  - lack of a good social support network to help with daily activities, e.g. shopping, cleaning, transport to appointments.

Many of these issues can be overcome with adequate family/carer support to assist with a home-based treatment, e.g. a PD.

- Important to make patients aware of access to assistance
- Although some of the barriers may also be contraindications to a home-based treatment, each patient needs to be individually assessed based on their own needs and support available in order to weigh up what is best for the patient and their family
- See Table 6.2 for advantages and disadvantages of HD and PD in the older person.

Table 6.2 PD vs HD—advantages and disadvantages in the older person

	Advantages	Disadvantages
PD	↓ BP episodes ↓ incidence of arrhythmias Better fluid balance Good blood BP control ↓ anaemia ∴ ↓ ESA use No vascular access needed Removal of B_2-microglobulins and other middle molecules Maintain RRF for longer Home-based treatment: no travelling, missed meals Maintain normal social routine Possibility of aPD to remain at home ↓ hospitalization rate	Protein loss—worsen pre-existing malnourished state Exacerbation of constipation Unable to perform technical aspects due to disability, e.g. problems with dexterity and impaired vision Difficulty lifting heavy bags of dialysate Problems with learning as result of cognitive impairment Longer training times and ↑ community support ∴ resource impact Social isolation → depression if house bound
HD	Does not require a large degree of participation and ability Intermittent in nature Potential to provide a social support structure ↓ problems with diabetes management	IDH Travel to dialysis unit 3 times/wk May require longer slower dialysis VA can be problematic with the ↑ use of temporary access → multiple complications

Assessment for dialysis

Medical considerations
- Presence of co-morbid conditions:
  - difficulty creating vascular access, e.g. diabetes and vascular disease
  - ↑ likelihood of hypotensive episodes and fluctuations in BP on HD, so may fare better on PD, e.g. IHD, angina, and hypotensive HF
- Contraindications to HD or PD.
- IS therapy, e.g. SLE or failing Tx:
  - potential for ↑ risk of peritonitis on PD, line sepsis with temporary HD catheter
  - corticosteroid use associated with delayed wound healing, e.g. may need to consider laparoscopic PD catheter insertion rather than surgical
- History of drug and alcohol abuse or poorly controlled mental illness
- Home adaptations such as rails.

Contraindications to HD
- Severe IHD/HF
- Severe vascular disease—no vascular access
- Central vein thrombosis
- HD unit a long distance away—unsuitable for home HD
- Active diabetic retinopathy.

Contraindications to PD
Absolute
- Previous abdominal surgery with adhesions, presence of a stoma or ileal conduit
- Recurrent and unresolvable hernias
- Unable to achieve adequate dialysis or UF
- No assistance available—physical or mentally unable to perform PD
- Homeless and those with poor social circumstances (e.g. living conditions). Unable to store fluid in home.

Relative
- Large renal cysts
- Skin or abdominal wall infection
- Inflammatory bowel disease, e.g. diverticulitis
- Morbid obesity
- Severe respiratory disease, e.g. COPD
- Chronic back pain
- Severely malnourished
- Uncontrolled incontinence
- Poor personal hygiene and care
- Unresolved impaired dexterity
- Poorly motivated and history of non-adherence problems
- ± large muscle mass and no RRF may not achieve adequate dialysis
- PD leaks
- Unable to tolerate required PD volumes.

Patient considerations

Where possible promote independent care and consider the following:
• Continence and level of hygiene
• Disability is not a contraindication to RRT, e.g. mobility, dexterity, eyesight and requires careful assessment by MPT:
  • requires a home assessment for home-based treatment
  • aids available to assist perform home-based treatment—adjustment to normal training tools and equipment such as talking clocks, weight scales, assisted PD devices
• Learning disabilities, e.g. lack of comprehension
• Family/social factors—can the family/carer provide the additional long-term support required for a home-based treatment?
• Lifestyle and normal routine—↑ flexibility of dialysis with home-based treatment → greater opportunity for employment, educational courses:
  • may require housing assessment housing, e.g. alterations may be required to the home, e.g. fitting a shower for PD or re-housing to accommodate storage and space to undertake PD/home HD. Financial support may be required
  • lack of cleanliness—not conducive to home-based treatments
• The risk of body image problems—younger patients may not wish to have a visible sign of their condition, e.g. fistula
• History of non-adherence and lack of motivation as these patients are not suitable for a home-based treatment.

When to start RRT

UK Renal Association 2011[3] recommendation:
- eGFR <10ml/min as there is no evidence of improved survival rates with starting RRT earlier.

European Best Practice (EBP) Committee[9] recommendations:
- eGFR <15ml/min/1.73m^2 and/or the presence of uraemic symptoms, uncontrolled BP and fluid overload or malnutrition which does not respond to medical treatment, or before eGFR <6ml/min/1.73m^2 in an asymptomatic patient
- Mean eGFR commencement on RRT in the UK is currently 8.6ml/min/1.73m^2 and has been stable for the last 3yrs (Renal Registry, 2010).[3]

The decision to commence RRT should not be based purely on eGFR but take into consideration:
- Patient's symptoms and wishes
- Nutritional status
- Physical and psychosocial status
- Presence of co-morbidities.

Uraemic symptoms are dependent on the individual and usually occur with an eGFR 15–20ml/min but may arise earlier. Some patients may benefit from starting RRT earlier if:
- Symptomatic of ESKD:
  - weight loss/malnutrition, anorexia, fatigue
- Unable to control BP, fluid overload, severe hyperkalaemia, and metabolic acidosis resistant to medical therapy
- Causing a significant impact on general health and well-being, QOL, and functional state of the patient
- High-risk patients, e.g. older person and diabetes as may become more symptomatic at a higher eGFR:
  - presence of vascular disease and potentially difficult access in case it fails and requires intervention—if performed at low eGFR temporary HD may be required.

▶ Some patients who are asymptomatic may have false expectations that they will feel differently once they have started RRT, so it is worthwhile discussing with them that they may not feel any changes to prevent any disappointment, increased anxiety, and depression.

Checklist for planning RRT

- Patient education and information on choice of RRT provided by
- MPT, e.g. nurse, medical staff, dietitian, social worker, pharmacist, counsellor, patient expert groups
- Refer to other members of MPT 6 months prior to requiring RRT or as required
- Organization of access surgery
- MRSA swabs:
  - AVF ideally 6 months prior to commencing dialysis
  - PD catheter minimum of 2–4wks prior, depending on type of catheter inserted
  - medical PD catheter insertion suitability if earlier start required
- Refer to renal dietitian if K^+ >5mmol/L, ↑ PO_4, ↑ lipids, weight control, low Alb, and/or weight loss
- Review anaemia treatment, e.g. type and dose of ESA
- Check serology up to date, e.g. HBsAg, anti HBsAg antibodies, anti-HCV antibodies:
  - HBV vaccination for all patients prior to starting RRT
- Check if HIV result up to date if considering transplantation
- Nephrology service visit by patient and family, e.g. tour of HD/PD units
- Arrange home visit to assess housing/storage for home-based treatments, e.g. PD, home HD:
  - assessment of nursing/residential home if assisted APD required
- Provide psychological support and refer to renal counsellor and social worker if required (see 📖 pp. 531–63)
- Agree RRT start date and location where possible
- Liaise with relevant dialysis unit
- Assess transport needs.

Further reading

Brown EA, Johansson L, Farrington K, et al. Broadening Options for Long-term Dialysis in the Elderly (BOLDE): differences in quality of life on peritoneal dialysis compared to haemodialysis for older patients. Nephrol Dial Transplant 2010; **25**(11):3755–63.

Daugirdas J. Handbook of Chronic Kidney Disease Management. Philadelphia, PA: Wolters Kluwer/ Lippincott Williams & Wilkins; 2011.

Davies S, Van Biesen W, Nicholas J, et al. Integrated care. Perit Dial Int 2001; **21**:S269–274.

Dimkovic N, Aggarwal V, Khan S, et al. Assisted peritoneal dialysis: what does it and who does it involve? Adv Perit Dial 2009; **25**:165–9.

Lamping DL, Constantinovici N, Roderick P, et al. Clinical outcomes, quality of life, and costs in the North Thames Dialysis Study of elderly people on dialysis: a prospective cohort study. Lancet 2000; **356**(9241):1543–50.

Levy J, Brown E, Daley C, et al. Oxford Handbook of Dialysis, 3rd edn. Oxford: Oxford Medical Publications; 2009.

Stanley M. Peritoneal dialysis versus haemodialysis (adult). Nephrology 2010; **15**:S24–31.

Tattersall J, Dekker F, Heimbürger O, et al. When to start dialysis: updated guidance following publication of the Initiating Dialysis Early and Late (IDEAL) study. Nephrol Dial Transplant 2011; **26**:2082–6.

References

1. NICE. Chronic Kidney Disease. Early identification and management of chronic kidney disease in adults in primary and secondary care. Clinical Guideline 73. London: NICE; 2008. Available at: ℜ <http://www.nice.org.uk/guidance/qualitystandards/chronickidneydisease/ckdqualitystandard.jsp> (accessed 2 November 2011).

2. Department of Health. The National Service Framework for Renal Services Part 1: Dialysis and Transplantation. 2004. London: Department of Health.

3. The Renal Association. Clinical Practice Guidelines, 5th edn. Available at: ℜ <http://www.renal.org/clinical/guidelinessection/guidelines.aspx> (accessed 6 May 2012).

4. The Renal Association. UK Renal Registry 13th Annual Report, December 2010. Available at: ℜ <http://www.renalreg.com/Reports/2010.html>

5. NHS Kidney Care. My Kidney Care Plan. Available at: ℜ http://www.kidneycare.nhs.uk/_Resourcestodownload-MyKidneyCarePlan.aspx>

6. NHS. Renal PatientView. Available at: ℜ <http://www.renalpatientview.org>

7. Department of Health. Mental Capacity Act, 2005. Available at: ℜ <http://www.legislation.gov.uk/ukpga/2005/9/contents>

8. NICE. Peritoneal Dialysis: Peritoneal dialysis in the treatment of stage 5 chronic kidney disease. Clinical Guideline 125. London: NICE; 2011. Available at: ℜ <http://www.nice.org.uk/nicemedia/live/13524/55517/55517.pdf>

9. European Best Practice Guidelines. The initiation of dialysis. Nephrol Dial Transplant 2005; **20**(sup 9):ix3–ix7.

Patient information websites

EdRen Info. Available at: ℜ <http://www.edren.org/pages/edreninfo/>

National Kidney Federation. Available at: ℜ <http://www.kidney.org.uk> (also provides details of local kidney patient associations)

NHS. Kidney Care. Available at: ℜ <http://www.kidneycare.nhs.uk/>

NICE Patient information. High blood pressure. Available at: ℜ <http://www.nice.org.uk/nicemedia/live/13561/56013/56013.pdf>

Patient.co.uk. Available at: ℜ <http://www.patient.co.uk>

The UK Renal Association. Available at: ℜ<http://www.renal.org/whatwedo/informationresources/>

Treatment of chronic kidney disease. Available at: ℜ <http://www.renalpatient.org>

Complications associated with chronic kidney disease

Uraemic pruritus

This is a very common and debilitating effect of the late stages of CKD and for those on RRT affecting 15–49% pre-dialysis and 40–50% of patients on HD (DOPPS study[1]). It can lead to sleep disturbance, stress, anxiety, and depression.

Clinical features

- The skin can become excoriated from chronic scratching and be a potential source of infection and dermatological conditions
- Pruritus is usually generalized, but is most common on the back and is worse at night, although this varies from person to person
- May be aggravated by heat, sweat, dry skin, and stress
- Alleviated initially by cool or hot showers, cool air, and activity
- Occurs only a few times a day or may be all the time.

Possible causes

- Dry skin (xerosis)
- Hyperparathyroidism, hyperphosphataemia, hypercalcaemia → calcium phosphate deposits irritating the sensory nerves in the skin
- ↑β2 microglobulin levels
- Peripheral neuropathy
- ↑ aluminium levels
- Hypervitaminosis A
- Immune dysfunction, chronic inflammation associated with ESKD
- Inadequate dialysis
- Anaemia
- ♂ gender.

Nursing considerations

- Discuss with medical staff, exclude a dermatological cause, e.g. allergy
- Advise the patient to avoid hot baths and soap that can dry out skin, wear gloves, and cut their nails to prevent excoriation of the skin if scratching excessively
- Treat anaemia if present
- Maintain normal serum calcium × phosphate product
- May require pharmacological interventions such as:
  - emollients, antihistamines (e.g. hydroxyzine), topical capsaicin, ultraviolet B light, gabapentin, evening primrose oil, ondansetron, topical tacrolimus ointment, acupuncture
  - experimental treatments include thalidomide, activated charcoal, omega-6 fatty acids
- Usually resolves with parathyroidectomy when tertiary parathydroidism is the cause (Ca^{2+} and PO_4 normal)
- If on dialysis—optimize adequacy of dialysis:
  - assess when itching occurs, e.g. only occurs on dialysis it may be a hypersensitivity reaction. Change to another form of heparin, dialysis membrane, or mode of sterilization and review efficacy
- Resolves post-kidney Tx.

Gastrointestinal problems

GI symptoms and disturbance are common in the advanced stages of CKD and those on RRT, which can lead to muscle wasting and malnourishment (see Table 7.1 for causes and management).

Table 7.1 Causes and management of GI problems

GI problem	Cause	Management
Constipation (most common)	Fluid restrictions, low K^+ diets, and inadequate exercise or side effect of medications More common in the elderly	Review medications and stop or switch to an alternative is possible Use of regular aperients, e.g. lactulose, senna ⚠ Avoid laxatives that contain magnesium, citrate or PO_4 Encourage ↑ exercise
Oral thrush/ candida May involve oesophagus	Antibiotics, IS, diabetes and the malnourished	Nystatin Good oral hygiene
Glossitis	B12, folic acid, and iron deficiency anaemia	Correct deficiency
Hallitosis	Unpleasant taste in mouth as a result of uaemia → ↓ appetite	Commence RRT Improve adequacy
Gingival hyperplasia	Medications, e.g. CCB/ ciclosporin	Review medications—stop or switch where possible
Nausea, vomiting, and anorexia	Uraemia Medications, e.g. iron supplement, PO_4 binders Need to prevent malnutrition	Review medications—stop or switch if possible Antiemetics, e.g. metoclopramide— ↓ dose dependent on GFR Commence RRT or improve adequacy of dialysis Refer to dietitian, suggest small frequent meals Assess foods which cause nausea, i.e. smell of certain foods and availability of foods which are palatable

Table 7.1 (Continued)

GI problem	Cause	Management
GI bleeding	Excess circulating urea which is broken down in the GI tract and forms ammonia → gastritis, peptic ulceration, and reflux Platelet dysfunction Medications, e.g. NSAIDs, heparin Angiodysplasia	Assess for ulceration and *Helicobacter pylori* infection Endoscopy/colonoscopy Treat with PPI, e.g. omeprazole for gastritis and antibiotics for *Helicobacter pylori* infection Review medications—stop or switch where possible Oestrogen therapy—side effect gynaecomastia, fluid retention and vaginal bleeding
Gastroparesis	Common complication associated with diabetes Causes feeling of fullness, nausea, and diarrhoea (see 📖 p. 338)	Use of antiemetics such as metoclopramide or ondansetron Erythromycin
Pancreatitis	Poor clearance of enzymes, e.g. amylase, lipase Associated with alcoholic liver disease	Usually conservative, e.g. nasogastric tube and NBM to resolve

Chronic pain

~50% of CKD patients complain of pain with the majority reporting it as moderate to severe. There is some under-reporting, which may be due in part to the effects of cognitive impairment in the later stages of CKD or an expectation that pain is normal with CKD. Chronic pain leads to problems with coping, sleep disturbance, depression, QOL, and psychological and physical functioning. There is an association between chronic pain and request to withdraw from treatment (see 📖 p. 520).

Types of chronic pain

- Nociceptive pain—related to tissue damage and results in the over-stimulation of sensory receptors:
  - patients complain of sharp, stabbing type pain at the site
  - responds well to opioids
- Neuropathic pain—involves nerve damage:
  - complain of burning, numbness, tingling
  - treatment options include; anticonvulsants, e.g. gabapentin, carbamazepine (⚠ ↓ dose as can cause toxicity); and antidepressants (⚠ side effects and requires observation)
- Some patients may only experience transient pain related to use which stops when they have completed the task, e.g. intermittent claudication when walking.

Renal-related causes

- Co-morbid conditions—diabetes, e.g. neuropathy, PVD, e.g. intermittent claudication, osteoarthritis, e.g. in knees, hips causing physical mobility problems
- Elderly, e.g. associated conditions such as musculoskeletal problems
- 1° condition, e.g. polycystic kidney disease (painful cysts), MM
- Altered perception of pain due to associated symptoms of kidney disease, e.g. fatigue, pruritus, depression, sleep disorders, RLS, nausea and anxiety
- Complications of CKD, e.g. MBD, gout
- Complications associated with RRT, e.g. back pain and abdominal distention, peritonitis in PD patients, steal syndrome in fistula, calciphylaxis, dialysis amyloid arthropathy.

Impact of living with uncontrolled pain

- Poor QOL
- Sleep disturbance
- ↑ levels of anxiety, depression, withdrawal from RRT
- Inadequate dialysis/fluid overload:
  - alteration of PD prescription by the patient, e.g. ↓ drain in volume if they are experiencing abdominal discomfort during the dwell period
- Stop dialysis early as unable to stay in chair/bed for complete session.

Assessment

- Undertake a pain assessment which includes:
  - history, e.g. when the pain first started, what makes it worse and what relieves it (e.g. moving or sitting/lying in a particular position)
  - location and type of pain (e.g. sharp/stabbing or burning)
  - impact on physical, social, emotional aspects of daily life
  - impact on QOL and sleep
  - previous treatments and effectiveness
- Various well validated pain score tools can be used within the clinical setting such as visual analogue scale, numerical rating, verbal rating tools, more formalized tools such as the McGill pain questionnaire, brief pain inventory (BPI), dialysis symptom index (DSI), and Edmonton symptom assessment system (ESAS).

Nursing considerations

- A good knowledge of pharmacokinetics when prescribing and administering analgesics by prescriber and nursing staff as the kidneys excrete many drugs (see 📖 pp. 566–7)
- Develop a treatment strategy in partnership with the patient, as there are both physical and psychological aspects involved in effective pain management:
  - information should include an explanation of the proposed treatment and side effects—check patient is taking analgesics as prescribed
- Provide realistic expectations as some pain conditions may not be resolved
- Be aware of the signs of depression and take into consideration psychosocial or spiritual issues and needs
- Use the World Health Organizations (WHO) principles for pain management to deliver pain relief:[2]
  - by mouth—where possible
  - by the clock—regular analgesia for continuous pain
  - by the ladder—to include breakthrough analgesia if required
  - for the individual
  - attention to detail—ongoing re-assessment for efficacy, side effects, adequacy of dose
- Medical staff will prescribe analgesia using the WHO analgesic ladder as a guide (see 📖 p. 519)[2]
- Consider practical solutions that may alleviate pain, e.g. switch from CAPD to APD—↓ abdominal discomfort if using larger volumes
- Consider home-based treatment if travelling to dialysis is aggravating pain, e.g. poor mobility.

Alternative complimentary therapies/non-drug related may also be considered

- Transcutaneous electrical nerve stimulation (TENS) machine
- Acupuncture
- Physiotherapy
- Relaxation therapy.

Sleep disorders

Sleep disturbance is a common and under-recognized problem in all stages of CKD with ~44–50% prevalence rate. However, this may be an underestimate, as patients may not complain of sleep disturbance unless prompted by healthcare professionals. The majority of CKD patients complain of difficulty falling asleep, maintaining sleep, daytime sleepiness, and fatigue.

- Assessment tools for screening include Epworth Sleepiness Scale and the Pittsburgh Sleep Quality Index (PSQI) or a referral made to a sleep specialist for sleep studies.

Types of sleep disorders
- Insomnia:
  - excessive sleepiness, e.g. daytime sleepiness
- Sleep apnoea
- Restless leg syndrome (RLS) and periodic limb movement disorder (PLMD).

Effects of sleep disorders
- Employment:
  - poor job satisfaction and work efficiency
  - ↑ accidents
  - ↑ absenteeism
- ↑ hospitalization rates
- More frequent visits to healthcare professionals
- Risk factor for anxiety and depression and impact on QOL
- ↑ mortality and morbidity.

Insomnia
Common complaint in dialysis patients (38–71%) which is associated with problems getting to or staying asleep, waking up very early which leads to poor daytime functioning.

Excessive sleepiness
A common complaint amongst dialysis patients, and causes difficulty staying awake during the day and lack of concentration.

Causes
- RLS or PLMD
- Sleep apnoea
- Metabolic factors
- Physical, e.g. pruritus, bone pain, polyneuropathy, cramps
- Depression
- Side effect of medication, e.g. corticosteroids
- Poor sleep hygiene (e.g. sleeping during dialysis sessions in the day)
- Alcohol, smoking
- Age, less with older age
- Psychological factors, e.g. anxiety, stress.

Nursing considerations
- Treat underlying cause, e.g. pruritus, RLS, sleep apnoea, depression, medications
- Good sleep hygiene and avoid sleeping during dialysis sessions
- CBT
- Medications, e.g. benzodiazepines (e.g. temazepam) or non-benzodiazepines (e.g. zolpidem)
- See p. 404 for treatment of cramps
- Transfer to nocturnal HD as less problems with RLS, if available may improve outcome.

Patient education on good sleep hygiene
Before bed
- Avoid alcohol, caffeine, smoking 6hrs before bed
- Avoid eating too much before bed or going to bed hungry
- Regular exercise is beneficial and should be encouraged:
  - no exercise within 4hrs prior to going to bed
- Go outside or be exposed to natural light for a period of time each day
- No stimulating activities before bed, e.g. playing a computer game.

Setting a routine
- Go to bed and get up at the same time each day
- After a poor night's sleep, avoid lying in to catch up on sleep
- Preferable not to take a nap during the day especially in the evening:
  - HD patients may need to engage in an activity to keep them awake on dialysis, e.g. reading, playing a game to prevent napping.

Environment
- Bedroom should be restful place used for sleeping or sex
- Avoid reading or watching television in bed
- Create a calm, restful, and comfortable place to sleep:
  - blackout curtains if waking up with the sun, use ear plugs if noisy etc.

Once in bed
- Don't clock watch
- If not asleep after 20–30mins, get up and do something in another room—keep it dimmed and try again once feeling tired and sleepy.

Sleep apnoea
Approximately 30–50% of ESKD patients (similar in HD, PD, and advanced CKD) suffer from sleep apnoea compared to 2–4% in the general population. Characterized by repeated episodes where there is cessation of breathing known as obstructive sleep apnoea (OSA).
- Repeated episodes of upper airway obstruction → ↓ blood O_2 saturation levels
- Further ↑ risk of CVD

- Symptoms include daytime sleepiness, fatigue, and impaired cognitive function
- Risk factors include older age, ♂ gender, and being overweight.

Causes
- Fluid overload and upper airway interstitial oedema
- Chronic uraemia (build-up of uraemic toxins) or DM can cause pharyngeal narrowing → neuropathy or myopathy
- Chronic metabolic acidosis
- Upper airway narrowing—e.g. enlarged tonsils
- Obesity.

Nursing considerations
- Lifestyle modification, e.g. weight loss, no alcohol near to bedtime, do not sleep in supine position
- Referral to sleep specialist:
  - dental appliance or continuous positive airway pressure (CPAP) machine
  - surgical removal of obstruction, mandibular splint/advancement
- Transfer from daytime HD to nocturnal HD or CAPD to APD as nocturnal treatments have been shown to have benefits possibly due to fluid removal
- ± resolves post transplantation
- ⚠ Avoid the use of sedatives.

Restless legs syndrome and periodic limb movement disorder

RLS is a common complication in advanced CKD with ~20–60% of CKD patients complaining of RLS compared with 5–15% in general population.
- Patients complain of sudden involuntary jerking leg movements with paraesthesiae:
  - may also occur occasionally in the arms
  - occurs at rest and relieved by moving
- Described as 'creeping', 'itching', or a 'creepy-crawly' feeling occurring every 20–30secs throughout the night
- Usually worse at rest, and most noticeable at night and in the evening
- PLMD disorder refers to involuntary jerking leg movements (may also occur in the arms) during sleep which occurs in >50% of dialysis patients.

Renal specific risk factors
- Anaemia and iron deficiency
- ↓ serum parathyroid concentration
- Calcium–phosphate imbalance
- Peripheral neuropathy
- DM
- Uraemia.

Impact of RLS/PLM
- Poor QOL
- Sleep disturbance, e.g. insomnia, daytime sleepiness
- Associated with ↑ mortality risk.

Nursing considerations
- Advise the patient to stop caffeine, smoking, and alcohol intake
- Review medications and stop if possible those that may be making it worse, e.g. antidepressants, metoclopramide, some antihistamines
- If symptoms are persistent—educate on posterior leg muscle stretching exercises before bed
- Alter dialysis time or frequency
- Correct anaemia and/or iron deficiency (see 📖 pp. 226–7)
- Medications that may be considered:
  - dopamine agonist (e.g. bromocriptine or levodopa) and antiepileptics (e.g. gabapentin and carbamazepine) have been found to be effective in the treatment of RLS
  - other drugs such as clonazepam can help—⚠ can cause drowsiness. Anti-Parkinson's drugs such as pergolide and pramipexole—side effects of nausea and drowsiness.

Cognitive impairment

Impaired cognitive ability has become more widely recognized as a major complication for CKD patients occurring in the early stages through to RRT and transplantation.

- 2–3 times more prevalent in the older person with an eGFR <45 ml/min/1.73m^2 compared to eGFR ≥60ml/min/1.73m^2
- Highly prevalent in HD patients 30–70%
- Tx does lead to improvement of cognitive function in many patients, in particular with memory and verbal learning
- History of stroke is a major risk factor; also associated with a low level of education.

Effects

- Poor memory
- Inability to concentrate, inability to make informed decisions, e.g. choice of treatment, finances, advanced directives
- Lack of an awareness of social and physical needs
- Poor comprehension of information provided on all aspects of CKD and treatment options
- Impaired visual-motor reaction times
- Altered intellectual and language skills
- ↓ QOL.

Renal-related causes

- Anaemia
- Uraemia
- Vascular disease
- Side effects of medications
- Sleep deprivation
- Depression
- Inadequate dialysis, dialysis related, e.g. hypotensive episodes on HD.

Nursing considerations

- Have a good understanding and awareness of cognitive dysfunction as it may affect the patient's ability to learn:
  - may be unfairly labelled non-adherent because of poor memory
- Those new to the nephrology service will have important decisions to make about their treatment options, choice of modality, or supportive care:
  - these need to made with the patient fully aware and understanding the implications to their decision
- In the AKCC, an initial assessment should be undertaken:
  - use of tools such as the mini mental state examination (MMSE) to enable early detection of high-risk patients
- Put strategies in place to assist with learning and comprehension of information
- Provide written information to take home to reinforce the education session and enable family to be involved
- Adapt training sessions to one-on-one or provide more frequent educational sessions if required
- Suggest a family member or friend attends education sessions and/or clinic appointments to re-iterate the information at home
- Encourage physical and cognitive activities which have been shown to help slow the rate of decline in the normal population
- Treat anaemia (see 📖 pp. 226–7)
- May improve changing to nocturnal HD
- ▶ If on HD, provide education before the HD session as cognitive impairment is worse during and immediately after treatment
- May have some improvement after a kidney transplant.

Depression

Depression is often unrecognized and untreated in the CKD population as the symptoms of a chronic condition and depression can appear very similar (e.g. anorexia, insomnia, tiredness). The prevalence of a major depressive disorder in ESKD is ~17–21% compared to 5% in the normal population.

- Suicide is more common in ESKD patients than the general population
- Depressed patients on dialysis see dialysis as more intrusive than those without depression:
  - ↓ QOL score and usually poor social support networks
- Successful transplantation can improve the patient's condition.

Clinical depression is associated with:

- ↑ mortality and death in some studies
- Non-adherence, e.g. failure to take medications or attend HD treatment sessions
- Inadequate nutritional status
- Chronic pain
- Immunological dysfunction, i.e. more prone to infections
- Abnormal glucocorticoid metabolism and pro-inflammatory: i.e. ↓ Alb, post-depressive illness
- ↑ risk of peritonitis in PD patients associated with less care taken when performing the exchange technique
- ↑ hospitalizations
- Relationship problems.

Independent predictors include:

- ♂ gender
- White or Asian ethnicity
- Recent hospitalization, alcohol or drug dependence
- Socio-economic status
- Poor social support and marital status
- Alcohol and recreational drug usage
- Recent bereavement
- Negative interaction and relationship with medical staff
- Tx status and dialysis modality.

Symptoms of clinical depression

- Loss of interest or pleasure in activities, low mood
- Feelings of sadness, helplessness, and guilt
- Physical changes such as:
  - change in appetite and weight, ↓ libido, altered sleep patterns (e.g. insomnia or hypersomnia), fatigue
- ↓ concentration
- Suicidal ideation
- Psychomotor changes (e.g. involuntary muscle twitching).

KDOQI[3] recommends screening all CKD patients for functional status and well-being at regular intervals. There are many validated psychometric assessment tools available such as the Beck Depression Inventory (BDI),

Cognitive Depression Index (CDI), and the SF-36 and KDQOL questionnaires both have sections on emotional symptoms.

Nursing considerations

- Good understanding of the symptoms in order to identify those at
  risk and recognize early signs and symptoms
- Identify any underlying cause, e.g. bereavement, chronic pain, transfer
  back to dialysis after a failed kidney transplant
- Provide psychological support to the patient, carer, family
- Discuss any concerns with the medical staff and counsellor—may
  require referral to a GP, psychiatrist, or psychologist to ensure
  clinical assessment undertaken
- Treatments for mild depression may include:
  - counselling
  - ↑ exercise where possible
  - self-help therapy, i.e. cognitive behavioural therapy (CBT)
- More severe cases of depression may require:
  - antidepressant medications such as selective serotonin re-uptake
    inhibitors, e.g. fluoxetine, sertraline
  - patients may be concerned about taking antidepressants and will
    require reassurance and information on side effects to promote
    adherence
- Knowledge of the side effects of antidepressants for those on
  dialysis.

Sexual dysfunction

Sexual dysfunction is common in both sexes with CKD, on RRT or post transplantation. It is either organic or psychological in nature (the causes and treatments are outlined in Tables 7.2 and 7.3). Sexual dysfunction has an impact on QOL, leading to stress, anxiety, depression, and difficulty developing or maintaining intimate relationships.

- >50% of ♂ with advanced kidney disease complain of erectile dysfunction (ED), ↓ libido, and less sexual intercourse
- ↑ incidence in ♂ on dialysis (reported as high as 82%), though less in kidney Tx patients as, for many, testosterone levels and sperm counts return to normal
- ♀ sexual problems include amenorrhoea, lack of sexual desire and arousal, unable to achieve an orgasm and dyspareunia:
  - few studies in ♀ but it is estimated that 44–75% of ♀ have some sexually-related problem. Symptoms tend to reverse with a successful kidney Tx.

Nursing assessment

- Good, open non-judgemental communication to ascertain the exact problem, is it organic or psychological in origin?
- Identify patient's perception of the problem (and their partner's):
  - if partner is present, find out what they feel about the situation
- ♂ assessment—identify the problem, e.g. ED, lack of desire:
  - absence of morning erections
  - normal libido and ejaculation
- ♀ assessment—identify the problem, e.g. lack of desire, amenorrhoea:
  - regular menses
- Questions for both sexes:
  - duration of the problem
  - was the onset gradual or sudden? e.g. sudden likely to caused by starting a new drug
  - what do they think is causing the problem?
  - have they tried any treatments?
  - do they use recreational drugs or drink a lot of alcohol?
- Investigations will include FBC, sex hormones, TFT
- Clinical observations should include BP and neurovascular observations, e.g. presence of pedal pulses
- Review latest adequacy results or organize if required
- Review medications and identify any that could potentially be the cause
- There are assessment tools available, e.g. International Index of Erectile Function (IIEF) and the Female Sexual Function Index (FSFI)
- Refer to medical staff as they will need to assess for normal 2° sex characteristics and normal sexual development.

Although there are treatment options available that medical staff may be able to commence, some patients may require a referral to a sexual dysfunction clinic, counsellor, psychotherapist, or back to the GP for ongoing management.

Table 7.2 Female sexual problems causes, clinical features, and treatment

Cause	Clinical features	Treatment
↓ oestrogen level → menopausal symptoms	Vaginal irritation, dyspareunia, mood swings	HRT can be effective in managing symptoms
No oestradiol-LH surge	Anovulation and infertility	Adequate dialysis
		Treat anaemia
↑ prolactin ↓ oestradiol levels	↓ libido, infertility and galactorrhoea	Adequate dialysis Bromocriptine, △side effect of hypotension
Diabetic neuropathy	↓ lubrication and genital sensation → dyspareunia and recurrent thrush	Advise the patient on the use of lubricants Treat yeast infection
Anaemia	↓ libido/fatigue	Correct anaemia
Psychological effects of living with a chronic condition	↓ libido/fatigue	Psychotherapy

Table 7.3 Male sexual problems causes, clinical features, and treatment

Cause	Clinical feature	Treatment
↓ testosterone → ↑ LH and ↑ FSH	ED and ↓ libido	Testosterone Optimize dialysis ED treatments
↑ prolactin as a result of endocrine dysfunction and ↓ clearance	↓ libido, galactorrhoea, gynaecomastia (30% in HD)	Adequate dialysis Bromocriptine, △side effect hypotension
Autonomic neuropathy Atherosclerosis	ED, anorgasmia	Optimize BP, DM Lipid control
Zinc deficiency	Low sperm count	Oral zinc supplements
Anaemia	ED, ↓ spermatogenesis	Treat anaemia
Medication side effects	ED	Review
Psychological effects of living with a chronic condition	ED, ↓ libido	Counselling Refer to ED specialist

ED treatment options

Referral to the sexual dysfunction clinic for assessment and ongoing management. May require psychosexual therapy, antidepressants, and/or testosterone supplementation.

Current medical treatments for ED

- Phosphodiesterase inhibitors, e.g. sildenafil, vardenafil, and tadalafil, which ↑ blood flow to the penis:
  - educate on the correct use and can be prescribed by GP or medical staff. ⚠ Should not be used in patients with a history of angina, recent MI, or those taking nitrates
  - advise patient to use on non-HD day to ↓ risk of hypotension
- Vacuum tumescence devices
- Intracavernosal injection prostaglandin E1 in to the shaft of the penis:
  - causes vasodilation and smooth muscle relaxation
  - ⚠ may cause bleeding, penile pain, and priapism
- Intraurethral alprostadil (MUSE, prostaglandin E1), delivers prostaglandin in to the corpus cavernosum
- Penile prosthesis.

Further reading

References

Patient information websites

Further reading

Barakzai AS, Moss AH. Efficacy of the World Health Organization analgesic ladder to treat pain in end-stage renal disease. *J Am Soc Nephrol* 2006; **17**:3198–320.

Castledine G, Close A. *Oxford Handbook of Adult Nursing*. Oxford: Oxford University Press; 2009.

Chambers EJ, Brown EA, Germain MJ. *Supportive Care for the Renal Patient*, 2nd edn. Oxford: Oxford University Press; 2010.

Chilcot J, Wellsted D, Da Silva-Gane M, et al. Depression on dialysis. *Nephrol Clin Pract* 2008; **108**:256–64.

Daugirdas, J *Handbook of Chronic Kidney Disease Management*. Philadelphia, PA: Wolters Kluwer/ Lippincott Williams & Wilkins; 2011.

Levy J, Brown E, Daley C, et al. *Oxford Handbook of Dialysis*, 3rd edn. Oxford: Oxford Medical Publications; 2009.

Madero M, Gul A, Samak MJ. Cognitive function in chronic kidney disease. *Semin Dial* 2008; **21**(1):29–37.

NICE. *Depression in Adults with a Chronic Physical Health Problem: Treatment and Management*. Clinical Guideline 91. London: NICE; 2009. Available at: ℘ <http://www.library.wmuh.nhs.uk/ pil/depression.htm>

Pierratos A, Hanly P. Sleep disorders over the full range of chronic kidney disease. *Blood Purif* 2011; **31**:146–50.

Pilling S, Anderson I, Goldberg D, et al. Depression in adults, including those with a chronic physical health problem: summary of NICE guidance. *BMJ* 2009; **339**:b4108.

Salisbury EM, Game DS, Al-Shakarchi I, et al. Changing practice to improve pain control to renal patients. *Post Grad Med J* 2009; **85**:30–3.

Tamura MK, Yaffe K. Dementia and cognitive impairment in ESRD: diagnostic and therapeutic strategies. *Kidney Int* 2011; **79**(1):14–22.

Tzeremas T, Kobrin S. *Uremic pruritus*, 2012. Available at: ℘ <http://www.uptodate.com/contents/ uremic-pruritus> (accessed 23 April 2012).

References

1. Pisoni RL, Wikströ B, Elder SJ, et al. Pruritus in hemodialysis patients: International results from the Dialysis Outcomes and Practice Patterns Study (DOPPS). *Nephrol Dial Transplant* 2006; **21**:3495–505.

2. World Health Organization (WHO). *Pain ladder*. Available at: ℘ <http://www.who.int/cancer/ palliative/painladder/en/>

Patient information websites

NHS Choices. *Treating insomnia*. Available at: ℘ <http://www.nhs.uk/Conditions/Insomnia/Pages/ Treatment.aspxa>

NKF. *Sex problems with renal failure*. Available at: ℘ <http://www.kidney.org.uk/Medical-Info/sex-problems/>

Chronic kidney disease, mineral and bone disorders

Introduction

Mineral and bone disorders are a common complication of CKD, resulting in both skeletal complications (e.g. abnormality of bone turnover, mineralization) and extra-skeletal complications (e.g. vascular or soft tissue calcification) as the eGFR falls <60ml/min (CKD stage 3A).

Different types of bone disease occur with CKD:

- High turnover bone disease due to ↑ PTH levels
- Low turnover bone disease (adynamic bone disease (ABD)) due to hypercalcaemia and suppression of PTH levels
- Defective mineralization (osteomalacia).

Secondary hyperparathyroidism (high bone turnover)

2° hyperparathyroidism develops in response to:

- Hyperphosphataemia
- Hypocalcaemia
- ↓ renal synthesis of 1,25-dihydroxycholecalciferol (1,25-dihydroxyvitamin D (calcitriol) → PTH
- Skeletal resistance to PTH.

High bone turnover (associated with 2° hyperparathyroidism) → weakness in bones due to ↑ reabsorption of mineral and the development of cysts within the bone tissues. ↑ bone turnover is associated with ↑ alkaline phosphatase enzyme level due to ↑ osteoblast activity within bone.

Adynamic bone disease (low bone turnover)

The prevalence of ABD varies from 15–60% in dialysis patients, characterized by a reduced ability to incorporate serum Ca^{2+} into the bone. Patients with ABD have lower blood levels of PTH than those with other forms of bone disease. The oversuppression of the parathyroid gland activity with high Ca^{2+} intake and/or administration of 1,25(OH)2D3 resulting in normal blood levels of PTH may be a factor in the development of ABD. Ca^{2+} uptake by the adynamic bone is reduced, and ∴ patients may develop hypercalcaemia if Ca^{2+} intake is increased or if dialysate Ca^{2+} is high.

Osteomalacia (defective mineralization)

Osteomalacia is due to a delay in the rate of bone mineralization resulting in unmineralized osteoid. The skeleton in osteomalacia is weakened, and patients with this bone disease have skeletal deformities, bone pain, fractures, and musculoskeletal disabilities. In CKD patients, the most important factor in the development of osteomalacia is aluminium overload and vitamin D deficiency. This is mainly seen in dialysis patients who have a large content of aluminium in bone due to the use of aluminium-based PO_4 binders. With a reduction in the use of aluminium the incidence of osteomalacia has decreased.

Calciphylaxis

- Calciphylaxis is a syndrome of extra-skeletal calcification, thrombosis, and skin necrosis as a result of abnormal bone mineral metabolism seen predominantly in patients with stage 5 CKD

- Clinical presentation includes necrotizing skin lesions (generally on the lower extremities) often with intense pain as a consequence of small vessel vasculopathy
- Pathogenesis of calciphylaxis is still uncertain but the factors implicated include:
  - CKD
  - DM
  - Obesity
  - Hypercalcaemia
  - Hyperphosphataemia
  - 2° hyperparathyroidism
  - Liver disease
  - Malnutrition
- Despite these factors being very common in ESKD the occurrence is very low, with a prevalence of 1–4%
- The mortality rate of patients that develop calciphylaxis has been reported to be as high as 60–80%, mainly due to sepsis from infected, non-healing necrotic skin lesions.

Pathophysiology

PO_4 retention begins in early CKD: as the eGFR falls, less PO_4 is filtered and excreted by the kidneys. Serum levels do not rise initially because of increased PTH secretion, which increases renal excretion. In advanced CKD stages 4 and 5, hyperphosphataemia develops because the kidneys are unable to excrete PO_4 adequately.

PO_4 binds to Ca^{2+} ions in plasma and reduces the ionized Ca^{2+} that is able to bind to the Ca^{2+} sensing receptor of the parathyroid chief cells. The result of this is an increased secretion of PTH contributing to hyperparathyroidism. The effects of PTH are to increase PO_4 excretion from the kidney and reabsorb Ca^{2+} from the bones to maintain a normal plasma Ca^{2+} concentration. In addition, in CKD the kidney fails to produce adequate amounts of activated vitamin D, causing hypocalcaemia and also contributes to hyperparathyroidism. Fig. 8.1 illustrates the pathophysiology of ESKD and Ca^{2+} and PO_4.

Signs and symptoms

Typically, most patients with hyperphosphataemia are asymptomatic, but the most common reported symptom by patients is itching, as a result of metastatic calcification of the skin. Long-term consequences may involve soft tissue calcification resulting from the precipitation of Ca^{2+} phosphates in non-osseous sites including heart (coronary artery and the valves), lungs, liver, muscles, joints, skin, or cornea and conjunctivae (resulting in red, sore eyes).

Key changes
- Ca^{2+} levels ↓ significantly between CKD stages 3 and 4 due to ↓ Ca^{2+} absorption from the gut
- PO_4 progressively ↑ during stage CKD 4 and 5 due to ↓ urinary excretion
- PTH levels ↑ early and progressively ↑ until CKD stage 5, → 2° hyperparathyroidism (SHPT)
- ↓ vitamin D levels contribute to ↑ PTH levels
- Hyperphosphataemia suppresses hydroxylation of inactive 25-hydroxy vitamin D to 1, 25-dihydroxy vitamin D (calcitriol, the active form of vitamin D)
- Vitamin D insufficiency and deficiency are common in patients with advanced CKD
- ↑ PO_4 levels, ↑ PTH concentration by direct effect of PO_4 on parathyroid gland
- Hypocalcaemia develops due to ↓ intestinal Ca^{2+} absorption, ↓ plasma calcitriol levels and binding of Ca^{2+} to excess levels of PO_4 in the blood
- Hypocalcaemia is a very potent trigger for secretion of PTH by parathyroid cells through the Ca^{2+} sensing receptor on the parathyroid cells
- ↓ serum calcitriol levels, hypocalcaemia, and hyperphosphataemia all independently trigger PTH synthesis and secretion
- Persistently elevated PTH levels exacerbate hyperphosphataemia from bone reabsorption of PO_4.

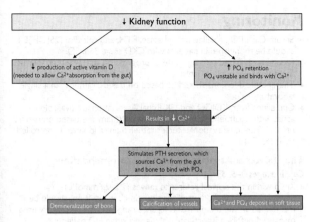

Fig. 8.1 Pathophysiology flow diagram.

Monitoring

- Serum Ca^{2+}, PO_4, alkaline phosphatase, PTH, and calcidiol (25(OH)D) should be monitored in patients with CKD stage 3–5, 5D
- Frequency is based on stage, rate of progression, and whether specific therapies have been initiated
- Therapeutic decisions should be based on trends, rather than a single laboratory values
- Guidelines from KDIGO and UK Renal Association are available to assist with treatment targets and decisions. (Many are based on expert opinion from observational studies rather than randomized controlled trials (RCTs).)

The UK Renal Association (2010) recommendations

Ca^{2+} in stages 3–5, 5T

- Keep within the normal reference ranges (2.2–2.6mmol/L)
- Stage 5D serum Ca^{2+} adjusted for albumin concentration, should be maintained within the normal reference range for the laboratory used, measured before a 'short-gap' dialysis session in HD patients
- Adjusted serum Ca^{2+} should be maintained 2.1–2.5mmol/L, with avoidance of hypercalcaemic episodes.

Ca^{2+} in HD

The choice of an appropriate dialysate Ca^{2+} concentration is crucial in the management of HD patients.

- ↑ Ca^{2+} load can be associated with vascular calcification
- Ca^{2+} ↓ can worsen 2° hyperparathyroidism.

In HD, Ca^{2+} transfer by diffusion depends on the concentration gradient between dialysate and blood, and a gain of Ca^{2+} is expected when the dialysate Ca^{2+} is >1.5mmol/L.

The choice of dialysate Ca^{2+} will depend on several factors:

- Parathyroid and vitamin D status
- Type and severity of concomitant bone disease
- Presence or absence of arterial calcification
- Dietary habits
- Concomitant medication.

Ideally the dialysate Ca^{2+} would be adapted to each patient's needs. From a practical point of view, a relatively high dialysate Ca^{2+} concentration in the range of 1.50–1.75mmol/L, should probably be preferred in HD patients with raised PTH levels who are not prescribed Ca^{2+}-based PO_4 binders or high doses of active vitamin D sterols, and in those who are receiving a calcimimetic. In those who are treated with high doses of Ca^{2+}-based binders and/or active vitamin D derivatives or who have a very low serum PTH level, the optimal dialysate Ca^{2+} concentration is probably lower, in the range of 1.25–1.50mmol/L.

PO_4

- In patients with CKD stage 3B–5, 5T maintain PO_4 0.9–1.5mmol/L
- In HD patients maintain PO_4, 1.1–1.7mmol/L.

PTH

- Treatment is considered in CKD stages 3B–5, 5D, 5T when serum PTH levels are progressively increasing and remain persistently higher than the upper reference limit for the assay, despite correction of modifiable factors
- The target range for PTH, measured using an intact PTH assay should be 2–9 times the upper limit of normal for the assay used
- Any marked changes in PTH levels in either direction within this range should prompt an initiation or change in therapy to avoid progression to levels outside this.
  Table 8.1 shows frequency of testing for MBD.

Table 8.1 Suggested frequency of biochemical testing in CKD–MBD

CKD stage	Ca²⁺	PO₄	PTH
3B eGFR 30–44ml/min	Every 6–12 months	Every 6–12 months	Baseline
4 eGFR 15–29ml/min	Every 3–6 months	Every 3–6 months	Every 6–12 months
5 eGFR <15ml/min	Every 1–3 months	Every 1–3 months	Every 3–6 months
5D	Every 1–3 months	Every 1–3 months	Every 3–6 months

Treatment

The management of CKD–MBD requires the skills of the multiprofessional team. Treatment includes:

- Dietary PO$_4$ restriction
- Maintenance dialysis
- Use of PO$_4$ binders
- Use of vitamin D sterols
- Calcimimetics
- Parathyroidectomy.

Dietary education

Dietary review, information, and early restriction in CKD (i.e. if serum PO$_4$ >1.6mmol/L) may prevent renal bone disease and 2° hyperparathyroidism. Patients with hyperparathyroidism require dietary advice regarding the avoidance of foods high in PO$_4$, in the context of any other dietary restrictions they might also be following. The need for dietary restriction needs to be balanced against the risk of malnutrition.

High dietary sources of PO$_4$ include:

- Milk
- Dairy products
- Cheese
- Eggs
- Chocolate
- Fish (bony)
- Shellfish and seafood
- Nuts, beans, pulses
- Meat and poultry.

Phosphate binders

- Used to reduce the absorption of PO$_4$
- Taken with meals and snacks to absorb dietary PO$_4$ in the gut
- Prescribed in patients whose serum PO$_4$ >1.6mmol/L
- Bind excess PO$_4$ in the gut and pass it out of the body in the stool, ↓ PO$_4$ available for absorption into the blood
- Depending on the type of binder used, usually taken just prior to, or immediately after meals and ↑ PO$_4$ snacks
- Dose and type of binders prescribed depends on amount of PO$_4$ eaten within the diet, serum PO$_4$ and Ca^{2+} levels, and individual patient preference
- Patient education is required to ensure PO$_4$ binders are taken appropriately.

Types of PO$_4$ binders

Ca^{2+}-based binders

Most commonly administered because they are cheap and help to maintain serum Ca^{2+}, e.g. Calcichew®, Phosex®. Tendency to be unpalatable and constipating, may cause hypercalcaemia.

Non-Ca²⁺-based binders

Generally prescribed for hyperphosphataemia not controlled by a Ca^{2+}-based binder or if hypercalcaemic, e.g. sevelamer and lanthanum. Sevelamer is a non-metal polymer-based binder that is not absorbed from the gut, while lanthanum is a rare earth metal which is minimally absorbed.

Aluminium based binders

Aluminium salts are effective PO_4 binders. Aluminium was limited in practice following the recognition of serious side effects associated with accumulation of aluminium, i.e. osteomalacia, encephalopathy, myopathy, hypoparathyroidism, and anaemia with resistance to ESA. Aluminium toxicity resulting in neurological complications is now rarely seen in clinical practice.

K/DOQI guidelines (2009) only recommend their use as a short-term therapy (≤4wk period) if serum PO_4 >2.26mmol/L. Plasma aluminium levels need to be monitored and the binders stopped if the serum aluminium concentration >2.2μmol/L (60mcg/L) or if the plasma aluminium concentration doubles. See Table 8.2 for PO_4 binders currently used in clinical practice.

Table 8.2 PO_4 binders currently available

Binder	Form	Advantages	Potential side effects
Calcium carbonate Calcichew® Titralac®	Tablet, Liquid	Effective, cheap, readily available	Hypercalcaemia, PTH suppression, GI side effects
Calcium acetate Phosex® PhosLo® Renacet®	Tablet, Capsule	Effective, less Ca^{2+} absorption than $CaCO_3$	Hypercalcaemia, GI side effects, most costly than $CaCO_3$
Magnesium carbonate/ calcium carbonate OsvaRen® Renepho®	Tablet		Hypermagnesaemia, GI side effects
Sevelamer-HCl Renagel®	Tablet	Effective, no Ca^{2+}, not absorbed, potential for ↓coronary/ aortic calcification compared to Ca^{2+}based binders, ↓plasma concentration of LDL-cholesterol	Cost, ↓ HCO_3 levels, GI side effects

(Continued)

Table 8.2 (Continued)

Binder	Form	Advantages	Potential side effects
Sevelamer carbonate Renvela®	Tablet, powder	Effective, no Ca^{2+} similar advantages to sevelamer-HCl, potentially improved acid-based balance	Cost, GI side effects
Lanthanum carbonate Fosrenol®	Tablet chewable	Effective, no Ca^{2+}, chewable	Cost, GI side effects
Aluminium hydroxide Alucaps®	Tablet, capsule, liquid	Very effective, variety of forms	Potential for aluminium toxicity, altered bone mineral mineralization, dementia, GI side effects

RRT

RRT removes PO_4, but not as efficiently as urea clearance, ∴dialysis patients are in positive PO_4 balance. PO_4 removal is enhanced if the duration and frequency of dialysis is increased.

Vitamin D analogues

Multiple vitamin D analogues include calcitriol, alfacalcidol, paricalcitol; vitamin D is mainly prescribed to suppress raised serum PTH levels. All vitamin D analogues can cause hypercalcaemia and hyperphosphataemia. Appropriate monitoring (i.e. 3-monthly serum PTH, monthly serum PO_4 and Ca^{2+}) and dose adjustment of PO_4 binders is required.

Other treatments

Cinacalcet is a Ca^{2+} receptor sensitizer (calcimimetic) that inhibits PTH release. It is usually used for patients receiving dialysis who have extreme plasma levels of intact PTH (defined as >85pmol/L (800pg/ml) which are refractory to standard therapy, and have a normal or increased adjusted serum Ca^{2+} level. Cinacalcet has the advantage of lowering PTH, serum Ca^{2+} and PO_4.

Surgical parathyroidectomy

This is indicated for severe 2° or tertiary hyperparathyroidism that fails to respond to optimum medical treatment, particularly if the patient is symptomatic or if there is coexistent hyperphosphataemia, hypercalcaemia, or evidence of high-turnover bone disease. Surgical parathyroidectomy is potentially avoidable with careful treatment of the mineral and hormonal disturbances in CKD.

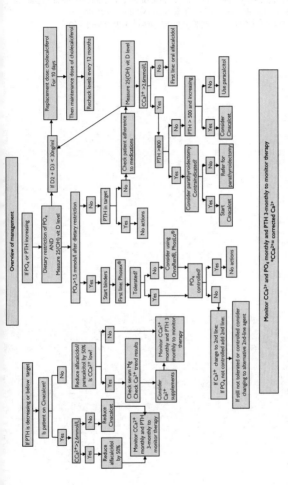

Figure 8.2 Mineral bone disease—suggested management protocol.

Management of PO_4 has to be in partnership with the patient as good control is achieved with adherence to dietary restrictions and pharmacological therapy. Many units have developed protocols to ensure appropriate and timely use of PO_4 binders and vitamin D analogues

Figure 8.2 shows a suggested protocol for managing MBD.

Conclusion

Renal bone disease is an important consequence of CKD. Frequent monitoring of the plasma concentration of Ca^{2+}, PO_4, and PTH is essential to minimize complications. Treatment includes dietary advice and titrated doses of oral phosphate binders and vitamin D analogues. For those on dialysis ensuring dialysis treatment is adequate. Monitoring and treatment by the MPT is recommended.

Further reading

European Dialysis and Transplantation Nurses Association/European Renal Care Association. *European Guidelines for the Nutritional Care of Adult Renal Patients*, 2002. Available at: ℘ <http://www.edtna-erca.org>

KDIGO. *KDIGO Clinical Practice Guidelines for the Diagnosis, Evaluation, Prevention, and Treatment of Chronic Kidney Disease-Mineral and Bone Disorder (CKD-MBD)*. Available at: ℘ <http://www.kdigo.org/guidelines/mbd/index.html>

Monthly Index of Medical Specialities website (providing information on prescription medicines). Available at: ℘ <http://www.mims.co.uk/MIMSPublications>

NICE. *The Effectiveness and Cost-Effectiveness of Cinacalcet for the Treatment of Hyperparathyroidism Secondary to Impaired Renal Function*. Available at: ℘ <http://www.nice.org.uk/nicemedia/live/11607/33855/33855.pdf>

The Renal Association. *CKD-Mineral and Bone Disorders (CKD-MBD)*, 2010. Available at: ℘ <http://www.renal.org/Clinical/GuidelinesSection/CKD-MBD.aspx>

Patient information website

UK National Kidney Federation website (provide information on bones, calcium, phosphate, and PTH in kidney failure). Available at: ℘ <http://www.kidney.org.uk/Medical-Info/Calcium-Phosphate>

Nutrition and chronic kidney disease

Introduction

Dietary treatment is one of the cornerstones of treating patients with ESKD. Historically, patients were treated with low-protein diets. The 'renal diet' was adapted to dialysis and Tx when RRT became available. Protein–energy malnutrition, hyperphosphataemia, chronic fluid overload, and obesity are the most common challenges leading to long-term complications. Nutritional support with advice tailored to the specific needs of the individual patient and continued monitoring are required. A renal dietitian will provide nutritional treatment plans following a full dietary assessment, medical history, and examination.

Nutritional assessment

Nutrition risk screening

Use of a simple nutrition risk screening tool such as MUST (malnutrition universal screening tool) uses 3 steps to identify adults at risk of under-nutrition, malnourishment, or obesity in the general population.[1]

Dietary assessment includes:

- Nutrition assessment tool: subjective global assessment (SGA) is a well-validated assessment tool for use in CKD patients[2]
- Diet history:
  - dietary interview or food diary: quantitative and qualitative assessment of nutrient intake
  - changes in food and fluid intake
- Weight history:
  - estimate % weight loss or gain
  - significant if >5% in 3-month period
- Uraemic symptoms:
  - GI symptoms including nausea, vomiting, food distaste (often described as bland, metallic, 'like cardboard'), early satiety
- Anthropometry:
  - height, weight, BMI, mid-arm circumference, triceps skin fold thickness, mid-arm muscle circumference
- Biochemistry:
  - serum Ur, Cr, K^+, HCO_3, Ca^{2+}, PO_4, Alb, chol, Hb, eGFR (see Table 9.1 for interpretation)
- Social/cultural factors
- Adequacy of dialysis:
  - inadequate dialysis is a common contributory factor to malnutrition
  - dialysis adequacy should be assessed in conjunction with normalized protein catabolic rate
  - when a patient is in a stable state, urea formation correlates with protein intake and protein breakdown
  - ▶ no single parameter should be considered in isolation.

Table 9.1 Nutritional interpretation of biochemistry

Parameter (serum)	Normal range	Nutritional interpretation
Ur	3.5–6.5mmol/L	Product of protein metabolism Low levels (<2.0mmol/L) reflect ↓ protein intake or absorption (e.g. Coeliac disease) and is a predictor of poor prognosis in dialysis patients ↑ levels associated with, and contribute to, worsening kidney function
K⁺	3.5–5.5mmol/L	Hypokalaemia rarely caused by ↓ intake alone, can be exacerbated by other causes, e.g. ↓ K⁺ diet, diuretics and diarrhoea Hyperkalaemia worsened by K⁺-rich foods, e.g. chocolate, fruits, tomatoes, liquorice, brassicas (cabbage) whole-grain breads/bar, medications, e.g. ACEIs, K⁺-sparing diuretics
HCO₃	22–30mmol/L	Acidosis results in a hypercatabolic state causing breakdown of skeletal muscle and a –ve nitrogen balance—worsened by ↓ protein diet
PO₄	0.9–1.5mmol/L	↓ may indicate an overall poor food intake due to the wide distribution of PO₄ in foods ↓ PO₄ occurs with intracellular shift in re-feeding syndrome ↑ PO₄—with processed foods, many food additives, dairy products, certain vegetables, and carbonated drinks. Protein-rich foods often high in phosphate—decision to limit these will be based on overall nutrition status of patient
Alb	35–45g/L	Hypoalbuminaemia is a late indication of malnutrition due to albumin's large synthetic reserve/long half-life ↑ in extracellular fluid or an acute phase response (↑ CRP) will result in artificially low levels
Total chol	<5.0mmol/L	↓ levels strongly associated with ↑ mortality, and is marker of poor nutritional status ↑ levels associated with ↑ CVD risk ↓ levels of LDL chol—↓ animal fats, increase HDL by ↑ fibre, seeds, nuts, oily fish
Hb	10–12g/dl	Anaemia may be caused/exacerbated by iron, folate or B12 deficiency (see 🛇 p. 223)

Nutritional requirements in advanced kidney disease

CKD stages 4 and 5

Energy
- Energy requirements are normal (i.e. 35kcal/kg)
- Those who are underweight require additional calories
- Energy intake to be reviewed in conjunction with protein intake to protect against energy and protein malnutrition.

Protein
- Protein intake should be maintained at 0.8—1.0g/kg IBW/day, especially in patients consuming ↑ protein
- Protein restriction (0.8g/kg/day) can be used to ↓ uraemic symptoms and rate of decline in RF:
  - benefits are minimal when associated with the ↑ risk of malnutrition
  - low-protein diets are difficult to maintain due to their complexity, palatability, and the need for nutritional supplements, including essential amino acid or ketoacid analogues
- Dietary protein intake ↓ spontaneously in patients as eGFR falls <25ml/min. Regular assessments of protein and energy intake are essential to prevent malnutrition
- Protein intake should be monitored in albuminuria to ensure dietary protein <1.0g/kg IBW.

Potassium
- K+ restrictions are usually unnecessary in CKD unless:
  - urine output is <1000ml/day
  - ↓ renal K+ excretion, e.g. use of ACEIs/A2RBs
  - BSL is poorly controlled in DM (insulin deficiency reduces K+ intracellular uptake).

Phosphate
- Dietary PO_4 restrictions may be required before serum levels rise >1.5mmol/L, especially if ↑ PTH:
  - may prevent MBDs, 2° hyperparathyroidism, and ↓ progression to ESKD.

Sodium and fluid
- Fluid restrictions not usually necessary unless urine output is markedly ↓. Na+ restriction (no-added-salt diet) if hypertensive or oedematous.

Renal replacement therapy

Once RRT commences and uraemic symptoms ↓, appetite and food intake gradually ↑. Some patients may have poor nutritional intake and malnutrition due to adverse effects of RRT, e.g. dietary restrictions.
- Where possible, general healthy eating guidelines are recommended, i.e. 50% energy from high complex carbohydrate, high fibre, and 30–35% from fats (poly- and mono-unsaturated fatty acid sources with low saturated fats).

Sodium and fluid in RRT

In ESKD, fluid management is influenced by RRF and mode of dialysis. Patients with a ↓ urine output should:
- Restrict intake to 500ml (insensible losses) + previous day's urine output/24hrs:
  - fluid intake may need to be ↑ during hot weather, e.g. excessive sweating, vomiting, diarrhoea
- Na^+ intake should be restricted to 80–100mol/day. As salt is a major driver for thirst, patients need to be educated about dietary salt intake and strategies to manage fluid restrictions
- Provide education about high-fluid foods, e.g. soup, dhal, jelly, custard, ice cream, yoghurt
- Management of fluid restriction includes: volume of cups, sucking ice cubes or ice lollies, chewing gum, or eating sugar-free sweets. Use of mouth wash or lip salves may be helpful
- Avoid salt substitutes such as LoSalt® due to its high K^+ content.

Haemodialysis
- HD patients are usually anuric and often require severe fluid restrictions (500ml/24hrs) and possible salt restriction (<6g/day).

Peritoneal dialysis
- Include 24hr UF volume when calculating fluid allowance (see 📖 p. 336).

Vitamins and minerals

Vitamin deficiencies can occur in CKD due to dietary restrictions, abnormal metabolism, and dialysate losses. Despite a lack of evidence, supplementary doses of H_2O-soluble vitamin B, vitamin C, and folate may be prescribed. Fat-soluble vitamins (A and E) are not routinely prescribed due to the risk of toxicity.

Haemodialysis

Energy
- Regular assessment by a specialist renal dietitian
- Advice is frequently aimed at ↑ energy intake, using energy-dense foods (high fat ± sugar) or prescribing nutritional supplements:
  - as there is an increasing tendency of obesity, dietary advice will depend on the individual patient weight trends and normal dietary intake.

Protein
- Recommended allowance is 1.1g protein/kg IBW/day.

Potassium
- Dietary K^+ restriction is usually required; level of restriction depends on RRF and serum K^+ levels.
- Restriction of dietary K^+ is reviewed according to serum K^+ levels
- Before dietary restrictions are instigated, exclude non-dietary causes e.g. ACEI (see 📖 p. 569)

- Limitation of K^+-rich foods, includes:
  - vegetables: potato (baked, chips, crisps), spinach, mushrooms, tomatoes, beetroot
  - fruit: bananas, dried fruit, rhubarb, apricots, avocado pears,
  - drinks: fresh fruit juices, coffee, drinking chocolate, malted drinks, blackcurrant cordials
  - others: chocolate, liquorice, evaporated and condensed milk, salt substitutes
- Advice on suitable cooking methods:
  - use large volume of H_2O for boiling vegetables
  - parboil vegetables before adding them to casseroles, soups
  - avoid using pressure cooker and microwave (re-heating is allowed)
  - limit portion size or quantity of high K^+ fruits and vegetables. 4 portions of low K^+ fruits and vegetables/day.

Phosphate
- Clearance of PO_4 is not particularly effective with conventional HD
- Daily/nocturnal dialysis ↑ PO_4 clearance; dietary restrictions can be relaxed
- Management of serum PO_4: low PO_4 diet, use of PO_4 binders and vitamin D analogues
- Dietary management: restrict PO_4 foods, reviewing protein portion size and foods with PO_4 additives (dicalcium PO_4, phosphoric acid, Na^+PO_4).

Peritoneal dialysis
Energy
- Energy restrictions required to compensate for the additional calories absorbed from dextrose concentration of the dialysate fluid
- Emphasize ↓ excessive intake of fats and sugar :
  - hypertonic dialysate solutions are sometimes used excessively to control fluid balance ∴ increasing energy intake
  - focus dietary advice on fluid and Na^+ management.

Protein
- 1.0–1.2g/kg/day assuming adequate energy intake
- Most patients will be in neutral or positive balance at a protein intake of ~1g/kg/day
- Those at ↑ risk of protein malnutrition include: the elderly, ↑ co-morbidities, ↑ protein loss, e.g. high/fast transport peritoneal membrane characteristics, frequent or prolonged episodes of peritonitis:
  - require ↑ prescribed intake of protein and nutritional supervision
  - ↑ levels are also needed for malnourished patients, those with intercurrent illnesses, e.g. sepsis
  - amino acid dialysate may be beneficial for high-risk or malnourished patients unable to eat sufficient protein, if it is used in conjunction with an adequate dialysis regimen.

Potassium
- Dietary restriction of K^+ is rarely needed in PD.

Phosphate
- See 📖 Haemodialysis, p. 205.

Food sources
- *Carbohydrates and fats:* breads, rice, pasta, legumes, grains, butter, margarines and other spreads, sugar, fizzy drink (lemonade), sweets, honey, jams, olive oil, double cream, fried foods, nutritional high energy supplements
- *Protein:* meat, fish, egg, milk, nuts, pulses, beans
- *Phosphate:* milk, dairy products, cheese, eggs, cereals, chocolate, fish (bony), shellfish and seafood, nuts, beans, pulses, meat and poultry.

Transplantation
Once kidney function has stabilized the aim is to achieve a healthy balanced diet and to reduce the risk factors for CVD (hyperlipidaemia, obesity) (see 📖 p. 76). The incidence of obesity (BMI >30kg/m²) can increase dramatically post-transplant due to appetite enhancing medications, e.g. corticosteroids.

Barriers to healthy eating
- Previous eating habits
- Previous advice given whilst on dialysis or in the AKC setting
- ↓ intake of fruits and vegetables due to previous K^+ restrictions
- Temptation to over-consume some of the previously restricted foods such as crisps, chocolate, alcohol, fruit juices, contributing to ↑ body weight and body fat.

Dietary management summary
- Monitor:
  - chol, triglycerides, blood glucose, K^+, bone minerals, PTH, Hb
- Aim for a healthy weight
- Patient education on healthy eating:
  - 'Eatwell plate' is an appropriate model to use[3]
  - eating a good variety of fruits and vegetables
  - ↑ fibre foods
  - fish, especially oily fish, lean meats, and pulses
  - ↓ fat dairy products
- Advise patients to:
  - minimize the use of foods ↑ in sugar, fat, and salt
  - keep alcohol intake within government recommendations
  - encourage physical activity
  - be aware of good food hygiene practices.

See Table 9.2 for a summary of dietary recommendations for CKD stages 4–5.

Table 9.2 Summary of dietary recommendations for CKD stages 4–5, 5D

CKD	Stages 4–5	HD	PD
Energy (kcal)	30–35kcal/kg IBW	30–35kcal/kg IBW	30–35kcal/kg BW
Protein	0.75–1.0g/kg IBW/day with adequate kcal intake	1.1g/kg IBW/day	1.0–1.2g/kg BW
K^+	If K^+ >6.0mmol/L limit intake to 1.0mmol/kg IBW/day	0.8–1.0mmol/kg IBW/day	Restriction only necessary if hyperkalaemic 1.0mmol/kg IBW/day
PO_4	Maintain 0.9–1.5mmol/L	Maintain 1.1–1.7mmol/L	Maintain 1.1–1.7mmol/L
Fluid	Individualized based on stage of CKD, oedema, and hypertension	500mL + PDUO	500ml + *PDUO + ultrafiltration volume
Na^+	<100mol if hypertensive	80–100mol/day	80–100mol/day
Nutritional therapy	Protein and energy intake	Protein and energy intake	Protein and energy intake
	Na^+, K^+, and fluid intake	Fluid and electrolyte management	Fluid and electrolyte management
	Weight control		
	Meal planning	Meal planning	Meal planning
	Recipe modification	Individual care planning	Individual care planning
	Physical activity	Self-care	Self-care
	Self-care		

*PDUO: previous day's urine output.

Nutrition and the older person

The elderly are at risk if they are in an acute hospital, nursing or residential care, or in their own homes. It is the health professional's responsibility to highlight nutritional problems and act upon them appropriately.

Nutritional requirements of older people are the same for any patient with CKD. Factors affecting nutritional status in the elderly are associated with the ageing process itself and are presented in Table 9.3.

Table 9.3 Factors affecting nutritional status

Factor	Problem
General health	Presence of other chronic conditions and/or disability, e.g. diabetes, COPD, rheumatoid arthritis
	Substance abuse, e.g. drug and alcohol
	Medication side effects, e.g. digoxin
Oral	Dysphagia, e.g. stroke, Parkinson's disease or other neurological disorder
	Dental-periodontal disease, poorly fitted dentures, e.g. mouth ulcers, problems chewing
GI	↓ immunity—more prone to infection and thus bacterial overgrowth
	↓ GI absorption and motility (e.g. constipation)
Alteration in senses	↓ sense of smell and taste, e.g. food tastes flavourless—do not enjoy food
	↓ appetite
Loss of muscle mass and strength	Poor grip/strength, e.g. open bottles/cans as a result of disability (e.g. osteo/rheumatoid arthritis, part of ageing process)
	Unable to use hand or tremor, e.g. stroke, Parkinson's disease or other neurological disorder
Psychosocial/ socio-economic	Social isolation—unable to access shops
	Financial constraints
	Bereavement/depression
	Loss of independence
	Disinterest in eating/forget to eat
	Apathy to cook or eat alone
	Unable to feed themselves
	Institutionalization

Management

Development of treatment plans should be discussed and negotiated with the wider healthcare team. This might include social services, carers, nursing or residential home staff. Information governance and current legislation protecting vulnerable adults, including issues such as mental capacity, should be taken into account.

Nutritional support

Develop action plans using information based on nutritional assessments.

- Nutritional support provided will vary between clinical cases, but may include the use of:
  - oral nutritional supplements and input from a dietitian or ↑ access to food and social support
- Those who are malnourished or unable to meet their dietary requirements from food should be assessed for:
  - access to food—additional support required at home for shopping or cooking. Suggesting the use of home delivered, ready-made meals; accessing luncheon clubs to improve social networks
  - unnecessary dietary restrictions being followed; advice is given on foods to eat and how to make food appetizing (e.g. use of herbs and spices/presentation)
  - how to supplement oral intake with ↑ energy foods
  - if required, provide nutritional supplements or enteral nutrition, e.g. via nasogastric, gastrostomy, and jejunostomy tubes; IV parenteral nutrition
  - assess for and, if appropriate, treat for depression
  - assessment and treatment of dietary nutritional deficiencies, e.g. Mg^{2+}, B vitamins, vitamin C.

Managing protein energy malnutrition

Malnutrition is common in CKD stage 5 affecting between 30–40% of patients and is a predictor of survival. Poor nutritional status prior to starting dialysis increases the odds ratio of mortality by 2.5.

Contributing factors

- Inadequate protein and calorie intake:
  - highly restrictive renal diet (Na$^+$, PO$_4$, K$^+$)
  - ↓ intake than normal, e.g. nausea
  - physical, e.g. elderly unable to feed self
  - social, low income
  - psychological, depression, stress, and anxiety
  - other conditions, e.g. diabetes ↓ gastric emptying
  - dialysis, e.g. PD, feeling of fullness ∴ ↓ appetite
- Protein loss:
  - persistent proteinuria
  - dialysis, e.g. particularly associated with episodes of peritonitis
- Uraemia:
  - metabolic acidosis
  - anorexia
- Catabolic state imposed by HD
- Chronic low-grade inflammation (repeated infections, oxidant stress, arteriosclerosis, malnutrition) associated with CKD
- Medication (PO$_4$ binders, oral iron).

Assessment

- Stage of CKD and severity of symptoms
- Severity of malnutrition by an experienced renal dietitian:
  - current nutritional intake
- Renal dietitian will design a specific treatment plan which might include the following:
  - supplementing diet with ↑ energy ± protein foods (milk, cream, sugar)
  - consideration of nutritional supplements, care must be taken to ensure that these are compatible with other dietary restrictions. A wide range is available including renal specific oral supplements
  - if enteral feeding is required, attention must be given to the total volume of the feeding regimen, ↑ HD may be required or ↑ hypertonic PD dialysate fluids usage.

Re-feeding risk

Metabolic adaptive changes occur to maximize use of available nutrients in a malnourished state. A re-feeding risk assessment is required prior to the commencement of feeding. The sudden provision of an excess of food, whether it is oral, enteral or parenteral does not allow time for the down regulation of metabolic changes to occur.

- Glucose, PO$_4$, K$^+$, and Mg^{2+} are rapidly taken up by the cells → ↓ serum levels
- ↑ extracellular fluid volume.

Those at risk[4]

- 1 or more of the following:
  - BMI <16kg/m^2
  - weight loss >15% within the last 3–6 months
  - little or no nutritional intake for >10 days
  - ↓ K$^+$, PO$_4$, Mg^2
- 2 or more of the following:
  - BMI <18.5kg/m^2
  - weight loss >10% within the last 3–6 months
  - little or no nutritional intake for >5 days
  - a history of alcohol abuse or drugs including insulin, chemotherapy, antacids, or diuretics.

Clinical features

- Cardiac: tachycardia, HF, arrhythmias
- Respiratory: dyspnoea, tachypnoea
- GI: abdominal bloating, nausea, diarrhoea
- Biochemistry: ↓ PO$_4$, Mg^{2+}, Na$^+$, K$^+$
- Neurological: seizures, coma
- Rhabdomyolysis
- Risk of AKI (may be missed as low muscle mass—↓ Cr).

Management

- Refer to renal dietitian:
  - assessment for malnutrition, e.g. screening tools such as MUST (see 📖 p. 202)
- ↑ intake gradually over a week
- Commence with 10kcal/kg/day, increase gradually
- Maintain accurate fluid balance chart
- Monitor—haemodynamic observations and ECG
- Check bloods daily for U&Es, Mg^{2+}, PO$_4$, glucose levels
- If abnormal, the use of oral or IV K$^+$, PO$_4$, Mg^{2+} to correct
- Use of strong vitamin B complex, thiamine, general multivitamin/trace elements.

Supplementation

- Gastrostomy (or PEG) feeding is ↑ used in HD patients at home when long-term nutritional support is required:
  - specific renal formulated feeds are available to provide nutrient dense, K$^+$, PO$_4$, and fluid-restricted options
- Parenteral nutrition should be reserved for those who cannot be fed enterally:
  - electrolyte quantities (particularly K$^+$, PO$_4$, and Mg^{2+}) should be ↓ and monitored daily
- Intradialytic parenteral nutrition (IDPN) involves infusing parenteral nutrition during dialysis:
  - many studies have evaluated the effectiveness and safety of IDPN which show a good safety profile and improvements in protein-energy status
  - ▶ clinical trials are limited and the results are not conclusive
  - the cost-effectiveness of the treatment is questionable

- IP amino acid dialysates solution may benefit malnourished PD patients:
  - use of 1.1% amino acid dialysate solution to replace one of the patient's normal dextrose exchanges/day
  - studies suggest small improvements in nutritional status in moderately to severe malnourished patients (see ▢ PD, p. 250).

Conservative management

For patients who opt not to have RRT, dietary control may contribute to symptom management and is ∴ individualized. It may include:

- Close monitoring to avoid complications of malnutrition
- K^+, PO_4, and Na^+ restrictions depending on serum levels
- Management of uraemic symptoms
- Use of dietary supplements, e.g. Calogen®, glucose polymer (eg Maxijul®).

Nurses' and dietitians' roles in nutritional management

The responsibilities of the team regarding management are outlined in Table 9.4.

Table 9.4 Roles of the nurse and dietitian

Nursing role	Dietitian role
Assessment—screening for malnutrition in new or existing patients: height, weight, mid-arm circumference. Referral to specialist dietitian where malnutrition is suspected	Assessment—assessment of malnutrition: triceps skinfold measurements, mid-arm muscle circumference, other assessments of body composition
Biochemistry and fluid—identifying abnormal PO_4, K^+ and → ↑ fluid gains	Biochemistry and fluid—provision of individual specialist dietary advice: renal specific diets, MBD, fluid gains
Eating and drinking: likes and dislikes, medical, cultural, ethical, and religious dietary requirements, e.g. diabetes, gluten free diets, halal, kosher Monitoring of dietary intake (food and fluid record charts)	Assessment of nutritional intake from food record charts. Information from patients including energy, protein, K^+, PO_4, Na^+, fluid. Devise an individual, holistic dietary treatment plan with the patient, which might include food fortification, nutritional supplements, enteral or parenteral feeds
Physical difficulties with eating and drinking, e.g. tremors, CVA	Liaising with MPT to ensure that nutritional requirements can be met, e.g. specialist feeding equipment
Supporting patients to follow the nutritional treatment plan devised by the dietitian	Responding to changes in clinical condition, e.g. biochemistry, general condition, to revise nutritional treatment plan

Further reading

Mitch WE, Alp Ikizler T. *Handbook of Nutrition and the Kidney*, 6th edn. Philadelphia, PA: Lippincott Williams & Wilkins; 2009.
Kopple JD, Massry SG. *Kopple and Massry's Nutritional Management of Renal Disease*, 2nd edn. Philadelphia, PA: Lippincott Williams & Wilkins; 2004.

References

1. British Association of Parenteral and Enteral Nutrition. Malnutrition universal screening tool (MUST) resources. Available at: <http://www.bapen.org.uk/musttoolkit.html>
2. Nutritional and inflammatory evaluation of dialysis patients: resources to use on subjective global assessment.
3. <http://www.nhs.uk/Livewell/Goodfood/Pages/eatwell-plate.aspx>
4. NICE. *Nutrition support in adults: Oral nutrition support, enteral tube feeding and parenteral nutrition.* Guidance CG32. London: NICE; 2006.

Useful websites

British Dietetic Association Renal Nutrition Group. *Evidence Based Dietetic Guidelines for Protein Requirements of Adults on Haemodialysis and Peritoneal Dialysis*, 2011. Available at: <http://www.bda.uk.com/publications/statements/RenalGuidelines.pdf>
European Dialysis and Transplant Nurses Association/European Renal Care Association. *European guidelines for the nutritional care of adult renal patients.* Available at: <http://www.edtnaerca.org>
European Society for Clinical Nutrition and Metabolism. Nutritional guidelines on enteral nutrition, parenteral nutrition and guidelines on nutrition in adult patients with renal insufficiency. Available at: <http://www.espen.org/espenguidelines.html>
The Renal Association. Clinical guidelines on nutrition and CKD. Available at: <http://www.renal.org/clinical/GuidelinesSection/Guidelines.aspx>

Patient information websites

British Journal of Renal Medicine. Available at: <http://www.bjrm.co.uk/patient-information.aspx>
Edinburgh Renal Unit dietary information for kidney patients. Available at: <http://www.edren.org/pages/edreninfo/diet-in-renal-disease.php>

Anaemia management

Introduction

Anaemia is one of the most common complications of CKD and develops early on in the disease process. Lower levels of kidney function are associated with lower Hb levels and an increased prevalence and severity of anaemia (CKD stage 3B onwards) It is also common in patients with diabetes and CKD (1 in 5 with stage 3 CKD and diabetes).

Anaemia in CKD is associated with increased mortality and cardiovascular events, increased hospitalization rates, and reduced QOL.

Anaemia in patients with CKD is usually normochromic and normocytic and develops in response to a variety causes. Non-renal causes of anaemia should be screened for and investigated before assuming that the cause is due to lack of erythropoietin production.

Causes of anaemia

Non-renal causes of anaemia
- Chronic blood loss
- Bone marrow infiltration, i.e. myeloma
- ↓ RBC survival
- Malignancy
- Red cell aplasia
- Hypothyroidism
- Chronic infection/inflammation
- Aluminium toxicity
- Haemoglobinopathies, i.e. thalassaemia, myelodysplasia, sickle cell disease.

Causes of anaemia associated with CKD
- Iron deficiency
- Vitamin B_{12} and folate deficiency
- Haemolysis
- Erythropoietin production
- Uraemic and cytokine inhibition of erythropoiesis.

Adverse effects of anaemia include:
- ↓ oxygen utilization
- ↑ cardiac output
- Left ventricular hypertrophy
- ↑ progression of CKD
- ↓ concentration
- ↓ libido
- ↓ cognitive function
- ↓ immunosuppressiveness.

Pathophysiology

Erythropoiesis

Erythropoiesis is the process by which red blood cells (erythrocytes) are produced. Erythropoiesis is stimulated by reduced O_2 delivery to the kidneys which then secrete the hormone erythropoietin. Erythropoietin is produced by the peri-tubular cells and is the hormone responsible for promoting the proliferation and differentiation of erythroid progenitor cells in the bone marrow. 90% of erythropoietin, is produced by the kidneys and 10% by liver.

Causes of failure in the autoregulatory sequence of erythropoiesis include:

- ↓ folate and vitamin B_{12} → macrocytic anaemia
- ↓ iron impairs erythropoiesis → hypochromic microcytic anaemia
- Inflammation/inflammatory cytokines.
  Other factors which affect normal Hb levels include:
- Ethnicity
- Smoking
- Age
- Gender
- Genetic disorders, i.e. thalassaemia and sickle cell disease.

Iron deficiency

- Iron plays an essential role in supporting erythropoiesis
- 65% of iron stored in the body is used to form Hb
- Iron deficiency is common in stages 3B, 4, and 5 CKD and is diagnosed when serum ferritin level is <100mcg/L
- 150mg iron is required to ↑ Hb by 1g/dl
- As red cell production ↑, iron stores ↓
- Iron stores need to be adequate otherwise red cell survival is reduced
- Normal red cell survival is 120 days, in CKD it is ~90 days
- Patients with CKD have a tendency to bleed due to platelet dysfunction which contributes to ↓ iron levels.

Types of iron deficiency are shown in Table 10.1.

Table 10.1 Types of iron deficiency

Absolute iron deficiency	Functional iron deficiency
Iron stores inadequate to support the erythropoietic needs of the bone marrow	Iron stores adequate but cannot supply marrow quickly enough with the iron required to support demands of erythropoiesis when stimulated acutely (e.g. with ESA therapy)
Serum ferritin <100mcg/L	Normal (30–200mcg/L) or ↑ serum ferritin levels (>800mcg/L)
% transferrin saturation <20%	% transferrin saturation <20%
% hypochromic red cells >10%.	% hypochromic red cells >10%.

Hepcidin

- Hepcidin is a peptide hormone which plays a role in the regulation of Hb production.
- Produced by the liver and controls iron absorption in the GI tract and iron release from reticuloendothelial tissue
- CKD is a chronic inflammatory condition and cytokines which are produced in response to inflammation are often raised
- ↑ cytokine levels are associated with ↑ levels of hepcidin
- ↑ iron levels promote the production of hepcidin which prevents the absorption of iron in the GI tract and the release of stored iron
- If serum iron ↓ → ↓ hepcidin production allowing more iron to become available.

Vitamin B_{12} and folate deficiency

- Vitamin B_{12} and folic acid are needed to maintain RBCs, DNA synthesis, and healthy nerve cells
- ↓ vitamin B_{12} → megaloblastic anaemia
- Lack of vitamin B_{12} in the diet → development of pernicious anaemia. Most susceptible: elderly, strict vegetarians
- Folate deficiency limits cell division, hinders erythropoiesis → megaloblastic anaemia
- Most common cause is poor diet and/or alcoholism
- Folate is plentiful in greens, yeast, and liver, but destroyed during cooking. Body stores are small (5–10mg).

▶ Both are water-soluble vitamins and are lost during HD which can result in dialysis-induced B_{12} and folate deficiency.

Haemoglobinopathies

- Those with CKD often have other haematological conditions:
  - myelodysplasia
  - sickle cell anaemia
  - thalassaemia
  - lymphoma
  - myeloma
  - uraemic bleeding.

Haemolysis

- The breakdown or lysis of RBCs and release of Hb can be caused by:
  - Drugs (penicillin, cephalosporin, methyldopa, quinidine)
  - Blood pump trauma to red cells during HD
  - Contamination of dialysate (chloramines, oxidants, copper, nitrates)
  - Overheating of dialysate
  - Re-use sterilants (formaldehyde)
  - Autoimmune haemolysis
- Causes should be investigated and where possible prevented.

Diagnosing anaemia of chronic kidney disease

Anaemia is defined by WHO as: Hb levels <11g/dl in pregnant ♀ and children aged 6 months to 5yrs, <12g/dl in non-pregnant♀, and <13g/dl in♂. NICE guidance (2006, updated 2011) suggests that an eGFR <60ml/min/1.73m² should trigger investigation into whether anaemia is due to CKD. In those with an eGFR ≥60 ml/min/1.73m² anaemia is more likely to be related to other causes.[1]

Investigation and management of ACKD should be considered if Hb ≤11g/dl or symptoms attributable to anaemia develop.

Signs and symptoms
- Fatigue and weakness
- Pale skin and mucous membranes
- Dizziness or light headedness
- Rapid heartbeat and palpitations
- Headache
- SOB on exertion
- Irritability
- ↓ exercise endurance
- ↓ cognitive function.

Screening investigations
- FBC: red cell indices (MCV, MCHC, MCH), reticulocyte count
- Serum ferritin
- % TSAT
- % HRC (where available)
- Serum B$_{12}$
- Red cell folate concentration
- Serum iron
- CRP
- Tests for haemolysis (haptoglobin, lactate dehydrogenase, Coombs' test)
- Assessment of occult GI blood loss
- Nutritional status.

Diagnosing iron deficiency
Serum ferritin
- Stored iron
- Commonly used as a standard marker for measuring iron deficiency
- Can be falsely ↑ in cases of infection and inflammatory conditions
- Measure CRP at the same time as ferritin
- ↑ CRP indicates infection or inflammatory condition, if ferritin also ↑ then not a true indication of the iron status at that time.% transferrin saturation (% TSAT)

- Transport system of iron
- Needs to be >20% to be effective
- Not a very reliable tool as %TSAT constantly alter
- More than one measurement required to ascertain an average reading.

% hypochromic red cells (% HRC)

- Defined as an individual cell with Hb concentration >28g/dl
- <2.5% of red cells are hypochromic
- ↓ iron stores ± mobilization of iron inadequate, HRC ↑ in number
- If >10% iron supplementation is required
- ► % HRC testing is not available in all laboratories.

Diagnosis of iron deficiency

- Serum ferritin <100mcg/L
- HRC >6%
- % TSAT <20%.

Optimal iron levels

People receiving erythropoiesis stimulating agent (ESA) maintenance therapy should be given iron supplements to keep:

- Serum ferritin 200–500mcg/L
- % TSAT >20% (unless ferritin >800mcg/L)
- HRC <6% (unless ferritin >800mcg/L).

---

1 The measurement of Hb levels is beginning to be reported in laboratories in g/L instead of g/dl. The conversion equates to 1g/dl = 10g/L, e.g. Hb 11g/dl = 110g/L.

Management of anaemia

Numerous national and international evidence-based guidelines are available from which local protocols are developed. When determining individual aspirational Hb ranges, patient preferences, symptoms and co-morbidities, and the required treatment should be taken into account. NICE guidance (2011) currently recommends a Hb range of 10–12g/dl.

⚠ The correction to normal Hb levels is not recommended in people with CKD.

▶ However, if absolute risk of cerebrovascular disease is low and the person might benefit (e.g. if they have a physically demanding job) then an Hb level above the aspirational range may be considered.

Benefits of treating anaemia

Improvements in:
- Mortality and morbidity
- Cognitive function
- Exercise capacity
- Sexual function
- QOL
- Nutrition
- Sleep patterns
- Immune responsiveness
- Cardiac status (↓ angina, improved cardiac output, ↓ LVH and LV dilatation).

Treating iron deficiency

Before initiating iron therapy, exclude any serious underlying cause of anaemia, i.e. GI bleeding. Prophylaxis with an iron preparation is justifiable in those who have additional risk factors for iron deficiency:
- Poor diet
- Malabsorption syndromes
- Menorrhagia
- Pregnancy
- Post subtotal or total gastrectomy
- HD patients
- ▶ Oral or IV iron can be given in HD patients.

Oral iron preparations
- Ferrous gluconate 300mg tablets (containing 35mg elemental iron)
- Ferrous sulphate 200mg tablets (containing 65mg elemental iron)
- Pregaday®* tablets (ferrous fumarate containing 100mg elemental iron with 350mcg folic acid)
- Ferrous fumarate syrup 140mg/5ml (containing 45mg elemental iron).

*Pregaday® is rarely used as the amount of folic acid content is not considered therapeutic for folate deficient anaemia.

Daily requirement to treat iron deficiency is ~200mg per day. For dosing of oral iron see Tables 10.2 and 10.3.

Table 10.2 Therapeutic doses of oral iron

Preparation	Dose	Frequency
Ferrous sulphate	200mg	2–3 tablets/day
Ferrous gluconate	300mg	4–6 tablets/day
*Ferrous fumarate syrup 140mg/5ml	10–20ml	Twice a day

*Ferrous fumarate syrup 140mg/5ml is generally used only in patients with swallowing difficulties.

Table 10.3 Prophylactic dosing

Preparation	Dose	Frequency
Ferrous sulphate	200mg	1 tablet daily
Ferrous gluconate	300mg	2 tablets daily before food.

Side effects of oral iron
- Gastric irritation
- Constipation
- Diarrhoea
- Black stools.

Choice of preparation is usually decided by the tolerability of side effects.
- ▶ If patients are taking PO_4 binders then ferrous salts should not be taken before food as PO_4 binders interfere with the absorption of the iron
- ▶ Modified-release preparations are not recommended as the majority of iron absorption occurs in the duodenum and proximal jejunum
- Oral iron has low efficacy in CKD, but might be used as a regular source of elemental iron, particularly in non-dialysis and PD patients.

Intravenous iron

- Parenteral iron is the iron supplement of choice for patients receiving HD and is given at regular intervals during dialysis
- Frequency, dosing, and choice of preparation will depend on local protocols, e.g. a bolus dose given fortnightly during dialysis, as a maintenance dose
- For those not receiving HD, IV iron is given to correct iron deficiency prior to commencing ESA therapy, or to maintain adequate iron stores whilst receiving ESA therapy
- Oral iron may also be used to maintain iron stores, with IV iron being given intermittently if ferritin levels <100mcg/L and Hb is below range, e.g. Venofer® given in divided doses over 3–5wks, or a single dose administration of Cosmofer®, Monofer®, or Ferinject® (these may also be given in divided doses if required)
- ▶ IV iron can be given to maintain Hb levels without the use of ESA therapy.

Side effects of IV iron
- Taste disturbances
- Nausea
- Vomiting
- Abdominal pain
- Diarrhoea
- Chest pain
- Headache
- Fever
- Myalgia
- Hypersensitivity reactions
- Injection site reactions
- Peripheral oedema
- Paraesthesia
- Fatigue
- Anaphylactoid reactions (rare)
- Staining of skin if extravasation occurs.

Administration of IV iron can take place in an outpatient setting or in the patient's own home. All patients receiving ESA therapy should receive iron supplementation.

Available IV iron preparations*

- Venofer® complex of ferric hydroxide with sucrose containing 2% (20mg/ml) of iron
- Cosmofer® complex of ferric hydroxide with dextrans containing 5% (50mg/ml) of iron
- Monofer® complex of isomaltoside 1000 contains 100mg/ml of iron
- Ferinject® complex of iron in a stable ferric state and a carbohydrate polymer containing 50mg/ml of iron.
- Rienso® complex of super paramagnetic iron oxide containing 30mg/ml elemental iron.

* Other preparations are available but not licensed in the UK.

Monitoring response to treatment

- Check Hb, serum ferritin, % TSAT or % HRC 1 month after treatment
- If Hb still ↓ and serum ferritin, % TSAT or ↓ %HRC consider a further course of IV iron
- If iron replete and Hb ↓ consider ESA therapy
- If iron replete and Hb within range monitor 3-monthly.

Treatment with erythropoiesis stimulating agents

- Treatment with ESAs should be offered to people with anaemia of CKD who are likely to benefit in terms of QOL and physical function
- Appropriateness of ESA use should be considered if co-morbidities or prognosis negate benefit
- A trial of ESA should be initiated if benefit uncertain
- An agreed review interval should be discussed with the patients
- Age alone should not be a determinant for treating anaemia of CKD.

Aims of treatment

- Maintain stable Hb levels 10–12g/dl for adults, young people, and children >2yrs
- Adjust treatment when Hb is within 0.5g/dl of the range's limits
- When determining individual aspirational ranges consider the following:
  - patient preference
  - co-morbidities
  - treatment required.

►ESA therapy should not be initiated without also managing iron deficiency.

Commencing ESA therapy

- Starting dose of ESA depends on Hb and underlying cause of the anaemia
- Several ESA preparations available (Table 10.4). Factors influencing choice of drug include:
  - route/frequency of administration (IV/SC)
  - pain on injection
  - patient choice
  - flexibility of dosing
  - cost
- Adjustment of ESA dose is determined by:
  - actual Hb level
  - aspirational Hb range
  - rate of ↑ in Hb level
  - clinical circumstances.

Contraindications to ESA therapy

Absolute contraindications
- Uncontrolled hypertension
- Previous anaphylaxis related to ESA use
- Pure red cell aplasia (PRCA) in relation to previous ESA treatment
- Patients who are unable to receive thromboprophylaxis.

Relative contraindications
- Hyperkalaemia
- Thrombocytosis
- Disseminated malignancy
- History of seizures
- Tenuous vascular access
- Sickle cell anaemia
- Chronic liver failure
- Ischaemic vascular disease
- Recent myocardial infarction, cerebrovascular accident, unstable angina
- History of venous thromboembolic disease.

⚠ Further caution
- Evidence of seizures in 3% of patients on ESA therapy. More common in children and related to rapid ↑ Hb often with poor BP control
- Small ↑ in thrombosis of synthetic vascular access grafts with ESA therapy. Not seen in native vascular access unless Hb >13g/dl
- Sickle cell anaemia. Painful sickling crises are more frequent with ESA therapy. Use in conjunction with haematological advice, ↓ than usual target Hb recommended.

ESA dosing
- Nephrology services independently decide which preparation to use for each modality
- Majority of HD patients receive their ESA IV during dialysis
- PD, transplant, and non-dialysis patients receive their ESA SC at home.
- Self-administration of ESA is encouraged. For those who are unable to inject themselves, carers or community nurses can assist.

▶All ESA can be given IV or SC. However it should be noted that some ESAs may require up to 20% higher dose if given IV.

Initiating dose of ESA
- Epoetin alfa, and beta 80–120 units/kg/week in divided doses
- Darbepoetin alfa 0.45mcg/kg/week in single dose
- Methoxy polyethylene glycol-epoetin beta 600ng/kg fortnightly/ monthly.

Table 10.4 ESA preparations

Name	Mode of action
Darbepoetin alfa (Aranesp®)	Longer acting, wkly/fortnight/monthly
Epoetin alfa (Eprex®)	Shorter acting 1–3 times/wk
Epoetin alfa (Binocrit®)	Biosimilar, shorter acting 1–3 times/wk
Epoetin beta (NeoRecormon®)	Shorter acting, 1–3 times/wk
Epoetin beta (Retacrit®)	Biosimilar, shorter acting 1–3 times/week
Methoxy polyethylene glycol-epoetin beta (Mircera®)	Longer acting, fortnightly/monthly

Titrating doses
- Aim to achieve desired Hb in 3–4 months
- If Hb ↑ too quickly:
  - withhold ESA dose until within required range
  - reinstate ~25% below previous dose
- ↓ dose by 25–50% if outside of range
- ↑ dose by 25% if below range.

Monitoring response to treatment

The frequency of monitoring will depend on
- Stage of anaemia treatment, i.e. initial correction or maintenance
- Frequency and mode of iron supplementation
- Modality
- Clinical situations, i.e. bleeding, surgery
- Availability of the patient.

Hb levels

- Every 2–4wks in the induction phase of ESA therapy
- Every 1–3 months in the maintenance phase of ESA therapy
- More actively after an ESA dose adjustment
- In a clinical setting chosen in discussion with the patient, taking into consideration their convenience and local healthcare systems.
  NB Monitoring may vary in practice, e.g. every 4–6wks if long acting ESAs are prescribed.

Iron status
- No earlier than 1wk after receiving IV iron and at intervals of 4wks to 3 months routinely.

ESA dose and frequency
- Adjust to maintain stable Hb between 10–12g/dl in adults, young people, and children >2yrs if Hb levels are within 0.5g/dl of the range's limits
- Review effectiveness of anaemia treatment in terms of rate of change of Hb levels.

Blood pressure
- Measure wkly for first 6wks of treatment, thereafter monthly in non-HD patients
- Hypertension is associated with
  - ↑ in Hb
  - vasoconstriction induced by treatment, arterial remodelling, and enhanced responsiveness to noradrenaline
  - change in fluid status, i.e. fluid overload
- Persistent hypertension should be treated with the relevant medication see 📖 p. 86.

Non-response/resistance to erythropoiesis stimulating agent therapy

Failure to achieve aspirational Hb levels using ESA therapy should be investigated, particularly if high doses of ESA are being prescribed.

Investigating ESA resistance
- Assess adherence
- Exclude:
  - concurrent illness
  - chronic blood loss
  - aluminium toxicity
  - chloramine toxicity (HD patients only).

▶ Consider patients resistant to ESAs when aspirational Hb range is not achieved despite treatment with:
- ≥300 units/kg/wk SC epoetin, or
- ≥450 units/kg/wk IV epoetin, or
- 1.5 µg/kg/wk darbepoetin (SC/IV)
- Or continued high doses of ESAs needed to maintain aspirational Hb range.

The most common cause of non-response is iron deficiency. Other causes include:
- Adherence
- Concurrent inflammation/infection
- Inadequate dosing
- Hyperparathyroidism
- Bone marrow fibrosis
- Aluminium toxicity
- Malnutrition
- Haemoglobinopathies
- Bone marrow disorders; myeloma, myelodysplasia
- Inadequate dialysis
- Blood loss
- Haemolysis
- Drugs, e.g. ACEI
- Carnitine deficiency
- PRCA.

Managing ESA resistance

- Identify cause
- Treat cause
- Chronic blood loss: investigate cause, if evidence of GI bleed consider use of PPIs, seek advice from gastroenterologist
- Revisit route of administration, check adherence, self-injection technique, dose being administered. Review dose as per unit protocol
- Iron deficiency: give IV iron and monitor response
- Aluminium toxicity: (HD patients) desferrioxamine test
- Improve dialysis adequacy
- Hyperparathyroidism: review PTH, bone profile, check appropriate medication being prescribed and patient taking correctly
- Review medication, e.g. ACEI dosing
- Review nutritional status
- Screen for bone marrow disorders, consider a bone marrow biopsy, refer to a haematologist for specialist advice.

If all possible causes of resistance to ESA therapy have been excluded and/ or treated with no response then PRCA should be considered.

Pure red cell aplasia

PRCA is a rare haematological condition where the bone marrow fails to produce RBCs.

Known causes

- Lymphoproliferative disorders (chronic lymphocytic leukaemia, bone marrow/stem cell transplantation)
- Infections: e.g. EBV, hepatitis, systemic autoimmune disease
- Drugs:
  - antiepileptic medicines
  - azathioprine
  - chloramphenicol
  - isoniazid
  - recombinant erythropoietin (rHuEPO)
  - mycophenolate mofetil.

PRCA induced by these drugs generally resolves within 1–2wks after the drug is withdrawn.

ESA-associated PRCA

- Leads to formation of antibodies to ESAs
- Occurs mainly with SC ESA administration due to the ↑ immunogenicity of proteins when SC injections are given
- Patient becomes ESA resistant and transfusion dependent
- Product-related factors that have the potential to impact on immunogenicity include:
  - sequence variations in proteins
  - the degree and nature of protein glycosylation
  - manufacturing process
  - handling and storage
  - components and properties of the product formulation.

Clinical features

- Rapid ↓ Hb
- Transfusion dependent
- Reticulocytopenia (<10 × 10⁹/L)
- ESA resistance (>300 units/kg/wk or equivalent)
- Bone marrow aplasia.

Patient-related factors associated with developing antibody-mediated PRCA include:

- Skin reactions
- Immune status
- Treatment history.

▶ ESA-induced PRCA should be confirmed by the presence of anti-erythropoietin antibodies together with a lack of pro-erythroid progenitor cells in bone marrow.

Treating ESA-induced PRCA

- Stop ESA
- Do not switch to another ESA preparation

- Consider commencing an immunosuppressive regimen to reduce erythropoietin antibody production, e.g. ciclosporin, prednisolone, mycophenolate.

⚠ Treatment may not be successful and some patients will remain transfusion dependent indefinitely.

▶ Drugs are currently being trialled which stimulate erythropoiesis, raise Hb, and eliminate the need for transfusions in patients with confirmed ESA-induced PRCA.

Adjuvant therapies

Therapies considered to optimize response to ESAs

Therapeutic doses of specific vitamins may improve control of anaemia when combined with ESA therapy.

- Vitamin C (ascorbic acid) can help mobilize iron stores and enhance the response to ESAs
- Folate supplementation for HD patients (5mg folic acid daily)
- Vitamin B_{12} injections (e.g. hydroxocobalamin 1mg every 3 months)
- Pentoxifylline—limited research has shown 400mg daily for 4 months in patients with ESA resistance resulted in an improvement in Hb levels.

Blood transfusion

►Where possible avoid blood transfusion particularly for those who are being considered for a kidney transplant.

If a transfusion is clinically indicated then it should be administered as per the British Committee for Standards in Haematology (BCSH) guidelines. The risk versus benefit ratio of the intervention needs to be analysed before prescribing a RBC transfusion to treat anaemia in patients with CKD.

Potential risks of transfusion

- Transfusion-acquired infections (HBV, HCV, CMV, HIV)
- Transfusion reactions
- Fluid overload
- Iron overload
- Accumulation of HLA antibodies which can reduce the success of kidney transplantation
- ↑ sensitization.

Indications for transfusion

- Acute blood loss
- PRCA
- Haemoglobinopathies, e.g. myelodysplasia.

► If HD patient requires a blood transfusion, the blood should be administered during dialysis and the volume included in the dialysis prescription for total fluid removal that session.

►Extra fluid removal may have to be considered for patients undergoing PD and their dialysis prescription reviewed accordingly.

In those not receiving dialysis, diuretics may be prescribed to be given during the transfusion to avoid fluid overload.

Patient education

- Practical information about management of ACKD
- Symptoms/causes of anaemia
- Associated medications
- Phases of treatment: iron management/ESA therapy why it is required, how it works, potential benefits, and side effects
- Importance of adherence and consequences of poor adherence—see p. 572
- Professional support, e.g. contact information, community services, continuity of care
- Monitoring, feedback on progress of results
- Lifestyle, diet, physical exercise, maintaining normality, meeting other patients
- Patient preferences: supervised or self-administration, dose frequency, method of supplying the ESA and its storage
- Safe and effective self-administration of ESA
- Providing ready, reasonable, and uninterrupted access to supplies.

Role of the healthcare professional

- Designated person(s) responsible for co-ordinating care whose principal responsibility is managing the anaemia. Usually a nurse or pharmacist
- Provide a single point of contact, to ensure patients receive a seamless service
- Monitor and manage a caseload of patients in line with locally agreed protocols
- Provide information, education, and support to empower patients and their families and carers to participate in their care
- Co-ordinate an anaemia service, working between 2° and 1° care
- Prescribe medicines related to managing anaemia and monitoring their effectiveness.

These roles and responsibilities vary depending on the anaemia management strategy of individual nephrology services.

Some services will have designated anaemia nurses or co-ordinators; others will integrate anaemia management into other roles such as advanced kidney care/pre-dialysis nurses, or pharmacists. HD, PD, and Tx each may have a designated anaemia link nurse or pharmacist who will be responsible for monitoring and auditing practice.

Further reading

British Renal Society/Anaemia Nurse Specialist Association. *A guide to community administration of intravenous iron for people with anaemia of chronic kidney disease*, 2012. Available at: <http://www.britishrenal.org/getattachment/AboutUs/Activities-(1)/IV-Iron-in-the-Community/CKD-Book-2012_revised-proof.pdf.aspx>

Bennett L Pickard S. *Haematology and the Patient with Chronic Kidney Disease; An Introductory Guide.* Luzerne: EDTNA/ERCA; 2009. Available at: <http://www.edtnaerca.org>

Mikhail A, Shrivastava R, Richardson R. *Clinical Practice Guidelines. Anaemia in CKD*, 5th edn, 2009–2012. Final Version (15.11.10). London: The Renal Association. Available at: <http://www.renal.org/Clinical/GuidelinesSection/AnaemiaInCKD.aspx>

NICE. *Anaemia Management in Chronic Kidney Disease: National Clinical Guideline for Management in Adults and Children.* Clinical Guideline 114. London: NICE; 2011. Available at: <http://www.nice.org.uk/guidance /CG114>

Useful websites

<http://www.anaemianurse.org>
<http://www.bcshguidelines.com>
<http://www.britishrenal.org>
<http://www.kdigo.org>
<http://www.renal.org>

Peritoneal dialysis

Peritoneal membrane structure

The parietal and visceral membranes are separated by the peritoneal cavity which contains 50–100ml of fluid (containing macrophages, polymorphs, and lymphocytes) acting as a lubricant preventing the membranes from adhering to the abdominal organs. The peritoneal membrane which has a surface area of ~1–2m^2 in adults, is made up of 60% visceral peritoneum (covers abdominal organs), 30% mesenterium and omentum, and 10% parietal peritoneum (lining of the inner surface of abdominal wall). The parietal peritoneum is where the majority of dialysis occurs as the visceral component has only 25–30% of the contact with the dialysate. The peritoneal membrane is a selective semi-permeable membrane and can act as a dialyser with solutes moving across from the peritoneal capillary blood to dialysate placed in the peritoneal cavity.

There are 3 peritoneal membrane layers
- Mesothelium
- Interstitium
- Capillary endothelium:
  - the capillary vascular surface area determines solute transport.

Blood supply
- Visceral peritoneum is supplied by the mesenteric arteries and drainage is via the portal circulation
- Parietal peritoneum is supplied by the epigastric, intercostal, and lumbar arteries and drainage is via the IVC (intraperitoneal (IP) drugs are metabolized in the liver)
- Estimated peritoneal blood flow rate is 50–100ml/min.

Lymphatic drainage
- There is some drainage of peritoneal fluid via the one-way lymphatic drainage system which drains peritoneal fluid and returns excess fluid and proteins back in to the blood circulation
- A small volume of fluid is reabsorbed from the peritoneal cavity into the lymphatic blood vessels. The rate at which it is absorbed is dependent on the intraperitoneal hydrostatic pressure (IPHP) which is affected by body position (e.g. supine ↓ IPHP), any active infection or inflammation, e.g. peritonitis, and respiratory rate
- Transport rate is ~1–2ml/min.

⚠ When calculating total fluid removal take into consideration that some fluid reabsorption will have occurred via the lymphatic system.

Principles of peritoneal dialysis

Solute and water transport

The 3 processes involved in H_2O and solute transport are:
- Diffusion
- Convection
- Ultrafiltration (UF).

Diffusion

The main process of solute transport across the peritoneum occurs by diffusion via the small pores or as a result of convection (solute drag). Diffusion occurs as solutes (e.g. Cr, Ur) move from a high to low conc as a result of random molecular movement and is dependent on the presence of a conc gradient. The speed of solute transport varies between individuals and can be measured by undertaking a peritoneal equilibration test (see 📖 p. 274). However, diffusion is at its highest at the start of dwell period in all patients when the conc gradient is at its highest and continues until equilibrium has been reached between the 2 solutions. It is important to note that diffusion can occur in the opposite direction, e.g. when using hypertonic dextrose dialysate where the conc in the blood compartment is lower than the dialysate. Table 11.1 provides an overview of substances either lost or absorbed via dialysate.

Factors that affect diffusion
- Solute conc gradient between the blood and dialysate
- Molecular weight, size, charge, protein binding, and H_2O/lipid solubility of the molecules:
  - smaller molecular weight solutes such as Ur diffuse more rapidly than larger molecules such as Cr
  - RBCs are too large to diffuse through the membrane
- Dwell time of the dialysate, i.e. time dialysate remains in the peritoneal cavity
- The effective peritoneal surface area and permeability
- The intrinsic peritoneal membrane resistance, dialysate flow rate, peritoneal blood flow rate
- Dialysate volume and temperature
- Vascular supply to the peritoneum (e.g. may be affected in vascular disease)
- The presence of infection and/or inflammation.

Table 11.1 Substances either lost or absorbed via dialysate

Lost	Absorbed
Protein, amino acids	Dextrose
H_2O soluble vitamins	Calcium
Hormones, e.g. parathyroid	Lactate
Trace elements	Drugs
Drugs	

Convection (solute drag)

An osmotic gradient is created by the use of dextrose or polyglucose dialysate which contain a higher conc of dextrose or polyglucose than in the peritoneal blood capillaries. Convection or 'solute drag' occurs when solutes which are dissolved in H_2O move through the small pores in to the dialysate. Middle molecules (e.g. β_2 microglobulins) mainly move via convection. Convection can be measured by the sieving coefficient(s) which represents the conc of the solute in the ultrafiltrate and its conc in the plasma, assuming the net diffusion is zero.

Osmosis

Osmosis occurs as a result of the movement of H_2O from an area of low solute conc to an area of high solute conc along an osmotic gradient. H_2O is pulled across the peritoneal membrane using a hypertonic dextrose dialysate creating an increase in osmotic pressure.

Ultrafiltration

UF is a term that refers to the movement of fluid across the peritoneal membrane via the small or ultrasmall pores as a result of a change in the conc gradient, i.e. high conc of dextrose in the dialysate and low conc in the peritoneal blood capillaries leading to an increase in osmotic pressure.
- 40–50% of total UF occurs via the aquaporin system and 50–60% via the small pores (see 📖 p. 246)
- UF is controlled by Starling's law:
  - UF is the total difference of the osmotic and hydrostatic pressures across the peritoneal membrane minus the net reabsorption by the lymphatic system
- UF is at its highest during the initial dwell time as the osmotic gradient is at its highest (see 📖 p. 246), however, if the dialysate remains *in situ* for too long, e.g. after osmotic equilibrium occurs, then fluid will be reabsorbed.

Factors that influence UF
- Total functioning peritoneal surface area
- Peritoneal membrane characteristics, i.e. permeability of the peritoneal membrane
- Osmotic pressure gradient, e.g. strength of dextrose dialysate
- Oncotic pressure—pressure exerted by larger molecules, particularly proteins
- Hydrostatic pressure gradient—pressure exerted by fluid at equilibrium as a result of gravity forces
- Length of the dwell time of the dialysate.

Theoretical concepts of solute transport

Currently the most widely used and accepted model is the 3-pore model. Peritoneal capillaries have 3 selective pores sizes which act as a barrier to solute and H_2O transport, see Table 11.2 for pore characteristics.

Table 11.2 Peritoneal capillary pore characteristics

Pore	Size (Å)	Density	Transport function
Large	>150	Small	Macromolecules, e.g. proteins, Alb
Small	40–50	Large	Small solutes dissolved in H_2O, e.g. Cr, Na^+, K^+, Ur
Ultrasmall	3–5	Large	H_2O only—barrier to solutes
Aquaporin-1			H_2O channels open when activated by a change in osmolality, e.g. dextrose dialysate

Å=Angstrom.

Aquaporin system

Aquaporin-1 pores are the main H_2O channels which are located in the endothelial cells of the peritoneal vasculature. Aquaporin-1 pores account for ~40% of the total volume of capillary UF. There are a small number of aquaporin-3 and -4 pores which are responsible for the transcellular H_2O transport created by an osmotic gradient, e.g. dextrose dialysate.

▶ Aquaporins are not activated by iso-osmolar solutions ∴ icodextrin is a suitable solution to use in patients with UF problems as it does not rely on the aquaporin system for H_2O removal (see 🕮 p. 250).

Sodium sieving

As only H_2O can pass through the ultrasmall pores of the aquaporin system, Na^+ is prevented from passing into the peritoneal blood capillaries and in effect is 'sieved'.

- Measuring Na^+ sieving can provide information on the UF capability of the peritoneal membrane
- The initial dialysate Na^+ conc is 132mEq/L and will decline in the initial phase of a hypertonic dwell to 120mEq/L, then gradually increase as a result of diffusion of Na^+ from the circulation
- If this does not occur then there is a failure in aquaporin function and ultrafiltration failure (UFF) should be investigated further (see 🕮 pp. 318–19 for more information on UFF).

▶ Consider the impact of Na^+ sieving when undertaking rapid exchanges, e.g. automated peritoneal dialysis (APD) to improve adequacy and remove fluid as it can → hypernatraemia. This results in excessive thirst negating the benefits of fluid removal as the patient will increase their fluid intake.

Peritoneal dialysate

The ideal dialysate solution should contain H_2O, an osmotic agent, minerals, and electrolytes providing:

- Solute clearance
- Adequate UF
- Minimal absorption of the osmotic agent
- Mineral and electrolyte replacement if required
- Correction of metabolic acidosis.

See Table 11.4, p. 253 for a summary of available dialysates.

Dextrose-containing dialysates

Dextrose dialysates are the most widely used solutions. Dextrose is metabolized to glucose, with ~100–200g/day of glucose absorbed using dextrose-containing dialysate (1.36% dextrose dialysate contains 108.4 kilocalories). See Table 11.3 for standard conc in dextrose-containing dialysates.

- Higher conc dextrose dialysates are used (e.g. 3.86% 'high bag') to provide greater osmotic pull and ∴ ↑ UF.
- Dextrose has a reflection coefficient (Rco) of 0.02 which means that it will be absorbed over time as the osmotic gradient diminishes (the ideal osmotic agent would have a Rco of 1.0)
- The standard volumes available range from 1.5–3L for manual exchanges (i.e. CAPD) and 5L for APD machines.

Advantages
- Inexpensive, easy to produce, and safe to use
- Provides effective UF.

Disadvantages
- Must be stored in a cool, dry place to prevent degradation
- Easily absorbed and can cause metabolic complications, e.g. hyperinsulinaemia, hyperglycaemia, weight-gain, diabetes, and dyslipidaemia
- Biocompatibility problems—the sterilization process can → formation of GDPs which are associated with the production of AGEs → changes in peritoneal defence mechanism and structure
- Exposure to high glucose conc over a long period of time → ↑ peritoneal membrane permeability, e.g. high transporter status.

Dialysate research
Low Na^+ dialysate:
- ↓ Na^+ conc to 100mmol/L in the dialysate → ↑ conc gradient between the peritoneal capillary blood and dialysate → ↑ Na^+ diffusion from the peritoneal capillary blood ∴ more Na^+ removed → improved BP control.

Table 11.3 Standard concentration in dextrose-containing dialysates

	Concentration	Rationale
Dextrose % dependent on manufacturer	1.36%–3.86% 1.25%–4.25%	Provide osmotic gradient
NaCl (mmol/L)	130–134	Prevent ↑ Na⁺/dehydration as majority of H_2O removed at start of dwell as ~ equal to the plasma serum level
Lactate (mmol/L)	35–40	Normalize acid–base balance Standard buffer—maintain stability of the dialysate
Ionized Ca^{2+} (mmol/L)	Standard 1.25	Use of lower conc as some Ca^{2+} absorbed Able to use Ca^{2+} containing phosphate binders/vitamin D to control PTH
	Lower 0.6, 1.0	↓ plasma Ca^{2+} level if high to normal range
	1.75, previous standard	Aim for plasma Ca^{2+} at upper limit of normal range
$MgCl_2$ (mmol/L)	0.25–0.75	≈plasma Mg^{2+}
K⁺ (mmol/L)	1.5	↓ plasma K⁺
pH	5.2–5.5 in dextrose dialysate	HCL—added during heat sterilization to prevent caramelization → acidic, inhibit the growth of bacteria

Non-dextrose based solutions

Icodextrin

Icodextrin is a glucose polymer solution which is 7.5% lactate buffered with a low GDP content and pH of 5.8. It is iso-osmotic having a colloidal osmotic effect (fluid is dragged through the peritoneal membrane) and has no effect on the aquaporin system, i.e. no H_2O moves across the capillaries $\therefore$ no Na^+ sieving effect. Na^+ removal occurs via convection through the small pores.

Advantages
- It has a relatively high Rco of 0.77 $\therefore$ can remain *in situ* for long dwells (8–12hrs) as not readily absorbed and maintains a conc gradient for longer, i.e. sustained UF:
  - UF volume is similar to a 3.86% dextrose bag at 8–12hrs
  - may improve UF in high or high average transporters
  - suitable for long night dwell in CAPD and day dwell in APD
- Absorbed via the lymphatic system and eventually metabolized to glucose with a calorie load equivalent to 2.25% dextrose dialysate
- Contains less GDP than other lactate buffered dialysate
- No glucose exposure, improved β microglobulin clearance
- No absorption of glucose $\therefore$ ↓ carbohydrate load and better diabetes control.

Disadvantages
- Expensive as only available from one company
- Adverse reactions as a result of ↑ serum maltose conc and other oligo/polysaccharides, e.g. skin rash (common to extremities and body) and culture −ve peritonitis (mononuclear WBCs)
- Once daily use to prevent a build-up of serum maltose
- Interferes with some tests, e.g. serum amylase levels are ↓ by 90% and masks the sign of pancreatitis
- Dialysate contains maltose and can affect glucometer readings resulting in false high reading. ▶ Ensure glucometer is compatible, do not use with a glucose dehydrogenase glucometer.

Nutrineal®

Originally developed to aid nutrition in malnourished patients; however, there is no firm evidence showing beneficial nutritional effect, improved survival, reduced peritonitis or hospitalization rates. Contains 9 essential and 6 non-essential amino acids with a total conc of 1.1% and comes as a single bag, is lactate buffered, has a pH of 6.7, and acts as an osmotic agent with similar effect to a 1.36% Dianeal® dialysate.

- Commonly used as an alternative to a dextrose-containing dialysate (e.g. ↓ glucose exposure, ↓ lipids), in those with recurrent peritonitis, malnutrition or diabetes.

▶ Must be used while eating a meal as calories are required for the amino acids to be taken up by the tissues. Dietetic input regarding supplemental feeding may be required if the patient is anorexic.

- CAPD patients—time exchange at a meal time, e.g. lunch or dinner
- APD patients are required to use higher dextrose dialysate strength bag to mix with Nutrineal®.

Advantages
- Amino acid supplementation—25% of daily protein intake with no PO_4
- UF equivalent to 1.36% dextrose dialysates
- No glucose ∴ no GDPs and no carbohydrate absorption
- More physiological pH 6.7
- Used for malnutrition, e.g. as a result of albumin loss 2° to PD
- Could be used as an alternative to using a dextrose-containing dialysate.

Disadvantages
- More expensive than standard dialysate
- >1/day usage associated with mild acidosis and worsening uraemia.

Biocompatibility and biocompatible solutions

The use of dialysate is known to cause physiological changes to the peritoneal membrane.
- Low pH and high lactate dialysate have been found to ↓ bactericidal capacity and phagocytosis and inhibit cell recovery
- Dextrose dialysates associated with ↑ levels of inflammation, angiogenesis, and loss of defence mechanisms:
  - exposure to glucose degradation products, e.g. AGEs which cause inflammation, fibrosis, and angiogenesis → UFF
- The ideal biocompatible solution would ↓ the exposure to glucose, have a low pH, GDPs, and AGEs.

Newer bag technology and the use of dual- or triple-chamber bags has enabled the use of HCO_3 solutions; while using a separate dextrose solution chamber prevents the formation of GDPs during the sterilization process. More research is needed into the long-term effects but initial studies suggest:
- Beneficial effects on preserving peritoneal membrane function and RRF
- Euro-balance study reported improved cell homeostasis with higher levels of CA-125.

Current solutions available
- Physioneal® (Baxter): lactate, mixed buffer, pH 7.4
- Stay-safe Balance®: neutral pH when mixed, dextrose and electrolytes separated from HCO_3 buffer
- BicaVera® (Fresenius): lactate free/pure HCO_3 buffer—not a neutral pH.

Advantages
- Physiological pH 7.4
- HCO_3 conc of 25mmol/L ∴ more physiological
- ↓ lactate conc (15mmol/L) and GDPs
- Better acid–base balance
- Theoretical and only observational evidence for:
  - ↓ peritonitis rates, inflammation, and improved technique survival
  - better UF and preserved membrane function and structure
  - ↓ systemic inflammation ∴ improved patient survival
- ↓ inflow/abdominal pain due to ↓ pH (shown in a RCT)
- Observational feedback from patients improved comfort levels.

Disadvantages
- No RCTs to support benefit claims
- Dextrose is still the main osmotic agent
- Expensive and more difficult to make
- More complicated—more connections to open
- May ↓ UF slightly >conventional dialysate
- Some contain lactate.

See Table 11.4 for advantages and disadvantages of different PD dialysates.

Table 11.4 Comparison of PD dialysates.

	Clinical use	Advantages	Disadvantages
Dextrose	Used as main PD dialysate in the majority of patients	Cheaper Made by all companies Good clinical experience/research on use Good for managing UF	Long-term effect on peritoneal membrane permeability ↓pH—GDPs formed during sterilization Absorb fluid in long dwells in H or HA*
Icodextrin	↑UF in H or HA* ↓glucose load (diabetes) Use for long dwell time, e.g. APD day dwell, CAPD overnight	↑and sustained UF ↓glucose load ↓GDPs ↓solute absorption	↓pH Lactate buffered Once a day use only Side effects e.g. rash, culture −ve peritonitis Need compatible glucometer for accurate BGL reading Expensive
Nutrineal®	Malnourished, diabetes and/ or recurrent peritonitis Alternative to dextrose dialysate as osmotic agent	↑amino acid ↓glucose load ↓GDPs	Lactate buffered Only use one/day ± worsen metabolic acidosis and uraemia Expensive
Bicarbonate/ lactate	Inflow pain Physician choice based on available evidence	pH equivalent to body ↓lactate ↓GDPs ↑instillation pain ± long-term benefits to membrane function, and ↓peritonitis rates	Osmotic agent is dextrose Need 2 or 3 chambers to produce Expensive More complicated for patent to use

*HA: high average transporter, H: high/fast transporter

Types and modes of peritoneal dialysis

PD technology has advanced over the years, from the use of glass bottles to plastic bags, the 'flush before fill', and development of biocompatible fluids using dual fluid chambers. The main route of infection is associated with the connection/disconnection in both types of PD. PD systems vary depending on the company supplying the product. The 2 main systems available are continuous ambulatory peritoneal dialysis (CAPD) and automated peritoneal dialysis (APD).

Modes of peritoneal dialysis

Maximizing the efficiency of solute clearance and/or fluid removal may require the use of different modes of PD. The choice of mode will be dependent on:
- Clinical requirement
- Patient choice and lifestyle
- Peritoneal membrane characteristics and transport status
- Physician choice
- Available resources, e.g. APD machines.

Continuous ambulatory peritoneal dialysis

Continuous ambulatory peritoneal dialysis

Most commonly CAPD consists of 3–5 exchanges per day, the majority of patients performing 4 exchanges. An example of a CAPD exchange can be seen in Figure 11.1.
- Regular exchanges throughout the day every 4–6hrs, with the overnight exchange having a longer dwell time of 8–12hrs
- Icodextrin can be used if absorbing fluid from overnight exchange.

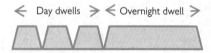

Fig. 11.1 CAPD exchange.

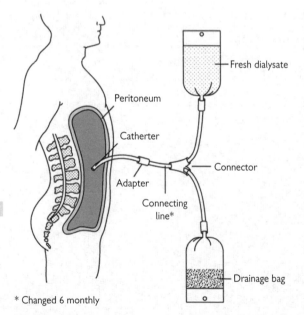

* Changed 6 monthly

Fig. 11.2 CAPD disconnect system. Reproduced with permission from Levy J, Brown E, Daley C, et al. Oxford Handbook of Dialysis, 3rd edn. Oxford: Oxford University Press; 2009.

The process of completing a drain in and out of dialysate is called an 'exchange' which is undertaken using a non-touch sterile technique. The system comes as two bags, with a 'Y'-shaped giving set. One bag contains the dialysate, the other is the empty drainage bag for the effluent. PD effluent is drained out initially, then, when complete, the 'flush before fill' is performed prior to draining in which also flushes away any potential contamination (i.e. new dialysate is drained straight in to the PD effluent bag). Once completed the new PD dialysate is drained in. The system is then disconnected using a non-touch sterile technique and a cap placed in the end of the PD catheter.

- The newer biocompatible solutions have more than one chamber for the dialysate which need to be mixed prior to draining in
- Normal drain out time = 20mins. Normal drain in time = 5–10mins.

▶ The total dialysate volume has an additional 100–200ml to allow for the 'flush before fill', e.g. the total volume of a 2L bag is 2.1L ∴ the patient still infuses 2L. This needs to be taken into account when measuring total UF volume—the flushes need to be subtracted from the total UF amount.

Automated peritoneal dialysis

APD is also commonly referred to as continuous cycling peritoneal dialysis (CCPD) involving the use of an automated machine. The machine warms and measures the correct amount of dialysate to be drained in, performs the 'flush before fill' and drains out the PD effluent usually whilst the patient is asleep. The patient then disconnects from the machine in the morning and the machine will deliver a last fill volume if required. It can also be used for intermittent PD (IPD) in cases where waiting for a training place and in the treatment of AKI.

- An example of a common prescription using continuous CCPD:
  - 9hrs, 2L fill volume (last fill 2L) = 10L
  - set machine for 10min drain out and 20min drain in (average times)
  - dwell time of 90mins
- Newer machines have data cards which are programmed to collect data from each APD session. This information can then be accessed remotely or via a USB stick by the PD team.

Intermittent peritoneal dialysis (IPD)

Historically IPD was used for AKI patients prior to the availability of HD and still remains an option (see Figure 11.3). However, it will not provide adequate solute clearance in the long term. It is now used in the following situations:

- Awaiting a PD training place and require dialysis in the interim and have no vascular access
- Dialysate leaks where dialysis is still required (e.g. low volume in supine position)
- Post abdominal surgery for small volumes
- Older patients who are unsuitable for HD (HF or no vascular access)
- Patients who are unable to attend to own PD or have a carer
- Uses short dwell times on APD machine for 1 day, e.g. 20–24hr session and then a rest day a few times a wk.

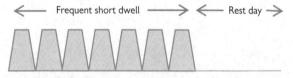

← Frequent short dwell → ← Rest day →

Fig. 11.3 Intermittent peritoneal dialysis.

Automated peritoneal dialysis (APD)

There are various regimens used within clinical practice which are dependent on the required fluid removal and solute clearance.

- Towards the end of draining no diffusion takes place which is lost time. It is possible using the tidal setting to start the re-fill process after the 'breakpoint' rather than leaving re-fill until completely drained.

- Night-time intermittent peritoneal dialysis (NIPD):
  - rapid exchanges overnight with a dry day
  - not frequently used, i.e. loss of dialysis time having a dry day.

Continuous cycling peritoneal dialysis (CCPD)

- Rapid exchanges overnight with a day dwell (last fill is the day dwell), see Figure 11.4
- Icodextrin can be used for long day dwell to prevent fluid absorption

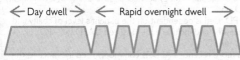

Fig. 11.4 Continuous cycling peritoneal dialysis.

Optimizing cycling peritoneal dialysis (OCPD)

Variations include performing additional 1 or 2-day exchanges, see Figure 11.5.

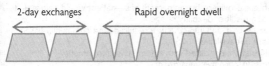

Fig. 11.5 Optimizing cycling peritoneal dialysis.

Tidal peritoneal dialysis (TPD)

Commonly used for the treatment of instillation/infusion pain of dialysate. ~20–30% of dialysate remains *in situ*, i.e. the peritoneum is not completely drained preventing any pulling effect experienced towards the end of draining (see Figure 11.6).

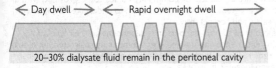

Fig. 11.6 Tidal peritoneal dialysis.

Assisted devices

UV flash™ is a germicidal assisted exchange device for those with visual impairment and dexterity problems. It provides an automatic connection and disconnection under UV light to avoid manual connect and the risk of touch contamination. The hospital occupational therapy department is also a good resource for adaptations at home.

Assisted peritoneal dialysis

The UK RA[1] recommends that aPD is made available for all patients wishing to undertake home dialysis who are unable to perform a self-care treatment themselves. This option should be explored with the patient and their family where PD could be performed at home or in a nursing home by a family member, carer, community nurse or nursing home staff.

- The uptake of aPD will be dependent on available resources and infrastructure of the nephrology service, e.g. availability of a community team and PD staff
- The type of PD used is dependent on the patient's level of ability and assistance required and include either assisted CAPD (aCAPD) or assisted APD (aAPD)
- aCAPD, and more recently aAPD, is commonly used in France as the main treatment option for the older patient using home care nurses rather than family members. aAPD has also been successfully used in Canada and Denmark. In some cases, assistance may only be needed during the initial set up period, e.g. while unwell or lacking confidence

Possible reasons for the low numbers of older patients on PD

- Healthcare providers' biased perceptions—patient would be unable to cope as a result of disability or age
- Resources, cost, and infrastructure required for a community-based team are not available
- Social isolation associated with a home-based treatment
- Depression, cognitive impairment
- No carer to assist with PD at home
- Nursing home staff not able to perform PD as part of their role
- Patient choice, e.g. opted for conservative management.

Training and education

In the UK, aPD is more likely to be performed by a healthcare assistance or family member, whereas in Canada and France it is carried out by registered nurses. Training and education for aPD requires nursing home staff, healthcare assistance, or community nurses to be provided with an educational programme which enables them to undertake PD in the community safely and competently.

- Time required to train the person is dependent on their level of nursing experience and training, e.g. a community registered nurse may only require 3 days, whereas a healthcare assistant or family member will need longer, e.g. 1–2wks
- Knowledge and understanding of PD, including technical aspects of the CAPD exchange or setting up and disconnecting APD
- Fluid management, e.g. prescription, IBW
- Troubleshooting guidance, e.g. alarms, poor drainage
- Complications and treatment, e.g. exit site infection, peritonitis
- Daily monitoring, e.g. weight, BP, blood glucose
- Medications, e.g. ESAs, use of IP heparin, antihypertensive medications
- Communication and documentation with the main PD unit.

Peritoneal dialysis access

The purpose of a PD catheter is to provide a safe and effective route to drain dialysate in and out of the peritoneal cavity, without causing pain/discomfort.

- Infection and PD catheter related problems account for up to 20% of permanent transfers to HD (excluding those on temporary HD for PD catheter-related problems)
- Overall PD catheter survival is 88% at 1yr with a removal rate of 15%.

Timing of PD catheter implantation

The UK RA,[1] ISPD,[2] and EBPG[3] recommend placement of the PD catheter should be timely and where possible inserted at least 2wks prior to use.

- May be used earlier if required with small volumes in supine position
- It is not recommended to create an AVF at the time of insertion of PD catheter unless there is a planned transfer time to PD organized.

PD catheter

Currently, no evidence favours one type of catheter, i.e. catheter function, survival and mortality rates are the same. Various PD catheters are available, see Table 11.5.

- A downward direction of internal and external segments of the tunnel, 2 cuffs, and a short sinus are associated with fewer complications and longer period of time to 1st episode of infection:
  - prevents debris and fluid collecting and ↓ risk of infection
- Shorter sinus tract (~5–7 cm long) promotes tissue growth around the tunnel segment
- SC cuffs placed ~2–3 cm from the skin, if closer may → an infection or cuff extrusion
- Pre-sternal catheters—longer tunnel (20–50cm) are used for obese patients or in presence of a stoma—not commonly used in the UK
- The exit site should be situated below the belt line to ↓ the risk of cuff protrusion and irritation
- ♀ tend to prefer the exit site above the umbilicus whereas ♂ prefer the site below the umbilicus

PD catheters consist of 3 segments:

- *Intraperitoneal*—within the peritoneal cavity with multiple small perforations → ↓ 'jet effect' of instilling dialysate. Sutured or positioned freely depending on implantation technique
- *Intramural*—1 or 2 cuffs placed within the abdominal wall tunnel:
  - double cuff, 1 cuff is embedded in to the abdominal rectus muscle. Provides support and anchors the PD catheter, prevents dislodgement and stops bacteria from travelling along the tunnel from the skin in to the peritoneum
  - single cuff PD catheters—SC cuff only
- *External*—exit site section can be seen. An extension line is used to add length for ease of use by the patient.

Table 11.5 Comparison of PD catheter types

Catheter type	Features	Advantage	Disadvantage
Straight Tenckhoff	0.5mm perforated holes 11cm from tip end of silicone catheter Overall length 40cm (adult) with double cuff	Can be inserted using various techniques Easy to insert	↑ risk of migration
Coiled	0.5mm perforated holes in the 18.5cm tip end of silicone catheter	Inserted using various techniques ↓ 'jet effect' and infusion pain Visualize placement on x-ray—radiopaque stripe	↑ risk of migration due to coil Pain if migrates More complex to insert
Swan neck	SC section has downward-pointing segment, e.g. 150° bend	Possible: ↓ exit site infections, ↓ cuff extrusion, ↓ outflow obstruction and catheter migration	Requires surgical insertion by trained specialist
Toronto Western, Oreopoulos	Catheter sutured into pelvis IP segment has 2 discs	↓ risk of migration—catheter tip placed in specific position ↓ exit site leaks	Surgical insertion GA: ↑ cost Abdominal incision: ↑ time until use Removal via laparotomy
Moncrief–Popovich	External segment buried SC until use (4–6wks), exteriorized using LA	Catheter ready for use when patient ready for training	No evidence ↓ infection or complications Need to wait 4–6wks to use catheter Involves 2 procedures
Upper abdomen/chest and presternal	Deep cuff is situated in the rectus muscle, the middle and superficial cuffs in the parasternal area	↓ risk of infection e.g. obesity, stoma, recurrent exit site infections, incontinent of urine or faeces, e.g. infants	Needs surgical insertion by trained specialist

Implantation technique

There are no RCTs that have found one implantation technique is superior to another. The choice of technique should be individualized taking into account past surgical/medical history, clinical condition, technique suitability, and the surgeon and/or nephrologist preference (see Table 11.6 for comparison of implantation techniques):

- In the UK some specialist PD nurses insert medical PD catheters
- Placement site: paramedian or lateral abdominal region provide good positioning into the abdominal rectus muscle and support for tissue growth around the catheter.

▶ Hospital stay is dependent on the choice of insertion technique. Laparoscopic and radiological techniques may be performed as a day case if the patient is suitable.

Calculating the insertion site

- Calculation undertaken by the PD nurse, nephrologist, or surgeon using the Crabtree guidelines[5]
- Selected PD catheter should produce a downward direction
- The PD catheter choice should be individualized to size and gender:
  - use of an inappropriate length can result in pain and ↓ function, e.g. too long or too short.

Prevention of MRSA

- Screen prior to PD catheter insertion for MRSA and nasal carriage *Staphylococcus aureus*
- Routine use of prophylactic antibiotics to help prevent *S. aureus* and Gram −ve exit site infections and peritonitis includes mupirocin and gentamicin applied topically to the exit site.

MRSA carriers

- Use mupirocin nasally
- If not using mupirocin to exit site routinely—regular nasal swabs
- 50% of dialysis patients are carriers of nasal *S. aureus*
- 2–3-fold ↑ risk of having an exit site infection and are 2–6 times more likely to have an episode of *S. aureus* peritonitis
- ↑ risk in diabetes and the immunosuppressed irrespective of being a carrier or not.

Current exit site treatment study pending results

The Honeypot study RCT is comparing the efficacy of Medihoney® antibacterial wound gel vs mupirocin in preventing exit site infections. Honey is known for its antimicrobial properties and its effectiveness against MRSA and VRE.

Table 11.6 Comparison of PD catheter implantation techniques

	Medical with trocar and guidewire	Laparoscopy peritoneoscopy*	Percutaneous guided fluroscopy	Surgical
Advantages	Small incision	Small incision	Small incision	Accurate catheter placement
	Quick and easy to insert	Immediate use	Immediate use	∴ ↓ tip migration
	↓ cost	Quick and easy to insert	↓ pain than surgical	↓ risk of perforation
	Immediate use	↓ pain	More accurate placement	Suitable for all types of catheters
	Good for AKI or high anaesthetic risk	↓ drainage problems	Less invasive	Need to use if history of adhesions
	↓ pain	↓ problems compared to surgical	No GA	
	Can be inserted by specialist renal team	± partial omentectomy or adhesiolysis if needed	Can be inserted by specialist renal team	
		Position catheter tip more precisely		
		Suitable for all types of catheters		
Disadvantages	Need virgin abdomen—no history of prior abdominal surgery or adhesions	Requires expensive equipment	↑ incidence of late fluid leaks	Requires GA—↑ associated costs, e.g. theatre/hospital
	↑ risk of organ or vessel perforation	Need specialized personnel	Risk of bowel perforation and incorrect position	More expensive
	↑ risk of poor catheter flow	Risk of bowel perforation, catheter migration, fluid leak		Larger incision
	No control over catheter position			Unable to use immediately
	Not suitable for more complex catheters, e.g. swan-neck			↑ risk of incisional hernia or fluid leak if catheter used too early
				No difference to infection rates

*NICE guidance[4] available.

Specific peritoneal dialysis catheter preoperative preparation

Routine pre-op management should be undertaken as per unit policy.
- On admission—PD staff will assess whether the patient remains suitable for PD as their condition may have deteriorated since they were assessed
- Bowel preparation completed as per unit policy, e.g. Picolax® for easier placement of the PD catheter and ↓ risk of bowel perforation
- Exit site marked and suitable PD catheter length organized by PD and/or medical staff:
    - ▶ only be performed by PD nursing or medical staff
    - patient should wear their normal clothes to assess position of the belt line
    - ask patient to sit and stand prior to marking the site to see where the belt line moves to
    - check that no skin folds/apron overlap the proposed exit site
    - avoid scars
    - ask the patient to hold a mirror and look at the exit site, check they reach to clean it effectively
    - mark the site with indelible ink
- Medical staff examination for presence of any hernias
- CXR and ECG required for GA
- Check screened for MRSA and nasal carriage of *S. aureus*
- Surgical site preparation as per NICE guidance and unit policy
- Patient to empty bladder to ↓ risk of bladder perforation
- Prophylactic antibiotics administered 1hr pre-op or in theatre as per unit protocol to ↓ risk of post-PD catheter insertion infection
- Use of vancomycin is associated with VRE—cephalosporin may be the choice of treatment (⚠ avoid use if the unit has a high prevalence of *Clostridium difficile*).

Appearance of PD effluent
- *Normal*—clear and contain no sediment. Place a newspaper or other printed paper under the drain out bag; it should be possible to read the print if the PD fluid is clear (useful when teaching patients to assess whether their drain out bag is clear)
- *Fibrin*—pieces of 'cotton wool' floating in the bag
- *Red*—blood (i.e. haemoperitoneum, see 📖 pp. 296–7)
- *Milky*—chylous peritoneum
- *Dark green*—possibly digested food, may be a ruptured duodenal ulcer, i.e. dark green is bile, or a ruptured gall bladder
- *Dark*—faecal with no green bile, large bowel perforation
- *Fluorescent green*—fluorescein dye used for fluorescein angiography, e.g. investigation for diabetic retinopathy.

Postoperative nursing considerations

Routine post-op management should be undertaken as per unit policy. See Table 11.7 for post-op complications <30 days.

- Exit site—non-occlusive dressing is applied immediately post-op and remains *in situ* for 5–10 days dependent on unit policy:
  - slight oozing—reinforce exit site dressing and leave undisturbed for first 48hrs
  - heavily blood-soaked dressing—must be changed by nursing staff (preferably PD) using aseptic technique and sterile saline
  - immobilize/anchor PD catheter to prevent trauma and ↓ the risk of infection
  - sutures should be avoided at the exit site; may be required as a result of excessive bleeding. ▶ Remove after 3–4 days to ↓ risk of infection
- PD catheter care:
  - catheter patency checked immediately post insertion by operator by instilling and draining 500ml–1L dialysate
  - some units may flush PD catheter with 500ml of 1.36% dialysate fluid until return is clear or very pale rosé in colour to prevent blockage as a result of blood clots
  - observe for signs of haemorrhage, e.g. frank blood loss and notify medical staff immediately
  - heparin 500–1000 units/L may be required if effluent has any clots or fibrin to prevent blockage of the catheter
  - cap off PD catheter and anchor securely to ensure it is completely immobilized.

Discharge advice
- Follow up appointment for training ~2wks
- Exit site dressing frequency dependent on unit policy, e.g. leave intact for a further week or change twice wkly for the first 2wks:
  - oozing from the exit site through the dressing, dressing falls off or is soiled—reinforce/replace and contact the PD unit
- Use of aperients as prescribed to avoid any straining/displacement of PD catheter, contact the unit if BNO within 3 days
- Educate on potential complications and action to take
- Exercise—advise patient not to lift any heavy objects, engage in strenuous exercise or sexual intercourse for 2wks
- No shower for the first 2wks until the exit site is healed. If wet and out of hours, replace and contact PD unit
- Swimming—no swimming until the exit site has healed (see 🕮 p. 327).

Table 11.7 Early PD complications usually seen <30 days postoperatively

Complication	Clinical feature	Treatment
Intraperitoneal bleeding	Frank or heavy blood loss in drain out bag	Normal to have some bleeding
	Signs of shock and haemorrhage	Return to theatre if bleeding excessive
		IP heparin to prevent clotting and blockage of PD catheter
Bladder perforation at time of insertion	Urine in drain out bag	Urinary catheter and PD catheter re-positioned
	Glucose ++ in urine following attempted exchange	
Intestinal perforation Immediate post-operatively <1%	Faecal effluent or blood in drain out bag	Return to theatre for urgent bowel repair
	Diarrhoea (+ve glucose after infusion PD dialysate)	Treat infection
	Abdominal pain	
	Gram –ve organism in PD fluid	
Fluid leak from exit site	Differentiate dialysate and serous exudate—test for glucose, +ve urinary dipstick if dialysate	Drain out and rest peritoneum for 10–14 days
		Urgent use, small volumes supine
		± prophylactic antibiotics
Exit site infection	Red/± purulent exudate	Swab exit site for MC&S
		Antibiotics
Internal kink in PD catheter	No inflow or outflow drainage	Return to theatre to correct
Omental wrap	No inflow/outflow	Surgical partial omentectomy
Abdominal adhesions	No inflow/ouflow drainage	Surgical adhesiolysis
Blood clot to the side holes of the PD catheter	No inflow/outflow drainage.	Flush PD catheter, IP heparin or may require urokinase
Constipation	No outflow	Aperients
Bladder obstruction	No outflow	If unable to void—insert urinary catheter

Adequacy of dialysis

Quantification of dialysis delivery can be performed by measuring small peritoneal solute clearance and RRF to give a total weekly amount. The use of urea kinetic modelling (UKM) computer programs is a widely accepted method of assessing the efficiency and adequacy of dialysis, modelling PD prescriptions and measuring protein intake.

Over the years the recommended targets for PD adequacy have changed as a result of 2 significant studies; CANUSA and AMEDEX. Prior to these studies the standard practice was to aim for a Kt/Vurea >1.7.

- CANUSA study: 1996, was a pivotal turning point for the clinical management of PD. The study found 2yr survival 78% with a Kt/Vurea 2.1 and a 5% ↑ in RR of death for every 0.1 ↓ in total Kt/Vurea:
  - conclusions drawn were 'more dialysis is better' and in 1997, KDOQI recommended higher adequacy targets, e.g. CAPD Kt/Vurea ≥2.1, ≥CrCl ≥60L/week
  - the inability to reach or maintain such a high Kt/Vurea, especially after the loss of RRF lead to the transfer of many patients to HD.
- Re-analysis of CANUSA results in 2001—indicated that for every 5L/week of residual GFR the RR of death ↓ by 12% and for every 250ml of urine output the death rate was ↓ by 36%.
  - total urine volume output was a significant predictor of mortality and RRF, rather than peritoneal solute clearance, predicted patient survival.
- ADEMEX study: found no difference in survival or QOL by ↑ Kt/Vurea >1.6
- Hong Kong study: found no significant improvement in patient survival but clinical problems were associated with Kt/Vurea <1.7
- NECOSAD study: showed significant RR of death associated with very low levels of dialysis, e.g. Kt/Vurea <1.5 and CrCl <40L/wk.

The current recommendation by the major renal associations (UK RA, EBPG, and ISPD[1-3]) is for a minimum
Kt/Vurea ≥1.7/wk and/or CrCl ≥50L/wk/1.73m²
UF = >750ml/day (ISPD recommend >1L/day)

Frequency of measurement
- Adequacy, check RRF and PET test <6wks for new patients
- 6-monthly adequacy and RRF check
- Annual PET test
- More frequent assessment if adequacy is reliant on RRF or clinically/biochemically indicated, e.g. uraemic symptoms.

Anuric patients with total UF <750ml (excluding the 'flush before fill' will require closer monitoring and possibly transfer to HD).

Calculating adequacy

Adequacy is determined by the calculation of Kt/Vurea which measures the amount of Ur removed during a 24hr period multiplied by 7 to give a total weekly Kt/Vurea. This is then added to the clearance via RRF to give a total Kt/Vurea.

$$\text{Wkly Kt/Vurea} = \frac{K \times t}{\text{Vurea}} \times 7$$

K = Ur clearance ml/min + Ur urine.
t = time on dialysis (mins/day).
Vurea = Ur distribution volume (volume of body H_2O or % body
weight).

▶ Inaccurate results can occur—consider protein intake, body size, e.g. very small, malnourished, amputee, or obese.

CrCl calculation

$$\text{Clearance}(C) = \frac{\text{dialysate Cr conc} \times \text{dialysate volume}}{\text{Plasma Cr conc}}$$

Normalized to 1.73m² BSA and multiplied by 7 for wkly CrCl.

▶ CrCl is affected by dialysate flow rate, UF, membrane surface area and permeability.
Regular measuring of CrCl can be used to assess loss of muscle mass associated with malnutrition, ageing, or amputation.

Output

Total output = 24hr adequacy collection + 24hr urine output—total 'flush before fill'.
• APD machine automatically calculates the total UF.

Adequacy collection procedure
• 24hr urine collection sample—measure Ur, Cr, and total volume
• 24hr PD effluent collection—discard the drain out effluent from the last exchange in the evening, e.g. 2200hrs and collect all PD effluent for the next 24hrs
• Patient brings all drainage bags or takes a sample from each drain out bag (APD—need to use overnight drain out bag) to the unit along with PD diary and the following:
  • time drain out started, time fill began
  • dialysate conc
  • drain out volume
• Blood samples are taken for Ur, Cr, and glucose
• PD effluent—measure Ur, Cr, and total volume instilled
• Measure total volume drained out and subtract the 'flush before fill' volume
• No morning exchange if PET scheduled for the next day—this will be added after commencement of PET.

▶ Potential errors can occur as a result of inaccurate collection of urine and PD effluent, e.g. not collecting all of urine output, not collecting the PD effluent and urine on the same day, recording an incorrect total volume from the APD machine.

Other methods of measuring adequacy of dialysis

Protein catabolic rate or urea generation rate

Measurement of adequacy does not take in to account protein intake from foods, protein catabolic rate, and urea generation rate. Evaluation of nutritional status is also important:

• Protein nutrition
• Serum Alb level
• Dietary protein intake (DPI)
• Protein catabolic rate—the estimated daily protein intake is calculated as part of the adequacy test using the loss of Ur in the PD effluent and urine (the assumption is the patient is in a nitrogen balance):
  • Ur generation rate is proportional to protein breakdown.

Residual renal function (RRF)

In the average patient for every 1ml/min of RRF there is an ↑ of 0.1 Kt/Vurea and 10L/week/1.73m^2 CrCl. RRF has a significant impact on total solute clearance and fluid removal and should be measured every 2–3 months in order to adjust the PD prescription with the ↓ in RRF.

Benefits of maintaining RRF

• Overall survival is improved
• Clearance of middle molecules, e.g. β-2 microglobulin
• Improved nutritional status, e.g. higher serum Alb levels
• ↓ anaemia and erythropoietin resistance:
  • good BP and fluid balance, e.g. less fluid overload and oedema
• ↓ risk of LVH.

Strategies to preserve RRF

• Avoid/caution with the use of nephrotoxic drugs and agents:
  • aminoglycosides, COX-2 inhibitors, NSAIDs, contrast media or iodinated contrast media, and gadolinium (see 📖 p. 569)
• Use of ACEI and ARBs to slow progression and time to anuria (see 📖 pp. 92–5)
• Use of diuretics, e.g. loop diuretics to improve urine output
• Good control of BP
• Avoid episodes of hypercalcaemia
• Avoid dehydration and hypovolaemia
• Avoid urinary tract obstruction/UTI
• Stop IS drugs in failing Tx recipients.

Determining peritoneal membrane characteristics

The peritoneal equilibration test (PET) is the most commonly used test for determining the peritoneal membrane characteristics. It was developed by Twardowski et al. in the late 1980s as a standardized method to measure solute and fluid transport across the peritoneal membrane and categorize membrane characteristics.

- Enables individualized prescriptions as transport status varies between patients (see Table 11.7 📖 p. 278 for membrane characteristics)
- Performed at 6wks for new patients then annually unless otherwise clinically indicated
- ► May be inaccurate if undertaken earlier as it takes a few wks for the peritoneal membrane to adjust and stabilize

PET procedure

- CAPD—normal exchange the night before (allow 8–12hrs dwell time) and no morning exchange:
  - results not affected by different strength or type of dialysate
- APD—normal routine and if possible start the programme slightly earlier in the evening in order to finish earlier
- Connect to a 2L 2.27% or 2.5% dextrose dialysate and drain out for 20mins (not >25mins):
  - stand to make sure completely drained out and record this volume
- Complete the 'flush before fill' and then start to drain in the dialysate with the patient supine:
  - if the patient is able, roll from side to side whilst infusing every 400ml to ensure good fluid mixing and peritoneal membrane coverage
- If completed an adequacy test the day before, ensure this drain out bag is added to the sample and volume recorded
- Once draining in complete, drain out 200ml and collect a 10ml sample, then return the 190ml into the peritoneal cavity and cap off, this is 0 hour sample. The patient can now move around
- Samples of PD effluent are then taken at 2hrs and 4hrs and all samples are sent for measurement of Ur, Cr, Na^+, and glucose:
  - Cr levels are corrected for glucose interference
- A blood sample is taken at 2hrs and sent for Ur, Cr, Na^+, and glucose.

► At 4hrs the bag is drained out and the total volume recorded minus the 'flush before fill' volume.

To obtain the most accurate PET
- Perform correctly according to local procedure
- Patient in optimum health
- A well-functioning PD catheter—no drainage problems
  (see 📖 p. 289):
  - a large residual volume will affect results
- No evidence of active peritonitis or fluid overload
- Good glycaemic control (↑ serum BGLs can affect the results)
- >1 month post peritonitis episode.

PET results

PET results are plotted into the PET template which identifies the peritoneal membrane characteristics (see Figures 11.7 and 11.8) which include:
- Dialysate to plasma ratio (D/P)—calculated for Ur, Cr, and glucose
- 4hr dialysate and plasma Cr levels—used to calculate the Cr D/P ratio
- Dialysate glucose conc at 0, 2, and 4hrs—used as an internal control which provides the amount of glucose absorbed.

The D/P Cr and D/Do glucose results should be equivalent in 90% of tests—if not, then the test may need to be completed as an error has occurred (see p. 275).

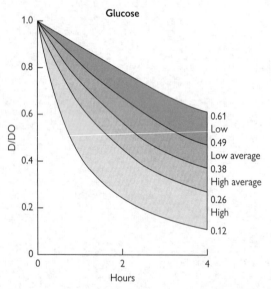

Fig. 11.7 Glucose test results. Reproduced with permission from Levy J, Brown E, Daley C, *et al. Oxford Handbook of Dialysis*, 3rd edn. Oxford University Press: Oxford; 2009.

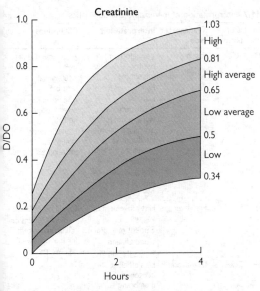

Fig. 11.8 Creatinine test results. Reproduced with permission from Levy J, Brown E, Daley C, et al. Oxford Handbook of Dialysis, 3rd edn. Oxford University Press: Oxford; 2009.

Interpretation of PET results

The most common membrane type is high-average and low average; 10% of the PD population are inherent high/fast transporters which can be difficult to manage. See Table 11.7 for peritoneal membrane characteristics and the most suitable mode of PD.

Table 11.7 Interpretation of membrane characteristics

D/P ratio creatinine	% of patients	Transporter type	Interpretation	PD options
0.82–1.03	10%	Fast/high	Very efficient peritoneal membrane Fast movement of solutes, ↑ absorption of glucose and loss of osmotic gradient—inefficient UF longer dwells and may absorb fluid May have poor UF Risk of low serum Alb	APD—need short dwell <180mins if possible icodextrin for day dwell if poor or no RRF Monitor serum albumin i.e. > protein loss
0.65–0.81	53%	High-average	Fast movement of solutes Efficient membrane Good UF and solute transport	CAPD or APD Avoid <120mins or >300mins, except for the long dwell, e.g. overnight
0.50–0.64	31%	Low-average	Less efficient peritoneal membrane Slow solutes transport Good UF	
0.34–0.49	6%	Slow/low	Inefficient peritoneal membrane Slow solute transport so osmotic gradient maintained for longer leading to very good UF	CAPD—need longer dwell time for solute transport >240mins ↑ volume rather than more exchanges APD is not suitable Very good UF—should not need icodextrin for long dwell

Modified PET test/simplified standard permeability analysis test

The modified PET test involves the use of a high strength dextrose dialysate, e.g. 3.86% or 4.25% left to dwell for 4hrs. Used if inadequate UF is suspected, e.g. in patients with high solute transport or UF <200ml to assess Na^+ sieving across the peritoneal vasculature by measuring the Na^+ D/P ratio at 1hr. Increasing the conc of dextrose in the dialysate does not affect the D/P Cr result.

Procedure

- Night prior:
  - CAPD patients: usual prescription (8–12hrs dwell)
  - APD: usual prescription, last fill with 1.36% (light) if they normally use icodextrin as interferes with the laboratory readings
- Pre-procedure assessment: BP lying and standing and weight, if signs of dehydration—refer to medical staff prior to commencement:
  - check BGL in diabetes:
  - standard permeability analysis (SPA) test documentation—record the strength of the high dextrose dialysate, e.g. 3.86% or 4.25% as the laboratory will need to correct for the measurement of Cr (dextrose interferes with the assay)
- Connect as per unit normal procedure
- SPA test commencement:
  - The procedure is the same as a PET, see 📖 p. 274
  - PD effluent samples are taken at 0, 1, 2hrs for Cr and glucose
  - 2hrs blood sample for Ur, Cr, glucose, and Na^+
  - at 4hrs drain out in a standing position, mix the bag and take a 10ml sample.

UFF is defined as <400ml/24hrs in the absence of any PD catheter malfunction or presence of a fluid leak[6].

Interpretation of SPA test

D/P ratio of Na^+ at 1hr after a 3.86% solution instilled
- Low ratio: 0.81–0.85 implies Na^+ sieving is occurring
- Higher ratio: 0.87–0.94 implies less efficient Na^+ sieving
- Total volume pre-flush <400ml = UFF.

Other methods for determining peritoneal membrane characteristics

FAST PET

A FAST PET can be started at home as it only requires one collection sample (for Cr and glucose) at 4hrs.

Mini-PET

Quantifies free water transport via the ultrasmall pores or aquaporin-1 channels.

Double mini-PET

Information on aquaporin function, i.e. free water transport. 2 PETs using a 1.36% and 3.86% dialysate with 1hr dwells. Gives initial UF volume, e.g. if shorter dwells are more suitable, however it does not provide an estimate of fluid reabsorption which can be the cause of UFF.

Personal dialysis capacity (PDC) test

Uses a kinetic modelling programme based on the 3-pore theory (see 📖 p. 246) and reflects available effective surface area for diffusion, reabsorption, and flow via the large pores and ∴ potential for inflammation. 5 exchanges of different dextrose conc in 24hrs (at 2, 3, 4, 5 10hrs). Blood samples are then taken for Ur, Cr, glucose, and albumin.

- Can be performed at home but patient performs 5 exchanges of different dextrose strengths at specific times, has to take a sample from each drain bag and collect a 24hr urine sample ∴ ↑ risk of inaccuracies
- Good prognostic tool for inflammation
- APD need to convert to CAPD for the test
- Labour intensive if performed within the clinical area
- ↑ cost as requires more laboratory tests
- Modelling programme assumptions may not be correct for patient
- Does not measure Na^+ movement, i.e. Na^+ sieving capacity.

Dialysis adequacy and transport test (DATT)

Requires sample from blood and 24hr dialysate of the patient's normal regimen. Calculates 24-hr D/P ratio, but only validated for $4 \times 2L$ CAPD (not APD). Similar to FAST PET, only provides solute clearance data.

Accelerated peritoneal examination test (APEX)

Gives a single number for both glucose and Ur peritoneal permeability, e.g. signifies the time glucose and Ur cross equilibration curves i.e. optimal UF dwell time. A shorter APEX time ≈high peritoneal membrane permeability. This test is quicker than a PET, but not often used clinically.

Peritoneal function test (PFT)

Involves the assessment of the total delivered treatment for Ur, Cr, protein, calorie intake, fluid balance, and peritoneal transport. Requires the use of Patient On-line™ kinetic modelling software. The results reflect the time taken for 50% equilibrium to have been reached between the dialysate and plasma (Pt50). Not commonly used in the UK.

Prescription management

In order to facilitate adherence with the new prescription regimen, and to ensure that any changes required have as minimal an impact on their life as possible, it is essential to involve the patient and family/carer in the prescription management process. There needs to be a balance made between the 'ideal' treatments and maintaining the best possible QOL for the patient/family/carer. In more complex cases decisions should be discussed at MPT meetings to find the best solution for the patient and family/carer.

Prescription regimens

When considering the most suitable CAPD and APD regimens, consideration should be given to various factors as outlined in Table 11.8.

Table 11.8 Factors to consider when prescribing PD

CAPD	APD
Exchange volume	Exchange volume
Size of the patient	Dwell time
Number of exchanges	Number of cycles
Timing of exchanges	Total number of hrs required
Total UF required	Dry or wet day
RRF	Any additional day exchanges required
	Total UF required
	RRF (may have dry day if high)

New CAPD regimen

- Exchange volume:
    - an average size person will require 2L, may require 2.5–3L for larger patients
    - smaller patients may need to start at 1.5L if unable to tolerate
- Commence 4 exchanges per day (3 during the day and 1 overnight), may ↓ 3 if good RRF
- Commence on all 1.36% dextrose dialysate, including overnight
- Peritoneal membrane characteristics are not known initially:
    - review of UF volume from each exchange to assess UF capability
    - check not absorbing from overnight exchange
    - if possible trial a medium exchange during training wk to assess response and UF volume

If commencing dialysis <2wks post insertion of a new PD catheter, commence with smaller volumes (e.g. 1L) as there is an ↑ risk of fluid leaks and gradually increase the volume as tolerated.

New APD regimen

Vary according to the amount of RRF, e.g. whether they require a 'wet' day for example:

- Commence on 10hrs if good RRF
  - 2L fill volume with 90mins dwell time, i.e. $5 \times 2L$
  - drain in 10mins and drain out 20mins.

The immediate use of a new PD catheter requires close monitoring, see Figure 11.9 for an example of immediate use of PD catheter using IPD.

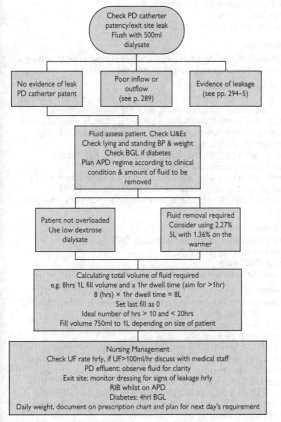

Fig. 11.9 Example of immediate use PD using IPD.

Inadequate dialysis and/or ultrafiltration

Possible causes

- Incorrect prescription for transport status
- Loss of RRF without altering prescription
- Mechanical problems, e.g. drainage problems
- UFF (see 📖 pp. 318–19)
- Unable to tolerate/cope with changes to prescription, e.g. social, hernia, leak, abdominal discomfort
- Large BSA and anuric
- Non-adherence to prescription regimen.

Assessment

Multiple factors need to be assessed and considered prior to making any changes to the PD prescription which includes:

General overall health

- The patient's perception of their health; for example, a 88yr-old man may have a poor adequacy result, yet he feels well in himself.
- Presence of uraemic symptoms, e.g. nausea, pruritus, uraemic breath
- Evidence of malnutrition, e.g. ↓ Alb, weight loss, muscle wasting, hypercatabolic state, e.g. sepsis
- Check serum Na^+, K^+ and HCO_3, Ca^{2+} and PO_4, e.g. acidotic, hyperkalaemic to exclude other causes
- Check serum Ur—↓ Ur adequate dialysis, ↓ protein intake, fluid overload or ↑ inadequate dialysis, catabolic state or ↓ RRF
- Cr is not a reliable indicator as varies depending on body mass (see 📖 p. 42).

Fluid status

- Undertake a fluid assessment (see 📖 p. 587)
- Lying and standing BP, weight
- Assess fluid intake
- Assess RRF volume—check 24hr urine volume, e.g. ↓ RRF.

Inadequate UF

- Review patients PD diary and prescription regimen, is there ↑ use of hypertonic dialysate?
- Assess for absorption on long dwell
  - review UF data on APD machine
  - CAPD—check volume drained from overnight exchange
- Patient may need to weigh drain out bags for 24hrs to assess UF of each exchange (▶ subtract the 'flush before fill' from each bag)
- Diabetes control, e.g. ↑ BGL affects osmotic gradient ∴ UF
- Loss of solute transport and UF capacity as a result of peritonitis, e.g. recent episode of peritonitis (<8wks) will affect the peritoneal membrane permeability and UF function
- Mechanical cause, e.g. loss of effective peritoneal membrane surface area as a result of adhesions, drainage problems, constipation.

PD prescription
- Assess adherence with the PD prescription, e.g. completing all of their exchanges, are they finishing early on APD, are they ordering enough fluid stock? Has the patient changed their dwell times, e.g. undertaking a different regimen from that which was prescribed?
- Inadequate prescribed time on APD machine
- Correct prescription for their peritoneal membrane characteristics
- Impact of long-term PD, e.g. fatigued with having to do exchanges often referred to as 'burn out'.

Prescription adjustment

With time on PD, membrane characteristics may change which, along with the loss of RRF, → inadequate dialysis and/or UF. This will require the adjustment of the PD prescription (see Table 11.9 for prescription changes to increase solute clearance and UF for both CAPD and APD regimens).

Key points
- If no PET result, experiment with different dialysates strengths
- Monitor adequacy and RRF regularly
- Dietary restriction of Na^+ and fluid restriction
- Preserve RRF—consider the use of diuretics (see 📖 p. 273)
- Check correct prescription to suit the peritoneal membrane characteristics
- The use of kinetic modelling programmes (e.g. Adequest 2.0™) provides options for prescription regimens, e.g. change mode from CAPD to APD for high/fast transporter status
- Predict UF and plan regimens using creative timing as not all high or high average can be switched to APD, e.g. use temporal profiles, e.g. 1.36% high/fast or high average start absorbing >2hrs, whereas a low or low average >4–6hrs
- Icodextrin provides sustained UF for all transport states
- ↓ calorie load by using icodextrin and/or Nutrineal® to prevent weight gain and unstable diabetes
- Use the whole 24hrs to maximize the dialysis time, e.g. preferably avoid 'dry days' or dry time, e.g. APD patients
- Review exchange drain volumes at clinic appointments, in particular if ↑ BP and fluid overload for early identification of absorption problems, e.g. APD day dwell and CAPD night dwell and switch to icodextrin
- Assess the impact of additional exchanges or time on APD, e.g. QOL, normal daily routine, on family/carers
- Early assessment and interventions for UFF, e.g. long-term damage which has altered peritoneal membrane permeability, defective aquaporin system, high/fast transporter
- ↓ cardiac output, e.g. HF or hypotension → circulatory blood flow → ↓ peritoneal capillary blood flow, ↓ perfusion of the peritoneal membrane ∴ ↓ solute clearance.

Table 11.9 Prescription adjustments for CAPD and APD regimens to increase solute clearance and/or UF

	Adjustment	Advantages/disadvantages
CAPD regimen		
↑ solute clearance	↑ exchange fill vol, e.g. 2L to 2.5L Smaller patients may only tolerate 1.5L Initially ↑ vol of overnight exchange e.g. ↓ IAP in supine position and less feeling of fullness and discomfort.	Flexible Less impact on normal routine, more likely to adhere to new regimen ↑ 3L risk of back pain, abdominal discomfort hernia and fluid leak
↑ UF and solute clearance	High/fast transporter may need to transfer to APD ↑ no exchanges, icodextrin overnight dwell and ↑ vol if large BSA	Patient may not wish to transfer Adherence problems due to impact on normal routine
↑ UF	Adjust the timing of exchanges to suit the peritoneal membrane characteristics e.g. high average transporter, use 3 exchanges 3–4 hrs apart and icodextrin overnight (8, 3, 15, 18 hrs)	± more problematic for patient to manage during the day Adherence problems
	Higher conc dextrose PD dialysate on 2nd or 3rd exchange (e.g. 2.27%). Do not use high conc overnight. Icodextrin for overnight especially if absorbing fluid	May affect BGL, ↑ calorie load, weight gain
↓ RRF ↑ UF (same for APD)	Diuretics Adjust fluid allowance rather than using high dextrose PD dialysate Consider icodextrin	Adherence problems to ↓ fluid allowance

Table 11.9 (Continued)

	Adjustment	Advantages/ disadvantages
APD regimen		
↑ solute clearance	↑ 2.5 to 3L fill volume	No impact on normal routine Less ↑ IAP as supine
	↑ dwell time e.g. 60–90mins e.g. low and low average transporters	± ↑ overall time required ±impact on normal routine
	↑ no of cycles e.g. high/fast transporter may improve solute clearance. May not be able to ↓ dwell time of each cycle →↓ UF volume	± ↑ overall time required and impact on normal routine
	Overall time on APD ▶ Check the drain time is not too long and set for 20mins e.g. and not 30mins Low average need more dwell time →↑ overall time	± ↑ overall time required and impact on normal routine
	Stop dry day—use the whole 24hrs for dialysis, last fill with icodextrin	No impact
	Additional exchange—perform CAPD exchange during the day, e.g. off machine at 7:30 am with last fill icodextrin, then evening exchange at 5 pm, back on machine at 10 pm. Could be ↑ to 2/day	Negative impact on QOL and cause adherence problems
↑ UF volume	Use icodextrin long day dwell	No impact
↑ UF and solute clearance— anuric	↑ vol, ↑ no. cycles, ↑ overall time and add day bag	↑ overall time required may impact on normal routine—possible transfer to HD if unable to manage

Case study 1

- A 83yr-old man with Kt/Vurea of 1.62, low-average transporter status who states he feels well in himself and has no symptoms of uraemia or fluid overload.
- To ↑ adequacy to reach a Kt/Vurea >1.7 would involve either adding an additional exchange or ↑ the exchange volume from 2L to 2.5L:
  - discussion at MPT meeting identifies he is also the carer for his wife who has early dementia
  - patient does not wish to undertake an additional exchange and does not feel an APD machine would be suitable as he cares for his wife who gets up at night
- The decision is made not to alter his regimen as it will negatively impact on his QOL by adding further burden of another day time exchange and the patient feels well.

Case study 2

A 48yr-old has been on CAPD for 2yrs with 2 episodes of peritonitis. He works 3 days a week and has 2 teenage children. He was a low average transporter, adequacy Kt/Vurea 1.89, CrCl 58L/week/1.73m². On his routine clinic appointment he states he is very tired and not feeling as well as previously. He has no RRF and his creatinine and urea levels have increased.

- His current CAPD prescription is 2 × 1.36% and 1 × 3.86% and a 1.36% overnight. His total UF is 400ml and he absorbing from his overnight exchange
- A repeat adequacy and PET is organized and the results show his Kt/Vurea is now 1.6 and CrCl 55L/week and now high average transporter:
  - option 1: ↑ volume to 2.5L × 3 1.36% to ↑ solute clearance and use icodextrin overnight to ↑ UF and ↓ glucose exposure
  - option 2: ↑ volume and number of exchanges to 5/day
  - option 3: switch to APD with icodextrin during the day as he now needs shorter dwell times
- Discussion with the patient he opts for option 3 as it will fit in better with his lifestyle.

Non-infectious complications

The most common non-infectious complications include:

- Drainage/outflow problems—occur as a result of an inability of the effluent to drain out (outflow) or to drain in (inflow). Drainage problems need to be rectified before instilling more dialysate as it may → ↑ IPP and cause leakage of the fluid into the SC tissue.
  - inadequate outflow (drain out time >20mins or incomplete) is a common complication and occurs in about 5–20%
  - assessment involves history taking, examination, AXR and a rapid exchange to check inflow and outflow
  - causes include: constipation, PD catheter malfunction, malpositioned PD catheter, kinking of the PD catheter, migration of the PD catheter tip
  - other causes—omental occlusion, adhesions, bladder distention, fibrin/blood clot
- Fluid leaks
- Haemoperitoneum
- Hernia
- PD-related pain
- PD catheter accidents
- Other problems
- Cuff protrusion
- Rectal and vaginal prolapse.

Constipation

This is a common complication often seen with a newly placed PD catheter, although it can happen at any time. Poor flow (usually slow and erratic) results from the inability of dialysate to drain freely as bowel full of faeces is pushed against the peritoneal cavity creating voids which fill with dialysate. If unresolved it can lead to movement of the PD catheter tip.

Assessment
- History, abdominal examination
- AXR is only required if constipation ruled out as cause.

Common causes
- Low-fibre diet, e.g. ↓ K^+ diet or poor appetite
- ↓ activity or exercise
- Dehydration
- Hypercalcaemia
- Drugs, e.g. phosphate binders, iron supplementation
- Elderly who are more susceptible
- Other conditions/diseases, e.g. CVA, diabetes, uraemia, systemic diseases such as SLE.

Nursing considerations
- Bowel preparation pre-insertion to ↓ risk of PD catheter migration
- Acute constipation—non-Mg^{2+}/PO_4 aperients, e.g. Picolax®, lactulose
- Provide dietary advice and/or refer to the renal dietitian
- ↑ fibre content of diet:
  - if on low K^+ diet, offer other alternatives
- Medication review
- Check Ca^{2+} level
- Assess for signs of dehydration and set fluid intake against IBW
- Patient education on the complications associated with constipation:
  - bowel action needed daily to maintain good drainage
- Use of regular aperients
- Encourage exercise.

Peritoneal dialysis catheter malfunction

Malpositioned PD catheter

Presents with poor fluid drainage (in and/or out) of a newly inserted PD catheter. An AXR will show the PD catheter out of position.

Kinking of the PD catheter

Usually presents soon after a new PD catheter is inserted with either poor drainage in and/or out, and is commonly positional, i.e. patient can drain out if lying on their side or standing.

▶Check that the external PD catheter segment is not kinked under the dressing.

Migration of the PD catheter tip

Usually seen soon after insertion and causes poor outflow (may also occur later); this may also be positional, e.g. the patient drains well only when lying on their side.
- Constipation due to the peristaltic action of the bowel
- Shoulder tip pain may occur if tip rubbing on the diaphragm
- An AXR will show whether the PD catheter tip is in the correct position in the pelvis or has migrated under the diaphragm
- ↑ residual volume on PET test >250ml.

Nursing considerations

PD catheter malposition or kinked
- Re-position PD catheter either surgically, laparoscopically or under fluoroscopy—a wire is used to move or straighten (if kinked) the PD catheter back into the ideal position
- It may be necessary to suture the PD catheter in place in the pelvic region to prevent further migration

PD catheter migration
Use of aperients, e.g. Picolax®, as the peristaltic action of the gut may move the PD catheter back in to position:
- May require re-positioning the PD catheter
- Prevention of constipation measures.

Other causes

Omental occlusion

Blockage of the PD catheter's small tip perforations can occur if the omentum sticks to the PD catheter leading to drainage problems. This may not be seen for some wks following insertion of the PD catheter.
- A laparoscopic or surgical omentectomy to free up the PD catheter tip.

Adhesions

Previous abdominal surgery or repeated episodes of peritonitis are predisposing factors for abdominal adhesions. If the PD catheter tip is placed in a position surrounded by adhesions it may reduce inflow and outflow and presents early.

- Contrast x-ray or CT scan may be required to visualize adhesions
- Adhesiolysis
- Surgical repositioning or stitching the PD catheter into pelvis
- If unable to resolve will require permanent switch to HD.

Bladder distention

Bladder distention can cause outflow problems as the fullness of the bladder may obstruct the tip of PD catheter. Review by medical staff to identify the underlying cause of bladder distention, e.g. prostatic hypertrophy and insertion of urinary catheter.

Fibrin/blood clot

Fibrin occurs as a result of protein formation from fibrinogen in the blood as part of the normal clotting cascade. Strands of fibrin lead to poor drainage (i.e. inflow and outflow) and is usually seen in the drain out bag as pieces of 'cotton wool'. This can also occur with blood clots.

Nursing considerations

- IP heparin (500 units/L) in subsequent exchanges for 3 consecutive days
- Milk the tubing to see if you can free up the PD catheter
- Some units may use a 5ml saline flush to forcibly flush the PD catheter directly into the tip
- Urokinase or alteplase may be used to dissolve fibrin clots which is instilled directly into the PD catheter and left for a minimum of 2hrs in order to breakdown the fibrin clot.

Fluid leaks

Early exit site leak

In a new PD catheter, a dialysate leak out of the exit site is usually a result of incomplete healing of the exit site prior to use, i.e. the cuffs have not fully embedded into the abdominal muscle. Weak abdominal muscles (e.g. prior abdominal surgery, multiple pregnancies) predispose to leak, i.e. weak muscles unable to cope with ↑ IAP.

• ↑ risk of an exit site infection.

Clinical features and assessment

• Visible staining on the removed dressing which may have a gold/yellow appearance
  • test the exit site fluid/exudate for the presence of glucose with a urinary reagent strip—+ve indicative of dialysate
  • low drain volume and overall total UFA peritoneal scintigraphy or CT scan after infusion of contrast dialysate to confirm location of the leak.

Nursing considerations

• Stop PD exchanges and rest for 2wks
• Regular checks of U&Es, frequency will depend on stability of the patient's condition
• May require temporary HD
• If temporary HD not an option and the patient cannot hold off PD, may require supine low fill volume APD/IPD with dry days
• ± prophylactic antibiotics to prevent any infection
• Re-starting PD
  • use small volumes ↑ gradually over a couple of wks to standard volumes
  • observe exit site routinely for signs of re-leaking
• Failure to heal may require surgery.

Later fluid leaks

Although the tissue around the exit site has healed preventing fluid leakage, dialysate may leak from the peritoneal cavity into the surrounding tissue. Fluid leaks can also be the result of poor drainage, e.g. 2° to continued instillation of dialysate, without draining out properly → dialysate leaks in to SC tissue.

Clinical features and assessment

• SC tissue of the abdomen and/or upper legs may have an orange peel 'peau d'orange' appearance
• Assess the genital region for any signs of swelling/oedema:
  • may appear as a hydrocoele or hernia in ♂ dialysate leaks into a patent processus vaginalis and down in to the scrotum. A hydrocoele may require a scrotal aspirate to test for the presence of glucose, i.e. dialysate

- scrotal leaks or recurrence of abdominal leak will need investigating for the presence of a hernia
- vulval region can become engorged with fluid and appears swollen. More commonly seen with newly inserted PD catheters
- ± CT peritoneogram with non-ionic contrast to locate the leak.

Nursing considerations
- Abdominal leak only—stop PD for 2–4wks, hold off dialysis if possible
- Regular bloods tests for U&Es, if unable to hold then re-start on low volumes
- Assess for an underlying problem of poor drainage (see 📖 p. 289)
- US with full dwell to show up leak site
- If leak not identified on US, CT with contrast or MRI
- Whilst waiting for surgical repair—use nocte APD only with low volume in the day dwell or CAPD low volume or continue rest if RRF is adequate
- Reposition PD catheter if continues to leak to a new site.

Pleuroperitoneal leak
Pleural leaks occur as a result of a defect in the diaphragm which allows dialysate to leak in to the pleural space with the ↑ IAP. This condition resolves spontaneously in 40% of patients.

Clinical features and assessment
- Present with pleural effusion which may require draining, test for the presence of glucose, i.e. dialysate
- Confirmation using a contrast peritoneogram or sulphur colloid instilled in to the peritoneum.

Nursing considerations
- May require pleurodesis
- Temporary HD to allow pleura to heal—requires regular check of U&Es
- ↓ IAP, e.g. switch to APD.

Haemoperitoneum

PD effluent can become blood stained when blood enters peritoneal cavity and appears pale pink in colour (rosé).

Causes
- Common post-op after insertion of new PD catheter or repositioning
- Menstruation (~50% of menstruating ♀ on PD), endometriosis or retrograde menstruation (at time of period) and ovulation (mid-cycle)
- Abdominal surgery, e.g. Tx nephrectomy
- Procedures, e.g. colonoscopy
- ↑ physical activity, e.g. straining and lifting heavy objects
- Consider possibility of underlying condition or disease, e.g. cyst rupture, polycystic kidney disease, ovarian, liver, kidney tumour (± haematuria present), pancreatitis, ruptured spleen
- Pregnancy (see 📖 pp. 545–6)
- Femoral or retroperitoneal haematoma, ruptured aneurysm
- Peritonitis (uncommon)
- Complications associated with long-term PD usage—encapsulating peritoneal sclerosis (EPS) (see 📖 pp. 320–1), peritoneal calcification.

Assessment

Patient assessment over the telephone
- Unwell—attend clinic
- Asymptomatic—save drain out bag and perform another exchange to check for presence of blood:
  - if no blood, then continue normal exchange regimen
  - if blood still present, complete the exchange and attend PD unit with the initial drain out bag.

In the PD unit
- Assess the severity and amount of bleeding, e.g. heavy or light in appearance
- Assess the frequency of bleeding, e.g. has the bleeding occurred before?
- Assess for the presence of other symptoms, e.g. pain with rupture cysts, other bleeding (e.g. rectal, spontaneous bruising)
- Do they have regular menses?
- Recent history of surgery or procedure, e.g. colonoscopy, trauma to patient or PD catheter. Sudden, lifting of a heavy object can result in a small peritoneal capillary trauma
- Review medications, e.g. aspirin or anticoagulants.

Nursing considerations
- Mild, blood-stained PD effluent:
  - send PD effluent for MC&S—RBC count
  - bloods for FBC, serum amylase (>40U/L may indicate perforated ulcer)
  - reassure patient, and perform rapid exchanges until the PD effluent is clear or light rosé in colour (may take 1–4 rapids to clear)
  - ± instillation of 500 units/L heparin/exchange to prevent clotting if heavily blood stained
- Heavily blood-stained fluid with symptoms of pain and fever:
  - refer to medical staff to assess for underlying intra-abdominal cause, e.g. ruptured cyst, kidney tumour, ruptured aneurysm
  - PD fluid should be sent for MC&S
  - PD HCT >2% requires urgent surgical referral
  - ± CT scan, US, or MRI to identify underlying cause.

The management is dependent on identification and treatment of the underlying cause:
- Menstruation—usually resolves quickly:
  - ± US if menstruating ♀ to check for ovarian cyst or tumour
  - recurrent problems, OCP can prevent ovulation and bleeding
- Anticoagulants—review aspirin or anticoagulant by medical staff
- Trauma—usually resolves quickly, use cooler PD fluid (i.e. room temperature) → peritoneal vasoconstriction and ↓ bleeding.

Hernia

The presence of a hernia is common (~9–20% of patients). Hernias are caused by the increase in IAP and/or high fluid dialysate volumes. Incisional hernias are the most common type and are associated with the PD catheter insertion or prior abdominal surgery. Inguinal and umbilical hernia are also common. If hernias are detected in the pre-dialysis stage they should be repaired prior to insertion of the PD catheter.

Clinical features
- Fluid leaks in to the subcutaneous tissue, e.g. genital oedema.

> **Nursing considerations**
> - Pre-surgical repair:
>   - ↓ fluid volume, APD nocte or IPD if there is a delay to correct with surgery, i.e. ↓ IAP when supine
>   - ± temporary HD if still continue to leak until repaired
> - Post repair:
>   - temporary HD or IPD postoperatively for a few wks as commencing PD too soon may cause the hernia to recur
>   - start with small volumes initially, gradually ↑ after 2–3wks as tolerated
> - Recurrent hernia:
>   - surgical repair using polypropylene mesh
>   - model for dry day and APD as this may be suitable, in particular with good RRF, i.e. no dialysate in situ standing which ↑ IAP. This will require close monitoring and repeat adequacies more frequently
>   - patient can wear a supportive girdle for abdominal hernia or truss for an inguinal hernia
>   - switch to HD permanently if continues to recur.

Specific peritoneal dialysis-related pain

The 3 most common types of pain are back, shoulder tip, and inflow which can significantly impact on the patient's QOL and ability to perform normal daily functions.

Back pain

The older person is especially at risk of back pain as a result of age-related degenerative changes as are those with a history of back problems, e.g. disc degeneration, osteoarthritis and spondylitis, prior abdominal surgery weakening the abdominal muscles, or the use of corticosteroids. If the abdominal muscles become weak a resultant lordosis occurs, which is exacerbated by the peritoneal fluid load, which further weakens the abdominal muscles.

Nursing considerations

- Analgesia and/or antispasmodics drugs
- Strengthen back muscles—refer for physiotherapy and back education
- Rarely may require blood tests, x-ray to rule out underlying diseases, e.g. tumour, inflammatory arthritis
- Review adequacy and PET results and assess whether PD regimen can be altered:
  - ↓ day PD dialysate volume if on CAPD
  - switch to APD, i.e. IAP ↓ when supine
  - ± consider switching to HD permanently if unresolvable and affecting QOL.

Shoulder tip pain

This can occur when infusing dialysate and is referred pain 2° to air trapped under the diaphragm or ↑ IAP. This is more common in new patients in the first few wks. It appears to occur less commonly in coiled PD catheters.

Nursing considerations

- Does not require any treatment as usually resolves after 10–20mins
- ± oral analgesia prior to starting exchange if the patient is finding the exchange distressing
- ± benefit from moving around whilst infusing the exchange.

Inflow pain

Inflow pain is a common problem for new patients caused by either the initial effect of acidic PD dialysate or the 'jet effect' of fluid exiting the small openings at the tip end of the PD catheter. Normally these symptoms settle and do not require any treatment. The PD catheter tip can get pushed up against the bowel wall (particularly if constipated) and lead to discomfort. Hot or cold PD dialysate will also cause some discomfort.

Nursing considerations

- Inflow pain as a result of acidic solution:
  - consider the use of a more biocompatible dialysate with a higher pH, e.g. Physioneal®
  - instil 1% lidocaine into dialysate prior to draining in
- Inflow pain as a result of the 'jet effect':
  - ↓ inflow rate, e.g. use a clamp on the inflow line to slow down the fluid
  - tidal APD—↓ tug/pull sensation close to completion of draining out
- Other causes:
  - constipation—treat with dietary advice and aperients
  - trapped wind can be very painful and may be relieved by peppermint oil, and review of medications, e.g. ↓ lactulose dose
  - AXR to check the PD catheter position is correct if pain persists
  - check dialysate is not too hot or cold
  - check patient is not putting the PD fluid in the microwave as it gives uneven distribution of heat resulting in potential pockets of hot/cold fluid
- If all treatment fails to resolve—need to consider replacing the PD catheter.

Other problems

Cuff extrusion

Caused by erosion of the catheter cuff through the skin as a result of an exit site infection or inadequate depth of placement of the cuff.
- Treatment involves shaving the cuff or, if repeated infections, removal of PD catheter. In this case, if there is no active infection, a simultaneous removal and replacement of PD catheter can be done

Rectal and vaginal prolapse

Prolapse is an uncommon complication of ↑ IAP. Treatment is surgical repair which will require temporary HD for a few wks. Once re-starting, commence with low volumes gradually increasing as tolerated.

PD catheter accidents

- Cut/break to the PD catheter—unintentionally cutting the PD catheter:
  - using scissors to cut tape or dressing too close to the PD catheter
  - shaving catheter cuff or during insertion of the catheter in theatre
- Contamination of the PD catheter:
  - touch contamination of PD extension line tip when removing or replacing the cap
  - attempted removal of blockage down the catheter using a foreign object.

Nursing considerations

Cut/break to the PD catheter
- Clamp the PD catheter above the break/cut using a blue plastic clamp (other clamping devices, with serrated edges, may cause trauma to PD catheter) and attend the PD unit as soon as possible
- *Sufficient PD catheter length left before the break:* the PD catheter can be cut and a titanium connector applied
  - *Only be undertaken by PD or medical staff*
  - the external segment can be repaired using a glue kit if there is sufficient catheter left to glue on the new segment (>15mm)
  - cut catheter and attach new segment, glue under sterile conditions as per local policy—remains in a special glue case until set (~24hrs)
  - IP prophylactic antibiotics—↓ risk of contamination peritonitis
  - cannot use PD catheter for 24hrs. There will be some absorption of the dialysate—monitor weight, BP, and check U&Es
  - unstable patients—discuss with medical team, e.g. if hyperkalaemic.
- *Insufficient PD catheter length to glue*—PD catheter will need to be removed and replaced

Contamination of PD catheter extension line
- Clamp the PD catheter as close to the exit site as possible without removing the dressing and attend the unit as soon as possible
- Line change, perform exchange and drain out PD effluent—any possible contamination will be drained out (see 📖 p. 332)
- Instillation of IP prophylactic antibiotics depends on local policy
  - if no fluid has been drained in or out, may not require antibiotics.
- ⚠ ► Advise patient to observe closely for next 24–48hrs for signs of peritonitis and contact the unit immediately.

Infectious complications: exit site infection

The three most common organisms associated with exit site infections (ESIs) are *Staphylococcus aureus* (50%), *S. epidermidis*, and *Pseudomonas* species.

- ESIs that lead to peritonitis, or present concurrently with peritonitis, will usually require removal of PD catheter, except for coagulase −ve *S. aureus* infections which often respond to treatment
- Aggressive treatment for *S. aureus* and *P. aeruginosa* is needed as associated with the development of peritonitis
- Replace PD catheter for recurrent, relapsing or refractory *P. aeruginosa* exit site infection to prevent peritonitis. Remove PD catheter if peritonitis develops and rest from PD
- Other causative organisms include diphtheroids, fungi, and streptococci.

The ISPD defines an exit site infection as:

The presence of purulent discharge, with or without erythema of the skin at the catheter-epidermal interface.

- Assessment requires good knowledge of the clinical features and appearance of both a healthy and infected exit site, e.g. differentiating between the presence of an infection or skin allergy (no discharge at the exit site with peri-catheter erythema)
- In a new exit site the early signs of an infection are:
  - lack of a normal healing process
  - purulent exudate
  - granulation tissue to the sinus tract by the 2nd wk.

Assessment and diagnosis

- Assess exit site for signs of infection, discharge, and pain:
  - check for pyrexia
  - check exchange effluent is clear if tunnel infection suspected
- If serous exudate, rule out PD fluid leak—tends to appear as a golden 'halo' on the old dressing (see 📖 p. 294)
- Swab exit site and send for MC&S prior to cleaning the exit site
- Score, and document on exit site chart, using the ISPD exit site scoring system[5] which calculates presence of infection (see Table 11.10).

Table 11.10 ISPD exit site scoring system.[7] Interpretation: infection if score ≥4; however, purulent discharge alone is enough to indicate infection. <4 may or may not indicate infection

Appearance	0 points	1 point	2 points
Swelling	No	Exit only <0.5cm	>0.5cm/or tunnel
Crust	No	<0.5cm	>0.5cm
Redness	No	<0.5cm	>0.5cm
Pain	No	Slight	Severe
Drainage	No	Serous	Purulent

Nursing considerations

- Clean exit site with normal saline or according to local policy
- Apply clean dry dressing, ensure PD catheter is securely anchored
- Commence empiric antibiotics (as per local policy) which should cover *S. aureus* and *P aeruginosa* organisms, e.g. ciprofloxacin, cefalexin, or flucloxacillin
- Check culture and sensitivities after 48hrs and that the correct antibiotics are prescribed according to sensitivities:
  - treatment is usually for 14 days
  - +ve exit site culture with normal appearance is likely to indicate colonization rather than an infection. This will involve thorough antiseptic cleaning
- *Pseudomonas* infections are more problematic to treat:
  - requires the use of 2 antibiotics, e.g. fluoroquinolones, aminoglycosides, ceftazidime
- Unresolved after 3wks—simultaneous removal and replacement of PD catheter (see 📖 p. 313)
- MRSA treat with clindamycin, doxycycline
- Re-educate and train patient if result of poor technique and care.

Tunnel infection

ESIs can track down the PD catheter and lead to a tunnel infection. The most common organisms are:
- *Staphylococcus aureus*
- *Pseudomonas aeruginosa*.

Assessment
- Assess the exit site track for signs of erythema, swelling, pain, and tenderness or any changes to the exit site itself, e.g. induration

Nursing considerations

- Oral or IV antibiotics
- May require removal of PD catheter
- If cuff protrusion occurs, it is possible to shave the cuff off using an aseptic technique
- ▶ Only to be performed by a specialist PD nurse or medical staff.
- Normal examination does not exclude infection, if tunnel infection suspected and there is no external evidence an US or CT scan may be required to assess for any SC tissue changes around the PD catheter.

Peritonitis

Early detection, diagnosis, and treatment of peritonitis is vital in order to preserve the effective functioning of the peritoneal membrane. Peritonitis rates have markedly reduced over the last 10yrs as a result of various improvements to the management of PD such as:
- Improved PD catheter materials and insertion techniques
- Connectology such as the 'Y' set providing a 'flush before fill' system
- Effective prevention management programmes
- Quality control and regular auditing, e.g. of causative organisms for peritonitis and route of infection to target changes in clinical practice:
  - computer software programmes are available which can be used to monitor and record infectious complications of PD.

In spite of all of these advances and improved preventative measures, peritonitis remains the most common and most serious complication of PD (see Table 11.11 for route of transmission and associated organism).
- Peritonitis accounts for 15–35% of renal hospital admissions
- Associated with high mortality rates
- Major cause of technique failure and transfer to permanent HD.

Higher peritonitis rates are associated with:
- Poor nutritional and/or inflammatory state—↓ serum Alb levels at the commencement of PD
- Use of IS
- HIV +ve patients—↑ rate of Gram −ve and fungal organisms
- Fungal peritonitis associated with previous treatment with antibiotics
- ↑ risk of Gram −ve peritonitis associated with constipation, use of gastric acid inhibitors
- Children (associated with URTI)
- Possible association with depression as a result of poor technique (e.g. loss of interest) altered immune system 2° depression
- Some ethnic groups, e.g. African Americans
- Substance abuse history
- Lower socio-economic groups
- Associated risk factors for age, gender, or diabetes.

Table 11.11 Peritonitis infection routes and causative organism

Route	Mechanism	Organism
Intraluminal Main cause of peritonitis Incubation period 24–48hrs	Touch contamination: bacteria from skin/surface transmitted via PD catheter	S. epidermidis S. aureus (~50% of cases) Pseudomonas Yeast Corynebacterium Bacillus Pasteurella (associated with cats) Proteus
Periluminal	PD catheter-related exit site and tunnel infections. *Biofilm formation from colonization of bacteria	S. aureus Pseudomonas Proteus Yeast
Transmural/enteric	Bowel, abdominal perforation ↑ risk with diverticulitis. Acute treatment of constipation	Gram −ve organisms, e.g. E. coli Anaerobes
Haematogenous	Bloodstream **Dental procedures **Sigmoidoscopy	Streptococcus, e.g. dental Mycobacterium
Ascending/vaginal	Vaginal via fallopian tubes Intrauterine devices **Gynaecology procedures Vaginal dialysate leak	Candida Pseudomonas

*Biofilm: bacteria become attached the surface of the PD catheter and in the long-term become resistant to antibiotics. May form a protective layer preventing adequate exposure to antibiotic, especially if the bacterium is slime producing, e.g. S. epidermidis, Pseudomonas.

• Can be penetrated by rifampicin, high conc antibiotic lock, and thrombolytic agents
• Replacement of PD catheter is indicated if repeated infections occur within a short period of time (common).

**Prophylactic antibiotics pre-procedure (see p. 266).

Other causes of peritonitis

Culture-negative peritonitis

Culture −ve peritonitis rates have declined with improved microbiology techniques. The culture −ve rate should be <20%, if >20% requires investigation and could possibly be related to culture technique.

- Present with the clinical features of peritonitis, with no growth or organisms seen on Gram stain after 3 days
- Send repeat sample for Gram stain, cell count, and differential:
  - PD amylase level (>100u/L consider pancreatitis)
- If still no growth and cell count indicative of infection then consider sending cultures for *Mycobacterium*, fungus, yeast, *Legionella*, *Campylobacter*, *Enterovirus*
- If responding clinically to current regimen, continue for 14 days and stop the aminoglycoside
- If no improvement, then the PD catheter will need to be removed
- Culture −ve results are associated with eosinophilic peritonitis from an allergic reactions, e.g. new patients reacting to plastic tubing, chemical, e.g. review medications (e.g. amphotericin), presence of endotoxins, icodextrin (± stop use and re-introduce), EPS (see 🔲 pp. 320–1), chyloperitoneum, specimen taken from a dry peritoneum, haemoperitoneum

Mycobacterial peritonitis

The causes are either TB or non-TB mycobacteria with a higher incidence in Asian and developing countries. Present with cloudy PD effluent, fever, weight loss, relapsing culture −ve peritonitis.

- No growth and will require specific staining and culture medium to identify organism
- Need to differentiate if it is miliary TB or TB peritonitis
- 4 drugs: isoniazid and rifampicin for 12–18 months, pyrazinamide and ofloxacin for 3 months. Use of IP rifampicin may improve efficacy
- ± PD catheter removal will depend on nephrologist decision
- Remove PD catheter if tunnel infection suspected.

Fungal peritonitis

Fungal organisms invade the catheter material very quickly. Associated with a high mortality rate of ~25% and requires admission. The most common organism is *Candida albicans*.

- ISPD 2010 guidelines[5] recommend:
  - removal of PD catheter immediately as there is a ↑ incidence of abdominal adhesions the longer the catheter remains *in situ*
- Treatment with antifungal medications such as amphotericin B and flucytosine initially until culture and sensitivities available. Other agents used include fluconazole, voriconazole, posaconazole:
  - IP amphotericin is very painful and can cause chemical peritonitis and will diffuse slowly into the peritoneum. ⚠ If RRF present as it is nephrotoxic
  - fluconazole is effective IP, IV or PO for the *Candida* species
  - flucytosine—⚠ monitor of serum levels as associated with bone marrow toxicity.

Clinical features of peritonitis

- Cloudy effluent (98–100%)—commence immediate treatment to prevent damage to the peritoneal membrane
- APD patients may not be aware of cloudy effluent at an early stage if drain line connected directly to a drain
- Abdominal pain—can be dependent on the causative organism with some patients not experiencing very much pain if at all
- Clear effluent and abdominal pain—advise patient to do another exchange to check for cloudy fluid:
  - if fluid remains clear and the pain continues, other causes need to be assessed, e.g. constipation, pancreatitis, peptic ulcer, acute intestinal perforation
- Rigors, sweating, fever
- Abdominal tenderness
- Anorexia, nausea, vomiting, and/or diarrhoea
- Drainage problems as a result of fibrin
- ↑ protein catabolic rate and protein loss in PD effluent.

Assessment of peritonitis

- Haemodynamic assessment to include TPR and BP—notify medical staff if febrile or signs of septic shock, e.g. ↑ pulse, ↓ BP
- Assess abdominal pain: usually described as tenderness and generalized pain with rebound. Liaise with medical staff if the patient is complaining of localized pain, e.g. ovarian, appendix
  - ± AXR if the bowel perforation or constipation is suspected
- Assess for any possible causes of peritonitis:
  - inspect exit site for signs of infection or tunnel infection, send swab for MC&S if any discharge present. If this is the source of the infection, the organism will be the same as the peritonitis organism
  - sensitively ask the patient if they could possibly have contaminated the line when connecting
  - peritonitis history, e.g. most recent episode
  - exit site history, e.g. most recent ESI
  - recent procedures, e.g. colonoscopy, gynaecological investigation, dental surgery (see 📖 p. 334)
  - normal bowel pattern, e.g. constipation, diarrhoea, other GI problems
  - check the patient is not on antibiotics as will affect culture results
- US may be required to diagnose a tunnel infection (see 📖 p. 305).

Specimen collection

- Send PD effluent for MC&S, Gram stain, differential, and cell count:
  - collect 50ml PD effluent and inject 5–10ml into blood culture bottles, remaining fluid should be placed in a sterile specimen container. Some units send the whole PD drain out bag to the laboratory
  - delivery to laboratory within 6hr, after hours place blood culture bottles in the incubator at 37°C
- ▶Dialysate needs to have dwelled for ≥2hrs prior to taking the sample
- APD dry day—instil 1L of dialysate, leave left *in situ* for preferably 2hrs
- If peritoneum has been empty for a sustained period of time (e.g. post-op/resting)—adequate flushing needed to remove any debris, then 1L of PD fluid should be instilled as previously described.

Confirmation of peritonitis

- Signs and symptoms of peritonitis, e.g. cloudy effluent, abdominal pain, nausea, fever
- Microscopy results show WCC >100 cells/μl, with >50% polymorphonuclear neutrophils cells present (low numbers in healthy peritoneum)
- Assess the % of cells rather than WCC if PD fluid has not been *in situ* >2hrs, e.g. APD
- Follow-up Gram stain and/or culture for identification of the organism ▶Gram stain may show no bacteria, but identify a yeast infection; if present commence antifungals and remove PD catheter early.

Patients in special circumstances

- Patients who are on holiday or who live a long way from the PD unit will require additional training in the assessment and management of peritonitis at home which may include:
  - collection and storage of PD effluent specimen
  - immediate treatment with IP antibiotics
  - how to reconstitute and draw up antibiotics, dosage, and route of administration.

Management of peritonitis

Day 1

- Commence 2–3 rapid exchanges to flush the peritoneum—may be soothing for the patient, prevents any blockage of PD catheter if fibrin present, and removes inflammatory mediators:
  - some units do not flush and go straight to treatment regimen
- Commence empiric IP antibiotic treatment as per unit policy (IP has better efficacy than IV in peritonitis)
- Antibiotics should cover Gram +ve and Gram −ve organisms, e.g. vancomycin and a 3rd-generation cephalosporin or aminoglycoside. ⚠ Aminoglycosides are nephrotoxic, caution with RRF
- Administer using sterile technique via the medication port of the bag
- Dwell for a minimum of 6hrs to maximize effect
- Full dose can be given in one exchange or divided doses as preferred by the patient
- ± IP heparin 500 units/L if evidence of fibrin present to prevent poor drainage
- Provide dietary advice and supplement to ↑ protein intake at risk of malnutrition—refer to renal dietitian, especially if Alb is <35g/L
- Usual treatment time is 14 days, *S. aureus* 21 days.

Patient well enough to be discharged home
- IP antibiotics may be dispensed in pre-prepared syringes which can be stored in the home refrigerator ∴ ↓ the risk of contamination
- Provide education and training on the instillation of the IP antibiotics and IP heparin if required
- Arrange community nurse/district nurse if patient/family unable to add IP antibiotics
- Telephone the patient daily for first 3 days to check effluent is clearing daily, if not arrange for review
- Check fluid balance as peritoneal membrane characteristics are affected ∴ more prone to fluid overload
- Organize follow-up appointment or home visit for review to check vancomycin levels, usually day 4 or 5 and day 10 and gentamicin daily:
  - check within therapeutic range and prevent toxicity
  - dependent on unit policy and dosage regimen.

If unwell—hospital admission
- IV fluids, IP antibiotics and analgesia, daily WCC, CRP to monitor efficacy of antibiotics, e.g. *S. aureus* peritonitis.

Day 2

- Contact the patient to assess response to the antibiotics if at home or assess on the ward if inpatient
- PD effluent should be clearing and the pain resolved
- If PD effluent is not clearing, re-send PD effluent for MC&S.

Day 3

- Follow up culture and sensitivity results to identify causative organism and ensure on the correct antibiotic (see Table 11.12, see 📖 pp. 315–16 for ISPD treatment regimens)

- Liaise with medical staff to alter antibiotics if required or a no growth found
- No growth cultures should remain on antibiotics that covers both Gram +ve, −ve and *Pseudomonas* organisms
- If responding to treatment, complete course of antibiotics
- Organize re-training if causative organism related to poor technique.

Day 5
- If no response to treatment, arrange PD catheter removal
- ▶ The ISPD define refractory peritonitis as failure of the effluent to clear after 5 days of appropriate antibiotics. The PD catheter should be removed to preserve peritoneal function and prevent mortality and morbidity associated with refractory peritonitis:
  - medical review and assessment for other causes
  - check the PD catheter for signs of tunnel infection (see 🕮 p. 305).

PD catheter removal

Early removal of PD catheter is associated with better membrane preservation and is performed under GA. Usually requires transfer for temporary HD. Non-infectious related reasons for removal include planned permanent transfer to HD or a successful kidney Tx.

PD catheter removal is required for:
- Refractory peritonitis—high risk of death and membrane failure associated with delay in removal of PD catheter >10 days
- Fungal peritonitis
- Relapsing peritonitis
- Refractory tunnel or ESI
- Peritonitis associated with bowel perforation
- Non-responding infection, e.g. *Mycobacterium*.

▶The PD catheter should not be re-inserted for 2–3wks post removal for refractory or fungal peritonitis.

Simultaneous PD catheter removal and replacement

Can be considered for the following:
- Refractory exit site infection—early use of PD catheter to avoid temporary HD with low volumes in a supine position
- Relapsing peritonitis with clear PD effluent—requires antibiotic cover
- No active infection present in cases of refractory or recurrent peritonitis where the WCC <100/μl (requires antibiotic cover post-op)

▶ Should not be done in refractory and fungal peritonitis—needs a minimum of 2–3wks (± >fungal peritonitis) between removal and reinsertion of new PD catheter, preferably using an approach to visualize for any adhesions.

Key points: prevention of exit site infection and peritonitis

- ↓ risk—appropriate patient selection and support
- ↓ contamination risk—use of 'flush before fill' systems, assisted devices for those with dexterity or visual problems
- ↓ risk of exit site and tunnel infections—prophylactic antibiotics pre-operatively
- Catheter design, location, sinus tract length, number of cuffs, and correct placement
- Correct insertion technique to ensure adequate tissue perfusion
- Good exit site management and early treatment of infection
- *S. aureus* screening and management
- Close monitoring in malnourished, diabetes, uraemia, hypothyroidism, obesity, IS and steroid medications → delayed wound healing
- Bacterial colonization of the sinus tract
- Use of prophylactic antibiotics prior to a non-renal procedures
- Avoid episodes of hypokalaemia which cause slowing of GI motility → excessive growth of bacteria in the gut
- Avoid episodes of constipation by regular use of aperients in those at ↑ risk. There is some evidence to support the use of lactulose daily (acidifies the stool ↓ bacterial growth)
- Maintaining healthy nutritional status as hypoalbuminaemia affects the immune system, e.g. malnourished
- Patient education programmes:
  - good knowledge, understanding and training in the care and management of exit site and competence in PD technique
  - minimum of annual re-training of patients/family/carers
- Staff education programmes to ensure all staff attain competencies in the care and management of PD
- Consider transfer to HD with repeated episodes of peritonitis.

Table 11.12 ISPD recommendations for peritonitis treatment regimen[5]

Organism	Treatment
Coagulase −ve *Staphylococcus* Most common *S. epidermis* by contamination Usually mild	Stop Gram −ve antibiotic IP cephalosporin or vancomycin for 14 days Removal of catheter if no response at 5 days Associated with relapsing peritonitis 2° to biofilm and colonization in the intra-abdominal segment of catheter Adjuvant use of rifampicin may avoid relapse (good biofilm penetration)
S. aureus (6–8%) Severe and difficult to clear. Usually due to catheter infection or possibly touch contamination	IP cephalosporin or vancomycin IP gentamicin and/or oral rifampicin Treat for 21 days Exit site and peritonitis less likely to respond to treatment
Meticillin resistant *S. aureus* (MRSA)	Vancomycin, teicoplanin for 21 days ± add rifampicin for 1wk (⚠ TB resistance with longer course). No response 5 days removal of catheter ↑ risk of transfer to HD
Gram −ve *E. coli, Proteus, Klebsiella*	Stop culture +ve antibiotic Cephalosporin for 14–21 days
Pseudomonas Biofilm—difficult to clear Severe—difficult to clear	Aminoglycosides, quinolones, 3rd-generation cephalosporins, e.g. ceftazidime. Combine 2 different antibiotics Treat for 21 days if responding Removal of PD catheter if no response at 2–4 days and continue treatment for 2 weeks
Enterococcal Gram +ve Most common *Enterococcus faecalis* or *faecium* Transmural (2–4%) Severe pain	Ampicillin ± aminoglycoside Treat for 3 weeks Vancomycin unless contraindicated in the unit e.g. VRE Intra-abdominal event—refer to surgeon Check technique

(Continued)

Table 11.12 (Continued)

Organism	Treatment
Corynebacterium (uncommon) Contamination (natural flora of the skin)	1st-generation cephalosporin or vancomycin for 2–3 weeks Associated with high refractory peritonitis
Streptococcal Severe pain—exit site or tunnel infection Check oral hygiene	Ampicillin or vancomycin for 14 days
VRE Presence of VRE in stools or use of broad-spectrum antibiotics	Ampicillin, if resistant quinupristin, dalfopristin, daptomycin
Polymicrobial +++ enteric organisms (especially with anaerobic bacteria) +++ Gram +ve organisms (associated with contamination or PD catheter infection)	Urgent referral to surgical team e.g. ischaemic bowel ↑ mortality risk Treat as for Gram +ve—usually responds well

Outcomes of peritonitis

The majority of peritonitis is treated effectively (i.e. 60–90% of cases) and →:

- Either permanent or temporary changes in peritoneal membrane permeability
- ↑ in solute clearance, glucose absorption, protein loss, and ↓ UF ability
- Severe and/or repeated episodes can lead to membrane failure which is the most common cause of technique failure.

Longer-term problems

- Development of adhesions—loss of effective peritoneal surface area, drainage problems (see 🕮 p. 289) and can → bowel obstruction
- PD catheter removal
- Abscess formation: <1%, usually fungal, Gram −ve or *S. aureus* organisms, diagnosed on CT scan or US. Drainage under CT/US guidance
- Transfer to HD—the major cause of technique failure is peritonitis which accounts for 30–80% of transfers
- Associated with the development of EPS (see 🕮 pp. 320–1)
- Death (defined as dying with active peritonitis or within 2wks of an episode of peritonitis):
  - death rate of 1–6% with mortality rates ↑ with Gram −ve or fungal peritonitis
  - 18% incidence of infection-related mortality as a result of peritonitis
- Severe episodes of peritonitis cause loss of protein and ↓ serum Alb levels → malnutrition (see 🕮 pp. 212–14):
  - mortality rates post transfer to HD in these cases is high which may be related to poor nutritional intake and protein loss
  - those with CVD are also at a higher risk of death.

Ultrafiltration failure

Solute and H_2O transport is dependent on the effective surface area of peritoneum available, intrinsic peritoneal permeability, and the presence of specific H_2O transport channels (see 📖 p. 245). Although effective surface area of the peritoneum increases over time, the peritoneal membrane loses capacity for UF. This is compounded by the ongoing loss of RRF with patients becoming totally reliant on the peritoneum for fluid removal. ~36% of patients will develop UFF after a prolonged period of time on PD

- Associated with recurrent episodes of peritonitis, long-term use of PD, and high use of high dextrose containing dialysate
- UFF is defined by the ISPD 2000,[6] as UF <400ml for 4hrs using a hypertonic dextrose dialysate (e.g. 4.25% or 3.86%).

Assessment and diagnosis

Usually present with fluid overload or drainage problems.

- *Determine if UFF or a treatable condition*—catheter malfunction, leak, drainage problems, incorrect prescription for membrane transport status, non-adherence (regimen too complicated, 'PD 'burn out'), ↓ RRF:
  - check PD catheter patency/fibrin—drain 2L of 1.36% dialysate exchange in and out
- *Drainage problems*—further investigation, e.g. constipation, AXR to check catheter position, peritoneoscopy to check for a leak or entrapped catheter
- *Normal drainage*—assess using modified PET to evaluate for UFF and Na^+ sieving capacity (see 📖 p. 279)
- *If modified PET <400ml*, assess small solute profile:
  - Low transport D/P Cr <0.5—disruption of peritoneal space, leaks, drainage problems, adhesions which will need HD or optimize RRF
  - High transport D/P Cr >0.81—inherent high transporter/recent peritonitis, long term PD
  - HA or LA D/P Cr >0.81 or <0.5—mechanical, enhanced absorption, e.g. lymphatic or tissue, aquaporin deficiency
- Assess Na^+ sieving, i.e. no ↓ in Na^+ levels in dialysate in the initial dwell phase indicates failure of aquaporin system (see 📖 p. 279).

Causes of membrane failure

High transport status

15% of all new PD patients will commence with a high transport membrane status associated with highly efficient small solute transport. However, there is a greater risk of protein loss and a higher mortality rate.

- Most common cause of UFF → large vascular surface area of the peritoneal membrane, with high D/P Cr or low D/Do glucose (see 📖 pp. 276–8)
- Avoid long dwells by using APD and the use of icodextrin for the day dwell
- May need to consider HD if anuric and <750ml UF/day.

Recent peritonitis
Peritonitis causes a temporary change in membrane status → a high transport status (i.e. loss of osmotic gradient as above) → membrane becomes hyperpermeable.
- Adjust prescription whilst the peritoneum settles and ideally repeat PET 8wks post infection to re-assess membrane function
- Use shorter dwell times and the use of higher strength dextrose dialysate and/or icodextrin to manage fluid balance
- Prevent malnutrition with the use of protein supplements to compensate for excess protein loss as a result of peritonitis and high transport status

Long-term use of PD and loss of functioning peritoneal membrane
As a result of the use of dextrose dialysate and accumulation of AGEs there are changes to the peritoneal vasculature → ↑ vascular surface area and high transport status (i.e. ↑ D/P Cr and ↓ D/Do).
- ↑ the incidence over time with a history of recurrent peritonitis and high usage of hypertonic PD dialysate
- There is no change in protein loss such as is seen in patients with high transport status post peritonitis
- Modified PET results <400ml UF and none or less change in Na^+ conc in the dialysate indicative of UFF
- May require adhesiolysis
- Transfer to HD will be required especially once anuric.

Aquaporin dysfunction
This condition is rare and difficult to assess in the clinical setting. If there is damage to the aquaporin system there will be a decline in H_2O removal by the ultrasmall pores (see 📖 p. 246). In those with severe UFF and no increase in solute clearance, aquaporin dysfunction should be suspected.
- Use icodextrin to remove fluid as does not involve the aquaporin system and avoid hypertonic dialysate
- May be some benefit from stopping PD for a short period, resting, and re-starting which may improve function
- No RRF, the patient may require HD.

Lymphatic reabsorption
To prevent excessive reabsorption, avoid using large volumes of PD dialysate and long dwells.

Prevention of peritoneal membrane failure
- Continuing education of patient/carer/staff to prevent episodes of peritonitis
- Aim of ↓ peritoneal membrane exposure to high dextrose dialysate as much as possible
- Consider other dialysate options, e.g. icodextrin or amino acid
- Initial results have been promising with more biocompatible solutions which may become an option in the future.

Encapsulating peritoneal sclerosis

Encapsulating peritoneal sclerosis (EPS) is a rare and life-threatening complication of peritoneal dialysis associated with significant mortality and morbidity. The incidence (0.5–3%) increases with time on PD and varies with country of origin. EPS can occur in transplanted patient, however only in those who were treated for several years on PD.

Pathophysiology

Sclerotic thickening of the peritoneum which surrounds either some or all of the small intestine, leading to partial or complete bowel obstruction and/or necrosis and encapsulation. Slow progression and usually asymptomatic until complications occur or may be acute as a result of severe peritonitis. Symptoms seem to appear when PD stopped and patient transferred to HD or transplanted.

Clinical features

- Bowel obstruction, e.g. partial, complete, or intermittent ileus, peritoneal adhesions, inflammation, or abdominal mass
- GI disturbance, e.g. abdominal pain, nausea, loss of appetite, constipation, diarrhoea, abdominal mass, ascites, weight loss, vomiting
- Malnutrition
- Loss of UF, peripheral oedema and fluid overload, ± haemoperitoneum
- Culture −ve non-resolving or recurrent PD peritonitis
- Inflammatory state, e.g. ↑ CRP, ↓ Alb, anaemia.

Diagnosis

- Clinical features of EPS—differentiate between EPS and other causes, e.g. paralytic ileus
- Use of diagnostic imaging:
    - most effective is CT contrast scan which shows peritoneal calcification, bowel thickening and dilatation and encapsulation (not reliable for early detection)
    - AXR may confirm or exclude bowel obstruction, however cannot be used for confirmation or exclusion of EPS
- Laparotomy or laparoscopy; however the patient is usually unwell and surgery may be too risky.

Potential risk factors

- Previous episodes of severe inflammation, e.g. peritonitis
- Biocompatibility, e.g. acetate buffered PD dialysate, low pH, ↑ GDPs
- Reaction to plastic of the catheters, antiseptics used during exchanges (e.g. chlorhexidine)
- Genetic factors
- β-adrenergic blockers ('beta blockers')
- Prolonged time on PD using high dextrose dialysate (e.g. 3.86%)
- Stopping PD may worsen EPS (e.g. transfer to HD or transplanted).

Nursing considerations

- Recovery is dependent on the severity of EPS
- Need to assess overall life expectancy and balance risks vs benefits, e.g. decision to switch mild EPS on PD to HD (QOL, life expectancy)
- Requires a MPT integrated approach.

Conservative management

- Bowel obstruction—NBM to rest bowel, NGT, and IV fluids
- Nutritional support—malnutrition is important factor in morbidity/ mortality associated with EPS ($\downarrow$ nutritional intake and inflammatory catabolic state)
  - Refer to dietitian for assessment, will require regular dietetic assessment (e.g. SGA, MAC, MAMC) as weight will not provide an adequate guide
  - Mild—oral supplements and anti-emetics
  - Nasogastric feeding or nasojejunal feeding tube if unable to tolerate oral feeding
  - Nutritional support, e.g. TPN if NBM (see re-feeding risk on 📖 p. 212–13).
  - Pharmacist review to ensure TPN prescription reviewed
  - Central venous access care and management
- Medications:
  - IS (e.g. azathioprine), corticosteroids and tamoxifen dependent on physicians preference.

Early referral to surgical team with expertise in EPS if does not respond to conservative management/nutritional therapy

- Preferably planned surgery as emergency surgery is associated with high mortality and morbidity rates
- Surgery management—peritonectomy
  - risk of bowel perforation, with temporary ileostomy or jejunostomy
  - high-risk surgery and usually requires ICU management post-op
  - treat anaemia—transfusion and RRT, i.e. HD
- 20% recurrence rate and require further surgery.

Prevention

- No evidence to support pre-emptive switching from PD to HD[8]
- Aim to preserve RRF and minimize the use of high glucose concentration (e.g. 3.86%) dialysate
- Minimize the number of episodes of peritonitis
- Aim to Tx PD patients within 3–4yrs to $\downarrow$ long-term use of PD
- Possibly biocompatible dialysate may be beneficial, however there is still no definitive evidence to support this
- Surveillance programmes   no recommendation at present
  - current techniques do not enable early diagnosis of EPS
  - consider monitoring patients on long-term PD (e.g. >5yrs), including transfer to HD or transplanted for monitor GI symptoms and investigate early
- Investigations being researched—new MRI procedure, interleukin 6 and Ca-125 as biomarkers and analysis of metabolomics profiles in PD effluent.

Structure and function of the peritoneal dialysis unit

The structure of the PD unit will be largely dependent on the number of patients on the PD programme and resources available.

- The PD unit should be managed by a dedicated MPT of PD nurses, a dedicated nephrologist with support of junior medical staff, renal dietitian, social worker, counsellor, and pharmacist services

Purpose of the PD clinic

- Training and re-training of patients/family/carers on all aspects of PD management
- 2-monthly routine PD checks (see pp. 334–5)
- 6-monthly clinic appointments with nephrologist, dietitian, nurse
- Drop-in appointments for acute complications:
  - peritonitis, ESI, drainage problems, contaminated line, fluid overload/dehydration
- PET/adequacy tests/line changes
- Telephone and follow-up contact providing advice on all aspects of PD, e.g. peritonitis, fluid overload, fluid and stock
- Community home visits (dependent on the unit infrastructure and staffing)
  - pre-dialysis home assessment or work/educational institution assessment if required
  - 1st CAPD exchange or set up APD machine at home post training
  - training at home, nursing home
  - high-risk patients who require more support
- Administration:
  - follow-up peritonitis and ESI results, modelling, and adjustment of PD prescriptions
- Liaison with fluid administrator
- Regular (e.g. wkly) MPT meetings:
  - review results of adequacy/PET tests, altering prescriptions and complex case management of those requiring additional support, e.g. district nurse, home services
- Annual PD audit to maintain quality and improve clinical practice and patient outcomes (see pp. 324–5).

Role of the peritoneal dialysis nurse

- Provide pre-dialysis information and education on PD as a treatment option:
  - assessment of suitability for PD (see 📖 p. 160)
  - undertake home assessment and assist social worker with re-housing or home adaptation if required
  - co-ordination of PD catheter insertion, training, and support in collaboration with AKCC nurse
  - provide patient/family/carer education and training on all aspects of PD, e.g. exchange procedure, exit site management, troubleshooting
  - nutrition and fluid management
- The management of PD on a day-to-day basis:
  - undertake, analyse, interpret adequacy and PET results
  - correct prescription of PD to maximize solute clearance and UF
  - exit site care and management
  - assessment and management of acute complications, e.g. peritonitis, exit site-related infections, malfunctioning PD catheter, fluid leaks, UFF
  - liaison with dietitian for dietary interventions (see 📖 p. 206, Nutrition for PD dietary advice, prevention, and treatment of malnutrition)
  - home visits to identify new problems, assess adherence and technique
- Liaison with ward staff for the management of PD inpatients
- Provide psychological support to patient and family
- Provide education and support to students and staff not working within the PD unit, e.g. ward staff, district nurses, nursing home staff
- Governance and audit
- Coordination of MPT meetings.

Clinical audit

PD audits should be completed annually in order to maintain quality and improve clinical practice and patient outcomes where possible. Clinical practice should be underpinned by evidence-based policies and procedures.

- The ISPD[2,6,7] and UK RA[1] guidelines should be used as a benchmark
- Audit results should be compared to registry results where possible
- More frequent auditing and the use of root cause analysis tools should be used if sudden change in clinical outcomes, e.g. ↑ peritonitis rates
- Audit data collection and review of results should involve the MPT inclusive of the surgical team undertaking the PD access surgery.

RA clinical areas of audit[1]

- Demographics of patients:
    - number of prevalent patients on PD and patient months on PD
    - type of PD, age, assistance required
    - number of patients stopping and starting PD
    - number of days of training required
    - location of training
- Availability of modality choice, monitoring of modality switching
- Patient to PD nursing staff ratio
- Availability of assisted PD, utilization and outcomes
- Audit of care pathway for dialysis preparation to include information given (including proportion of patients offered PD), when and who delivers it
- Audit of information on modality options provided to patients presenting who urgently require RRT, and both initial and subsequent modality of RRT selected by these patients
- Audit of care pathway for catheter insertion to include timeliness and need for temporary HD
- PD catheter complications and outcomes:
    - cause of technique failure in patients stopping PD
    - 1° catheter patency 80% at 1yr (censor for death and elective modality change)
    - bowel perforation <1%
    - significant haemorrhage <1%
    - ESI within 2wks of catheter insertion <5%
    - peritonitis infection within 2wks of catheter insertion <5%
    - functional catheter problem requiring manipulation or replacement or leading to technique failure <20%
    - fluid leaks
- Type of system used—non-standard systems and clinical indication
- PD dialysate fluid:
    - number of patients using hypertonic PD dialysate (e.g. 3.86%) to maintain fluid balance
    - fluid absorption in long dwell, e.g. overnight (CAPD) or day (APD)
    - use of biocompatible solutions
- Adequacy, PET status, and RRF:

- frequency of solute clearance (residual and peritoneal) estimation cumulative frequency curves for the total solute clearance
- frequency of measurement of membrane function, residual urine and peritoneal ultrafiltration volume
- number and type of membrane characteristics
- RRF and UF volume/day
- identify patients with a total fluid removal <750ml/day
- Kt/Vurea >1.7 and CrCL >50
- Cumulative frequency curves of plasma bicarbonate
- Routine annual audit of infection outcomes—prevalence of peritonitis:
  - number, causative organism, sensitivity, and outcome of all episodes of peritonitis and ESIs
  - peritonitis rates of <1 episode per 18 months
  - a 1° cure rate of ≥80%
  - a culture −ve rate of <20%.

Calculating peritonitis rates

Peritonitis rates need to be calculated and reviewed by the PD team at least annually to assess, monitor, and evaluate peritonitis rates and maintain quality. This allows the PD unit to investigate any rises in rates and implement prevention strategies.

ISPD[7] and UK RA[1] recommendations/standards
- Peritonitis rates ≤1 episode every 18 months and no growth <20%.

ISPD 2010[7] guidance on calculating and reporting peritonitis rates
- Rate is calculated for all infections and each organism:
  - months of peritoneal dialysis at risk, divided by number of episodes, expressed as interval in months between episode
  - number of infections by organism for a time period, divided by dialysis-years' time at risk, and expressed as episodes per year
- As % of patients per period of time who are peritonitis free
- As median peritonitis rate for the programme:
  - calculate peritonitis rate for each patient and then obtain the median of these rates.

New patient training and education

Preferably a new PD catheter should not be used for 2wks unless the patient cannot hold off dialysis and has no other access. During this period, patients need to attend the PD clinic for dressings or follow-up when attending for dialysis.

Preparation for training

If possible check the PD catheter is working and the exit site is clean and healing a few days prior to when training is scheduled to avoid lost time if the catheter is not functioning.

- Check PD catheter patency by draining in and out 1L dialysate
- Laxatives 1–2wks prior to commencing training
- Liaise with patient or family member(s) to be trained for time/date of training and organize hospital transport (and accommodation if available) if required
- If training at home, liaise with patient/family with date and time of training and ensure fluid stock and equipment have arrived
- Preferable to undertake training in a single designated room or area
- Home training is advantageous as the patient is familiar with the home setting and will not need to make a transition from hospital
- A single PD nurse should complete the teaching programme to provide continuity. If not possible good handover is essential
- Training usually takes 3–5 days depending on the health and ability of the patient/family member.

Training period

- Check exit site is clean and healing
- Check patency of PD catheter if not already checked
- Commence with 1st exchange of 1–1.5L, adjust initial volume according to the patients size and comfort, gradually ↑ to desired fill volume, e.g. 2L
- Undertake assessment and plan training week in partnership with the patient/family member—set achievable goals (see 📖 pp. 605–6)
- Sessions should be no longer than 15mins; it is within the first 5mins that most information is absorbed.

General theory content

- Review function of the kidney, CKD, and the need for dialysis
- Basic principles of PD, purpose of the PD catheter, function of the peritoneum
- Management of CKD complications, e.g. ESI, peritonitis, fluid overload, dehydration, renal bone disease, anaemia
- Suitable PD locations—no windows open, pets in the room, keep clean and dust free, small children
- Importance of personal hygiene and effective handwashing—use of antibacterial hand rub
- Principles of aseptic technique
- Demonstration of the system to be used to talk through technical aspects (e.g. consider use of DVD)

- Troubleshooting, e.g. problems draining in or out, fibrin, pain on inflow, blood in PD effluent, contamination of line
- Management of peritonitis and ESI, i.e. action to take—emergency contacts and when and where to call
- Daily routine, weight, BP, PD dialysate used and volume, colour of fluid, BGL (i.e. diabetes) documented in PD diary
- Discuss the importance of clinic appointment attendance:
  - bring PD diary, medication list, adequacy and PET information
- Fluid stock ordering and storage: check delivery of stock prior to completing training
- Review medications and send copy to GP. Educate patient on medications, e.g. dose, route, side effects, mechanism
- Tx issues discussed and follow up Tx work-up if required
- Discuss aspect of living with CKD (see 📖 pp. 531–63)
- Provide psychological support to patient and family: observe for any signs of depression, anxiety, and adherence problems
- Schedule an appointment with social worker and counsellor for initial assessment and support
- Community services—liaise with district nurses, practice nurse/GP to co-ordinate care in the community, e.g. weight/BP/ESAs.

Care and management of exit site—observe performing dressing
- Assessment and procedure to perform exit site dressing (see 📖 p. 330):
  - action to take, e.g. signs of infection, crust formation
- Position and anchoring the catheter, check not kinked under dressing
- Not to use scissors in close proximity of the catheter in case they accidently cut the tubing or insert anything down the extension line to clear blockage, e.g. fibrin
- Information and advice on exercise and activities, e.g. they should not play any contact sports or strenuous lifting, e.g. rugby and weight lifting. Sports such as scuba diving need to be discussed with medical staff
- Swimming—preferably should only swim in chlorinated H_2O (e.g. rivers/lakes may have stagnant water $\therefore$ ↑ bacteria count) with the use of a H_2O resistant occlusive cover to prevent the exit site from getting wet, e.g. stoma bag, re-dress immediately
  - discuss with nursing staff prior to access correct equipment/location
- No baths—shower daily, re-dress the exit site immediately afterwards.

Fluid and diet management
- Definition of IBW
- Managing fluid balance daily and use of different dialysate strengths
- Fluid overload or dehydration complications and signs/symptoms
- Importance of using prescribed prescription and preserving RRF
- Education of fluid allowance and foods containing water
- Ensure patient has been seen by a dietitian, i.e. ↑ risk of malnutrition (see 📖 p. 206, Nutrition for nutritional requirements).

PD prescription and use of different dialysates
- Check dialysate bag prior to use, e.g. correct strength, volume, expiry date, colour and no signs of leak
- Understanding the different strengths and use and monitoring UF.

Practical aspects of CAPD training
- Patient should observe CAPD procedure, connecting/disconnecting prior to 1st attempt
- During this time, explain the different aspects of the procedure:
  - use of bag warmer and not to use a microwave (37°C)
  - preparation for exchange, e.g. set up, equipment, surface cleaning
  - connection technique/flush before fill/disconnecting
  - disposal of waste, e.g. effluent, bags, lines/sharps
  - observation of adequate drain out and record UF volume
- Observe patient performing CAPD exchange.

Practical aspects of training APD patients
- Technical aspects of the APD machine—mechanics of the APD machine, e.g. how it works, how the fluid is warmed (location of the warmer and which bag to place on the warmer):
  - talk through the mechanical process of each cycle
  - preparation of machine, e.g. set-up, cleaning, lining and priming the machine/connecting and disconnecting
  - temporary disconnection, e.g. to go to the toilet if the extension line is not long enough
- Emergencies and who to contact, e.g. power failure, machine errors
- Troubleshooting—alarms, how to bypass or stop early
- Settings on the machine—check the correct program is set:
  - make adjustments if required
  - check initial drain volume adequate
  - review at the end of program and document total UF volume
  - perform safety check of the machine
- Collecting drain out fluid for adequacy test
- Prescription:
  - number of cycles and the fluid volume per cycle
  - strength of dialysate fluid required
  - location of last fill if it is a different strength/solution, e.g. icodextrin
  - if performing additional daytime exchange, aware of the strength, volume, time of the exchange

It may be useful to have the written instructions printed in large font on the wall for them to follow or they may prefer that they are talked through the procedure by the nurse step by step

Checklist prior to discharge home
- Competent and safe at performing a CAPD/APD and exit site management
- Fluids and supplies have been delivered
- Medications with up-to-date list
- Aware of the need to prevent episodes of constipation and actions to take to maintain RRF
- Transport arranged if required

- Summary letter sent to GP including up-to-date medication list.
- Referral made to district nurse/practice nurse if required, e.g. BPM
- Home visit organized for 1st PD exchange or setting up APD machine
- Review and medical clinic, adequacy, and PET appointments booked.

Exit site care and management

New exit site

- The exit site dressing should be left intact for 5–10 days. Dressings should not be changed immediately postoperatively unless they are blood soaked and preferably changed by PD staff (see 📖 p. 268)
- Assess at wk 1 and if clean and dry and no signs of infection, then leave for a further week (see ISPD exit site scoring tool, 📖 p. 304)
- Clean with normal saline for the 1st 2wks and then with antiseptic wipe/solution as per local policy
- The patient should not shower until the exit site is healed which is usually at the 3rd wk as the exit site is colonized at this stage.

Nursing considerations

- When removing the old dressing, ensure catheter is not hanging and is in a safe position to prevent trauma
- Observe for the following prior to cleaning the exit site:
  - check for any staining on the old dressing
  - observe exit site for signs of infection, e.g. redness, pain, swelling
  - check for signs of catheter erosion or crusting
  - if exit site infection suspected, take a swab and send for MC&S prior to cleaning (TPR after completing the dressing)
- If crust present, do not use force to remove it, it will come off itself when ready—will cause trauma
- Always clean in one circular direction with antiseptic wipe or solution, e.g. clockwise or anticlockwise
- Clean around the catheter with the gauze and complete this 3 times. Checking the wipe for signs of exudate
- Place only a small amount of antibiotic topical cream/ointment on to the gauze and apply around the exit site
- Allow the catheter to fall in its natural direction; do not force the catheter to sit in a position as it will cause trauma to the exit site
- Ensure catheter is not kinked
- Apply the new dressing over the exit site, pinching the end to secure the catheter.

▶Always ensure the PD catheter is anchored securely

Patients transferred to HD or post Tx should be advised to continue caring for the exit site until PD catheter is removed, e.g. transfer to permanent HD or successful Tx. The extension line can be removed and the PD catheter capped off by nursing staff using aseptic technique to reduce bulk.

1st **home visit**

A home assessment is usually undertaken prior to acceptance on to the PD programme, which ensures the home environment is appropriate.

- General assessment of the home, e.g. cleanliness
- Assess the room where the PD is being undertaken, e.g. spare room, kitchen or bedroom (e.g. APD) for cleanliness, window closed, no pets in the room, no fans, able to wash hands and walk to dialysis area without having to touch anything, somewhere to hang fluids (CAPD) or a table for the APD machine
- Check fluids have arrived and stored appropriately
- Check patient can carry fluid from storage area to dialysis area
- For APD machines, drainage bags are required if there is insufficient access to a drain, e.g. sink or toilet. If possible, request a sink to be installed via the social worker
- Observe patient/family member undertake PD exchange or set up APD machine/connecting and disconnecting
- Review troubleshooting, alarms for APD machine and potential complications
- Ensure patient aware of telephone numbers and contact persons if required in an emergency
- Observe patient perform exit site dressing
- Observe patient taking weight, BP, completing PD diary, and understands PD regimen
- Discuss any issues/problems the patient/family member may have and action on return to the unit
- Feedback at the next MPT meeting the patient/family's progress.

▶ If patient also performing a PD exchange at work/institution, arrange for a visit to assess the patient in that environment. This will require liaison with the employer or institution.

Subsequent home visits

May be required or may be routine, e.g. annual home assessment, dependent on the infrastructure of the renal unit. Some units will organize home visits for the older person or immobile patients to reduce the need to travel to hospital.

1st peritoneal dialysis check

- Assess for any change in well-being, in particular if the patient has suffered from uraemic symptoms
- Identify any problems, e.g. poor drainage, constipation, fibrin
- If absorbing any dialysate fluid, check for signs of leaks, e.g. scrotal, abdominal area
- Check they have sufficient supplies and equipment
- Lying and standing BP, TPR
- Fluid review:
  - check weight and complete weight assessment if required, setting new IBW and confirm dialysis prescription with the patient
  - review patient's PD diary and prescription, is it completed?
  - type and number of exchanges, in particular are they using heavy bags already to remove fluid?
  - how much UF from each bag if the bags are being weighing? UF volume form APD machine
  - are they maintaining their IBW?
  - good understanding of fluid management
- Review medications
- Blood tests for U&E, Hb, BGL (i.e. diabetes)
- Observe patient attending to exit site dressing if possible to assess technique, signs of infection and trauma (e.g. not anchored well):
  - re-educate and schedule review if required
- Check wounds for infection and remove sutures/staples if required
- Review and evaluate the patient's knowledge, understanding, e.g. aware of action to take, e.g. peritonitis, ESI
- Discuss any concerns with the patient
- Check date is booked for adequacy and PET
- Offer praise and support to boost self-esteem. Reinforce achievements, e.g. completing training and getting home and the importance of self-management
- Discuss the patient's blood results and if possible demonstrate using the computer if there has been an improvement in blood figures, e.g. Ur, Cr, K$^+$—this provides positive feedback and reassurance that dialysis is working and further empower self-management
- Provide information about patient support groups.

Line change

The external segment of the PD catheter is connected to an extension line via an adaptor which provides additional length for easier patient management.

- A line change should be performed every 6 months as it ↓ the risk of cracks and breaks from continuous use
- Place a blue clamp to the external segment
- Wear sterile gloves and use an aseptic technique, soaking the adaptor section for 2mins with antiseptic solution soaked gauze prior to changing:
  - use sterile gauze to grip the adaptor end may if it is difficult to open
  - the old line is removed and new line immediately connected.

Routine peritoneal dialysis check

Frequency of routine PD checks is dependent on clinical condition. If the patient is stable and PD is working well, most patients will attend clinic every 2–3 months and usually see the PD nurse.

- Use as an opportunity to assess the patient's technique at performing exit site dressing if possible, re-educate if required
- Check integrity of PD catheter
- Identify any patient/family/carer concerns
- Weight, lying, and standing BP, temp:
  - BP and cardiovascular risk management, see 📖 pp. 84–90
- Review patients PD diary—check home weight vs IBW, home BP:
  - check current prescription the patient is using at home
  - check total UF, RRF (urine output)
- Assess for any problems with drainage, absorbing fluid, constipation
- Refer to renal dietitian re: weight loss/gain (see 📖 p. 202)
- Blood tests: U&E, FBC, HCT, glucose and HbA1c (i.e. diabetes), Ca^{2+}, PO_4, ALP (PTH every 6 months)
- Anaemia management
- Check for acidosis especially if malnourished, may need to adjust dialysis dose and/or dialysate buffer conc
- Alteration of Ca^{2+}, PO_4, PTH (see 📖 pp. 192–6)
- Liaison with transplant team as required
- Check adequacy and PET results are up to date
- Review and adjust prescription as needed
  - ongoing psychosocial support, refer to MPT as required, e.g. dietitian, social worker, counsellor, refer to patient support groups
- Update patient's care plan, e.g. My Kidney Care Plan.[5]

Management of non-renal invasive procedures

PD patients invariably require tests and procedures outside of the nephrology service. Requires pre-procedure prophylactic antibiotics to ↓ the risk of peritonitis and should be performed with an empty peritoneal cavity. Common procedures include colonoscopy, gynaecological, dental, angiography, PEG feeding tube: may need to rest for 4–6wks with appropriate antibiotics and antifungal drugs as risk of leakage.

Undertaking a telephone assessment

PD is a home-based treatment and so such much of the contact with the PD unit is via the telephone. It is important to assess patients effectively and safely over the telephone in order to problem-solve and plan any specific treatment that may be required.

- Give your name, designation, and organization
- Confirm patient's name, date of birth, and unit number
- Access records if possible
- Identify who are you talking to if it is not the patient, preferably speak to the patient directly
- Identify the problem, use open-ended questions at the beginning, then closed questions to gather more specific details

- At the end of the call, recap what you have discussed and understand as the problem and the agreed action plan
- Check the patient/family/carer is happy with the action plan and ask them to repeat it back to you. Outline action to take if condition worsens, i.e. they have been asked to attend the PD unit
- If the patient is not to attend the unit, make sure you are confident and happy with this decision. It is better to review the patient in person if in doubt
- Document in notes and arrange follow up to check progress.

Non-PD related surgery on a non-renal ward

Patients admitted to a non-renal ward require management by PD staff.

- Liaise with the ward nursing staff as to patient's condition and treatment. Discuss with renal team and refer to MPT if required, e.g. renal dietitian, assess if any social services are required for discharge or if the renal social worker is required for any change in circumstance, e.g. post CVA
- Request daily weight, lying and standing BP, fluid balance chart and advise on patient's fluid allowance
- Contact details for PD/renal ward staff for out of hrs troubleshooting
- Review medications and check for any potential nephrotoxic drugs if the patient has RRF or contraindicated in ESKD (see 🕮 p. 569)
- Provide education and support on managing a PD patient
- If blood transfusion required—accurate fluid assessment and fluid removal
- Liaise with medical and nursing staff as to time of surgery, check FBC, U&E, CXR and ECG (if GA) taken preoperatively:
  - fluid assessment to ensure not fluid overloaded and preserve RRF
  - IV cannula in forearm to preserve access
  - drain out PD effluent
- Postoperatively re-start PD if appropriate
  - abdominal surgery—rest for 2wks and recommence on low volumes. Stoma formation is contraindicated and will require HD
  - check K^+, e.g. K^+ released from cells, blood transfusion
  - discuss management plan and potential discharge date
- Liaise with renal team daily basis for ongoing management issues
- If patient unable to manage own PD, arrange for PD staff or after hrs ward staff to perform PD and exit site dressing.

Fluid management

Fluid overload

Patients presenting with fluid overload require a thorough assessment. It is common for most PD patients to present at some point.

- ↑ 1kg above the agreed IBW ~additional 1L of fluid in the circulatory volume

Possible specific PD-related causes of fluid overload

- Loss of flesh weight, but still aiming for old IBW
- Non-adherence
- Alteration in peritoneal membrane permeability, e.g. changed from low average to high/fast transport status and still using long dwell times
- Episode of peritonitis which alters peritoneal membrane permeability for a short period of time
- ↑ salt intake
- ↑ fluid intake
- Loss of RRF without adjusting fluid intake and/or PD prescription
- Incorrect PD prescription, e.g. PET results not used to prescribe ideal prescription to match peritoneal membrane transport characteristics
- Catheter malfunction, e.g. catheter migration, poor drainage from constipation
- Lymphatic/tissue reabsorption → ↓ drain volume even using high dextrose dialysate to create the osmotic gradient (see 🕮 p. 242)
- UFF (see 🕮 pp. 318–19).

Clinical assessment to determine cause of fluid overload

- Assess whether this is a short-term or long-term problem
- Undertake a fluid assessment (see 🕮 p. 587)
- Compare of IBW, current clinic and home weight
- UF (exclude 'flush before fill') + urine output + 500ml insensible loss—oral intake
- Refer to renal dietitian for assessment of salt intake
- Review last adequacy and PET results, organize if no up-to-date result available
- PET residual volume >250ml will need AXR to check PD catheter position
- ↓ drain volume and overall fluid volume removal, e.g. leak, adhesions
- ↓ UF and low transporter, i.e. advanced stages of peritoneal sclerosis
- Modified PET test, bioimpedence measurements
- Measure drain out volume for each exchange if absorption of PD fluid suspected
- Check diabetes control
- Assess PD catheter function, e.g. poor or positional drainage, e.g. adhesions, migration of catheter tip, constipation:
  - if patient in clinic, drain in and out a 2L 1.36% and check for patency of catheter
- Assess and identify any adherence issues.

Nursing considerations are dependent on underlying cause

Initial management will include removal of fluid to achieve IBW, e.g. use of hypertonic dextrose dialysate, fluid restriction, ± ↓ dwell time in acute phase

Fluid and salt restriction

- Non-adherence to prescription regimen—discuss with patient if suspected to identify underlying cause, e.g. impact of ↑ number of exchanges on QOL, misunderstanding regarding fluid allowance
- Agree IBW and fluid allowance with the patient
- Provide advice on low salt diet and refer to renal dietitian
- Educate on fluid management and the complications associated with the inappropriate use of high hypertonic dialysate
- Adjust prescription to suit transport status and for loss of RRF
- Consider loop diuretic if significant RRF to ↑ urine output volume
- Consider the use of icodextrin for sustained UF, particularly in diabetes, absorbing from overnight exchange (CAPD), day exchange (APD)
- Manage catheter malfunction (see 📖 pp. 292–3)
- Good diabetes control (see 📖 p. 338)
- ± assess for UFF (see 📖 p. 318)
- Develop action plan and follow-up evaluation.

Dehydration

PD-specific causes

- Incorrect IBW, e.g. gained flesh weight and still aiming for IBW
- Inadequate oral and food intake, e.g. anorexia
- GI illness, e.g. diarrhoea, vomiting
- Peritonitis affects peritoneal membrane permeability in the acute phase
- Inappropriate use of too many high dextrose-containing PD dialysates
- The result of a high UF with the use icodextrin.

Nursing considerations

- Identify the cause and treat if appropriately
- If due to volume depletion, e.g. diarrhoea, IV fluids may be required if unable to ↑ oral intake in the short term:
  - the patient will continue to lose fluid as a result of UF so will need to compensate in the interim
  - use of all low dextrose conc dialysate initially, may need to consider ↓ number of exchanges if good RRF
- If RRF, immediate action to prevent loss of kidney function
- Incorrect IBW, undertake a weight assessment and set new IBW
- Loss of flesh weight, refer to dietitian for assessment as may require supplements
- Review prescription and adjust, e.g. stop icodextrin or heavy bags if causing large UF volume
- Educate patient on the correct prescription if using incorrect dialysate.

Diabetes management

The permeability of the peritoneal membrane in diabetes has a tendency to be higher → use of more hypertonic solutions to maintain the osmotic gradient and subsequent required UF.

Advantages of PD

- Fewer haemodynamic changes (e.g. ↓ BP episodes)
- No vascular access required
- Less heparin exposure
- Option of IP insulin administration
- Preservation of RRF for longer
- Relatively constant state of electrolytes.

Disadvantage of PD

- ↑ glucose load.

Nursing considerations

Management under joint renal/diabetes clinic if available

Diabetes: aim for HbA1c <53mmol/mol (7.0%)
- Monitor BGL: closely initially—may ↑ oral hypoglycaemics or insulin requirements due to ↑ glucose load, additional calories if previously anorexic (e.g. ↑ appetite)
- ↓ requirements if switched to icodextrin ∴ ↓ calorie load if using hypertonic dialysate previously
- May need to convert to insulin
- Ensure regular foot, eye and dental examinations organized

Diabetes agents: avoid oral hypoglycaemics with a long half-life, e.g. glibenclamide switching to, e.g. glipizide, as is short acting and mainly cleared by the liver
- ⚠ Metformin is best avoided as associated with lactic acidosis
- Thiazolidinediones associated with ↓ insulin requirement and resistance. ± due to anti-inflammatory effect. ⚠ use with HF associated with oedema and CCF
- IP insulin can be used, however need to adjust dose in liaison with the diabetic team and pharmacist
- Tend to require a higher dose, more complex to manage in APD
- Potential source of contamination, i.e. injecting the PD dialysate port and associated development of hepatic subcapsular steatosis.

Prevent obesity: monitor and aim for healthy weight, advise on weight reduction— ↓ cardiovascular risk (see 📖 p.77)
- Prevent the effects of ↑ calorie load—avoid the excessive use of hypertonic PD dialysate.

GI symptoms: exacerbation of gastroparesis and gastric reflux (common complications associated with diabetes) as a result of the large volume of fluid in the abdomen or ↓ gastric motility as a result of ↑ calories → slow gastric emptying.

- May complain of a feeling of fullness and ↓ appetite
- Use of smaller volumes at mealtimes and compensate with larger volumes at night which may help (as in supine position ∴↓ IAP)
- ± oral erythromycin
- Metoclopramide—⚠ side effects
- Suggest small, frequent meals.

PD prescription: effective UF—maintain plasma: dialysate osmotic gradient by good blood glucose control and monitor RRF. Loss of RRF occurs more rapidly possibly due to the presence of a chronic inflammatory state, ↑ cytokines levels.

- Icodextrin, APD—long day dwell and CAPD—icodextrin as overnight dwell as does not affect BGL as gives sustained UF
- Amino-acid PD dialysate, Nutrineal® as an alternative and avoid glucose exposure or solutions which contain ↓ GDPs (see 📖 p. 250)

▶ Patients should carry alert cards if using icodextrin in case of hospitalization in other units to ensure correct glucometer (see 📖 p. 250).

Prevention of hypoalbuminaemia in high transporter: monitor serum Alb levels—liaise with the renal dietitian for adequate protein intake

↑ *risk of infection*: discuss the need for meticulous exit site care.

Transfer from peritoneal dialysis to haemodialysis

The use of an integrated approach to RRT facilitates the flow of patients from one modality to another. Discussing and preparing the patent in the pre-dialysis stage to expect HD as a treatment option at some point can assist to reduce the stress and anxiety associated with the transfer. The expected length of time on PD averages 3–7yrs at which time if the patient has not received a successful transplant, consideration will need to be given to switching to permanent HD.

Temporary HD
- Abdominal surgery
- Acute pancreatitis
- Catheter removal and awaiting new catheter, e.g. peritonitis, tunnel infection
- Bowel leak
- Fluid leak
- Hydrothorax
- Severe malnutrition.

Permanent transfer to HD
- Loss of effective peritoneal membrane efficiency
- Loss of RRF or due to large body size, e.g. once anuric unable to maintain solute clearance
- Inadequate fluid removal and solute removal
- Uncontrolled hypertriglyceridaemia
- Unresolved mechanical problems, e.g. hernia, adhesions
- Repeated episodes of peritonitis
- Non-adherence and patient choice
- Patients inability to cope and manage home-based treatment:
  - deterioration in health and physical functioning, e.g. incontinence
  - patient unsuitable in the first place, but may have wished to try PD
  - no family member/carer or assisted PD service available to take on treatment at home
- Severe malnutrition.

Nursing considerations for the transfer process
- Information and education on HD to the patient and family, e.g. process, complications etc.
- Location where they will be dialysing, options for the future once stable on HD of a satellite unit or possibly home HD:
  - type of HD will need to be assessed by the HD staff along with the lifestyle, employment situation etc. of the patient
- Visit the HD unit and meet the staff and other patients
- Organize appointment with vascular access surgeon/nurse to arrange access, e.g. arterio-venous fistula
- Liaise with MPT and notify them of the patients transfer
- Organize removal of fluid boxes/equipment from their home.

Further reading

General

Bernardini J, Price V, Figueiredo A. ISPD guidelines/recommendations: Peritoneal dialysis patient training, 2006. *Perit Dial Int* 2006; **26**:625–32.

Guest S. *Handbook of Peritoneal Dialysis*. Lexington, KY: CreateSpace Independent Publishing Platform; 2011.

Khanna R, Krediet R (eds). *Nolph & Gokal's Textbook of Peritoneal Dialysis*, 3rd edn. New York, NY: Springer; 2009.

Levey J, Brown E, Daley C, et al. *Oxford Handbook of Dialysis*, 3rd edn. Oxford: Oxford University Press; 2009.

Adequacy/PET

Jansen MA, Termorshuizen F, Korevaar J, et al. Predictors of survival in anuric peritoneal dialysis patients. *Kidney Int* 2005; **68**(3):1199–205.

La Mila V. Peritoneal transport testing: thorough critical appraisal. *J Nephrol* 2010; **23**(6):633–47.

Lo WK, Ho YW, Li CS, et al. Effect on Kt/V on survival and clinical outcome in CAPD patients in a randomized prospective study. *Kidney Int* 2003; **64**(2):649–56.

Paniagua R, Amato D, Vonesh E, et al. Effects of increased peritoneal clearance on mortality rates in peritoneal dialysis: ADEMEX, a prospective, randomized controlled trial. *J Am Soc Nephrol* 2002; **13**:1307–20.

Van Biesen W, Heimburger O, Krediet R, et al. Evaluation of peritoneal membrane characteristics: a clinical advice for prescription management by the ERBP working group. *Nephrol Dial Transplant* 2010; **25**:2052–62.

Dialysis-related infection

De Vin F, Rutherford P, Faict D. Intraperitoneal administration of drugs in peritoneal dialysis patients: a review of compatibility and guidance for clinical use. *Perit Dial Int* 1009; **29**:5–15.

Encapsulating peritoneal sclerosis

Brown E, Van Biesen W, Finklestein F, et al. Length of time on peritoneal dialysis and encapsulating peritoneal sclerosis: position paper for ISPD. *Perit Dial Int* 2009; **29**:595–600.

Woodrow G (Chair). UK *Encapsulating peritoneal sclerosis clinical practice guideline*. UK EPS Clinical Guideline Group; 2009. Available at: ℘ <http://www.renal.org/pages/media/Guidelines/EPS-Guideline-4.pdf>

Kawanishi H, Moriishi M. Epidemiology of encapsulating peritoneal sclerosis in Japan. *Perit Dial Int* 2005; **25**:S4, S14–S18.

Kawanishi H, Moriishi M. Encapsulating peritoneal sclerosis: prevention and treatment. *Perit Dial Int* 2007; **27**:S2; S289–S292.

Summers A, van Dellen D, Birtles L, et al. Why we need increased surveillance of encapsulating peritoneal sclerosis. *Eur Nephrol* 2012; **6**(1):61–4.

References

1. Woodrow G, Davies S. *Clinical Practice Guidelines: Peritoneal Dialysis*. London: UK Renal Association; 2010.

2. Figueiredo A, Goh BL, Jenkins S, et al. Clinical practice guidelines for peritoneal access. *Perit Dial Int* 2010; **30**:424–9.

3. European Best Practice Guideline Working Group. European best practice guidelines for peritoneal dialysis. *Nephrol Dial Transplant* 2005; **20**(supp 9): ix8–ix12.

4. NICE. *Laparoscopic insertion of peritoneal dialysis catheter. Interventional procedure guidance 208*. London: NICE; 2007. Available at: ℘ <http://guidance.nice.org.uk/IPG208/Guidance/pdf/English>

5. Crabtree JH, Burchette RJ, Siddigi N. Optimal peritoneal dialysis catheter type and exit site location: an anthropometric analysis. *ASAIO Journal* 2005; **51**(6):743–7.

6. Mujais S, Nolph K, Gokal R, *et al.* Evaluation and management of ultrafiltration problems in peritoneal dialysis. *Perit Dial Int* 2000; **20**(supp 4):S5–21.
7. Li P, Szeto CC, Piraino B, *et al.* ISPD Guidelines/Recommendations. Peritoneal dialysis-related infection recommendations: 2010 update. *Perit Dial Int* 2010; **30**:393–423.
8. NICE. *Peritoneal Dialysis: Peritoneal dialysis in the treatment of stage 5 chronic kidney disease.* Clinical Guideline 125: London: NICE; 2011. Available at: ℘ <http://www.nice.org.uk/nicemedia/live/13524/55517/55517.pdf>

Patient information websites

℘ <http://www.kidney.org.uk/Medical-Info/pd.html>
℘ <http://www.kidneypatientguide.org.uk/site/adequacy.php>
℘ <http://www.patient.co.uk/doctor/Peritoneal-Dialysis.htm>

Patient information

Stein A, Wilde J. *Kidney Failure Explained*, 4th edn. London: Class Health; 2010.

Haemodialysis

Definition of haemodialysis

Haemodialysis (HD) is one of a number of therapies collectively known as RRT. HD is used for 2 distinct categories of kidney disease management—those who have ESKD sometimes known as stage 5 CKD and in AKI.

In common with all RRTs, HD is not a cure for kidney disease; it is used to manage the signs and symptoms of CKD or AKI and is in that sense a palliative procedure. Generally speaking, HD is life saving/preserving whether it is used in AKI or ESRD, as it is used to remove the toxic by-products of protein metabolism along with excess body fluid. Sometimes HD is used purely to remove certain drugs from the circulation (e.g. lithium) or to control severe electrolyte disturbance.

It is called HD because it is a process which accesses the patient's blood (haem) via an extracorporeal (outside the body) circuit and passes it through a filter (dialyser) where dialysis (diffusion across a semipermeable membrane) takes place.

Principles of haemodialysis

HD describes the process by which blood is filtered across a semiper-meable membrane (see 'The dialyser') in order to remove both toxins and excess fluid. The movement of electrolytes and toxins occurs according to the biological principle of diffusion while fluid removal is achieved via a process often called ultrafiltration.

Diffusion

Diffusion is the movement of solutes (substances dissolved in a fluid) from an area of high concentration to an area of low concentration until the two concentrations are equal (Figure 12.1). Importantly in HD, a semiper-meable membrane separates the two concentrations of fluids (blood and dialysate); hence strictly speaking dialysis and not diffusion occurs.

The semi permeable membrane prevents large molecules and blood cells crossing from the blood into the dialysate fluid (see 📖 p. 354).
Since diffusion occurs across a gradient:
- Urea and Cr (waste products of protein metabolism) move from the blood into the dialysate
- High levels of electrolytes (e.g. K^+) move from the blood to the dialysate
- HCO_3 ions move from the dialysate into the blood
- Physiological levels of core electrolytes (Na^+, Ca^{2+}, Mg^{2+}) move in relatively equal amounts both ways.

To maintain the diffusion gradient blood and dialysate flow in opposite directions through the dialyser—this is called the counter-current.

Ultrafiltration

Ultrafiltration (UF) is the term used for the removal of fluid during dialysis. In HD, UF is achieved by the mechanical creation of hydrostatic pressure across the dialysis membrane (Figure 12.2). On the blood side of the dia-lyser there is a positive pressure as H_2O and small solutes are forced across the semipermeable membrane. Large molecules do not pass through the membrane. On the dialysate side a negative (sucking) pressure is applied by pumping less fluid into the dialyser than the dialysate effluent pumps out; generating a transmembrane pressure (TMP). The UFR is dependent on the pressure gradient. For example, to remove 600ml of fluid an hour the dialysis machine may introduce 490ml/min of dialysate to the dialyser but the pump at the distal side will pump out 500ml/min (60min × 10ml/min = 600ml).

Diafiltration

Simultaneous use of dialysis and ultrafiltration to provide water and solute clearance.

Convection

Some small solutes (usually electrolytes) dissolved in the water are removed in solution as the water is removed. This process is called con-vection or solvent drag but is not an important aspect of solute removal during normal dialysis (Figure 12.3).

Diffusion

Movement of solutes from an area of high concentration to an area of low concentration until the concentrations are equal.

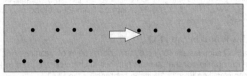

Fig. 12.1 Diffusion.

Ultrafiltration.

Pressure applied by mechanical forces across the membrane (TMP).

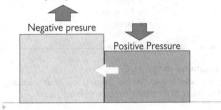

Fig. 12.2 Ultrafiltration.

Convective Transport

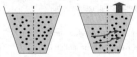

Fig. 12.3 Convective transport.

Water quality

The average adult drinks 10–20L of fluid a week. This fluid is taken in orally and enters the acidic environment of the GI tract which kills most pathogens. A person dialysing for as little as 3hrs thrice wkly is exposed to ~270L of H_2O/wk. This H_2O is only separated from their blood by a thin semipermeable membrane.

Impurities found in tap H_2O

Domestic H_2O supplies are subjected to various stages of cleaning prior to being safe for human consumption. A number of chemical are used to kill micro-organisms. See Box 12.1 for the contents of tap H_2O.

Box 12.1 Contents of tap H_2O

- Chloramine
- Arsenic
- Fluoride
- Aluminum
- Trihalomethanes
- Barium
- Hormones
- Cadmium
- Nitrates
- Copper
- Sand
- Mercury
- Clay
- Radium
- Silica
- Microbial pyrogens
- Endotoxin
- Pesticides
- Lead.

Effects of contaminants in the H_2O

Many H_2O impurities have known serious impacts on health, although these are usually the result of long-term exposure (Table 12.1).

Table 12.1 Effects of contaminants

Contaminants	Toxic effect
Aluminium	Bone disease, dementia, encephalopathy, microcytic anaemia
Calcium (Magnesium)	Hypertension, nausea, vomiting, headache, weakness
Chloramine	Haemolysis, anaemia, methaemoglobinaemia
Copper	Nausea, headache, haemolysis, hepatitis
Fluoride	Osteomalacia
Lead	Neurological disorders
Microbial pyrogens, endotoxins	Nausea, vomiting, fever, shock, hypotension, enhanced dialysis amyloid formation
Nitrate	Cyanosis, methaemoglobinaemia, hypotension, nausea
Sulphate	Acidosis, nausea, vomiting
Zinc	Anaemia, fever, nausea, vomiting

Carbon filters remove chlorine

- Reverse osmosis (RO) removes salts, bacteria, and endotoxins
- Ultraviolet lamps, used in some systems, remove bacteria post RO
- Ultrafilters remove residual endotoxins and bacteria post RO both within water systems and also in HD machinery.

Microbial purity of the H_2O is measured by taking a count of the live bacterial colonies level in the H_2O, measured as colony forming units per millilitre (CFU/ml).

A high microbial content ↑ the risk of infection and chronic inflammation which is associated with malnutrition, amyloidosis, and reduced response to ESA and hence anaemia.

Gram −ve bacteria release endotoxins when they are growing and upon organism death. In some circumstances these endotoxins are able to pass through the dialyser membrane. Exposure to endotoxins can cause symptoms including: pyrogenic reactions (see 📖 p. 405) appetite suppression, extended clotting, and a dulled response to ESA therapy (see 📖 p. 234). Measuring endotoxins levels (in EU/ml) is an important aspect of managing water quality and safety.

H_2O quality standards

Creating H_2O of suitable quality to be used in the preparation of dialysis fluid is important. Various bodies define standards to safeguard the routine production of H_2O for use for HD and HDF. The maximum contaminant levels allowed are given under these standards, for both regular and ultrapure H_2O as well as concentrates used in dialysate production.

Testing guidelines

Each unit should have standard operating procedures in place for sampling, monitoring, and recording of H_2O quality; the minimum requirement for testing include:

- Wkly chlorine levels
- Monthly endotoxin and microbiological content
- 3-monthly chemical contaminants.

It is important that the microbiological sampling takes account of the various points in the dialysis process that contaminants may enter the process:

- The various stages of H_2O treatment
- All points of connection on the dialysis machine
- The dialyser (at the dialysate ports).

Where microbiological contaminant levels are in excess of 50% of the maximum permitted levels for bacteria and endotoxins (e.g. 50CFU/ml and 0.125EU/ml for 'regular' H_2O) vigorous disinfection is needed.

Nursing considerations
- Internal and external machine disinfection at each use
- Microbiological testing, as per unit policy and procedure
- Daily chloramine testing in some units
- Being alert to pyrogenic reactions
- Being alert to possible ESA resistance.

Best practice dictates all new water treatment plants should provide ultrapure H_2O to avoid the complications which arise as a result of poor H_2O quality.

Dialysate

Dialysate is made up of 3 components:
- Purified H_2O
- Electrolytes (of various concentrations)
- A buffer (usually HCO_3, lactate/acetate are rarely used).

See Box 12.2 for composition of dialysate.

Dialysate is mixed inside the dialysis machine where H_2O is added to the electrolyte concentrate and buffer. Dialysate is used in the HD process to provide the diffusion gradient by which dialysis occurs. Dialysate contains:
- No, or ↓, level of solutes which should be removed/reduced in the patient's blood
- Physiological, or near physiological, levels of electrolytes which need to kept at ↔ levels in the patient's blood
- ↑ concentration of solutes which are needed in the patient's blood (usually HCO_3).

▶ Levels of some electrolytes may be altered in order to achieve specific effects e.g. ↓ K^+ levels or ↑ Ca^{2+}.

Box 12.2 Composition of dialysate
- Na^+: 132–155mmol/L
- K^+: 0–4mmol/L
- Ca^{2+}: 1.25–1.75mmol/L
- Mg^{2+}: 0.75–1.5mmol/L
- Cl^-: 90–120mmol/L
- Dextrose: 0–5.5mmol/L
- HCO_3: 27–40mmol/L
- Acetate: 30–45mmol/L (in acetate-based dialysate only)
- pH: 7.1–7.3.

Sodium

Na^+, usually found in the extracellular plasma, plays the leading role in controlling the homeostasis of H_2O (acting as an osmotic agent). Disruption of the body's Na^+ balance in CKD means plasma Na^+ levels often have to be corrected during HD. High plasma Na^+ contributes to HPT and ↑ thirst (and hence fluid intake).

Recent observations of the effects of dialysate Na^+ levels indicate a standard of about 136mmol/L may be associated with lower incidence of IDH since the patient is less thirsty between HD sessions and drinks less necessitating less fluid removal on HD.

Na^+ profiling
For patients in whom it is difficult to remove fluids during HD the use of Na^+ profiling is widely used to help maintain their intradialytic BP (see 📖 pp. 394–5).

Calcium

Plasma Ca^{2+} levels are frequently affected by CKD. The majority of HD patients will use a dialysate with Ca^{2+} of 1.25–1.75mmol/L. Patients with hyperparathyroidism, and subsequently hypercalcaemia, will benefit from dialysate with lower Ca^{2+} concentration.

Evidence suggests low Ca^{2+} dialysis may help in the control of hypertension but it is also associated with an ↑ incidence of sudden cardiac death. Patients with hypocalcaemia may benefit from dialysate with Ca^{2+} at the higher level; however, the risk of over suppression of PTH and subsequent adynamic bone disease needs to be considered.

Potassium

K^+ levels are often disrupted in CKD patients. Dialysis patients can become hyperkalaemic due to the inability to excrete dietary K^+. Normal dialysate has a K^+ concentration < normal physiological levels in order to reduce plasma K^+ (1, 2, or 3mmol/L).

▶ Caution with altering K^+ doses should be exercised as both hypo or hyperkalaemia ↑ the risk of cardiac arrhythmias.

▶ Individuals with CKD adapt to ↑ K^+ levels and may not need such vigorous treatment for hyperkalaemia as the general population.

Magnesium

Mg^{2+} is necessary in the activity of >300 body enzymes. In some patients Mg^{2+} may need to be supplemented either intravenously or by changing the dialysate dose.

Chloride

Cl^- is the body's main anion found in extracellular fluid. It is ingested as NaCl (table salt). The control of Cl^- levels through HD contributes to the management of the body's acid status.

Glucose (Glu)

Glu-free dialysis is associated with asymptomatic hypoglycaemia in patients with diabetes and should be avoided. Glu is itself a strong osmotic agent and its use in dialysate fluid and subsequent diffusion into the patient's circulation aids in plasma refill during fluid removal; however high levels of dialysate glu may leave diabetes patients hyperglycaemic.

Phosphate

Regulation of serum PO_4 can be problematic for patients on HD. While the level of PO_4 in the dialysate undoubtedly plays a role in PO_4 control it is not as important as dialyser size, dialysis frequency, or the use of HDF. (For more information about electrolytes see 📖 pp. 593–601.)

Dialysate options

Individual patient's dialysate prescriptions reflect clinical need.

Dialysate options
- Ca^{2+} >2.8mmol/L ↓ Ca^{2+} dialysate (1.0–1.25mmol/L)
- Ca^{2+} <2.0mmol/L ↑ Ca^{2+} dialysate (1.50–1.75mmol/L)
- K^+ >6.0mmol/L ↓ K^+ dialysate (0–2.0mmol/L)
- K^+ <3.5mmol/L ↑ K^+ dialysate (3.0–3.5mmol/L).

NB: dialysate containing glu 1.0–2.0g/L is used in diabetes patients to minimize risk of hypoglycaemia.

Buffer

A buffer, almost exclusively HCO_3, is used in dialysis to counteract the acidity of the electrolyte concentrate and helps reverse acidosis.

HCO_3 in the dialysate is much higher than the physiological level and passes across the dialysis membrane into the patient's plasma. Lactate levels will be raised post dialysis where lactate is used as the buffer. Where there is liver damage or other reasons to suspect an impairment of lactate clearing, its use should be avoided.

Dialysate delivery

Dialysate, HCO_3, and purified H_2O are mixed individually for the patient or through a machine which performs this centrally and distributes pre mixed dialysate to several dialysis machines (Figure 12.4). It is the responsibility of the nurse to ensure each patient receives the correct dialysate.

Dialysate temperature

In recent years the role of dialysate temperature in the management of intradialytic hypotension has received increasing attention. There is a balance to be achieved between a dialysate temperature which helps maintain BP and patient comfort. It is now usual to set the dialysate temperature between 35.5–36.5°C to mimic usual body temperature.

Dialysate flow rate (DFR)

The DFR is essentially read as the rate at which dialysate is drawn through the dialyser. Many practitioners believe dialysis clearance is directly proportional to the DFR, so the faster the flow rate the better the dialysis; recent studies suggest this may only be the case up to fairly modest rises in DFR of around 600ml/min for low-flux dialysers. Usual practice in the UK is for the DFR to be set at around 500ml/min for low-flux and 800ml/min for high-flux dialysers.

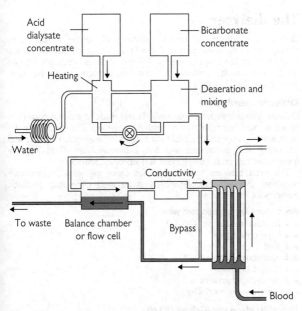

Fig. 12.4 Dialysate delivery in HD machines. Reproduced with permission from Levy J, Brown E, Daley C, et al. *Oxford Handbook of Dialysis*, 3rd edn. Oxford: Oxford University Press; 2009.

The dialyser

Dialysers are tubular and contain thousands of hair-like hollow fibres through which the blood passes. These fibres are surrounded by a space through which the dialysate passes. The use of fibres within the dialyser maximizes the surface area over which dialysis can occur across the membrane (typically 0.5–2.1m^2).

Dialyser membranes

Dialyser membranes are semipermeable and made of either natural (cellulose or modified cellulose) or synthetic polymers. The synthetic polymers are biocompatible to avoid inducing an inflammatory response and adsorbing both endotoxins and beta-2 microglobulin (B$_2$m).Cellulose membranes can cause complement and leucocyte activation.

The most biocompatible membranes cause the least inflammatory response; the best biocompatibility is achieved using fully synthetic membranes.

Biocompatibility is associated with:
- ↓ amyloid (see 📖 pp. 410–11)
- ↓ hypersensitivity
- ↓ IDH
- ↓ infectious episodes
- ↓ malnutrition
- Improved lipid profiles
- ↓ mortality and morbidity.

Ultrafiltration coefficient (KUf)

The hydraulic permeability of the semipermeable membrane is defined as a single value for the dialyser and indicates its ability to allow fluid removal during dialysis.
- Modern synthetic dialysers are highly water permeable
- Volumetric dialysis machines control water removal
- The KUf of a dialyser is determined by:
  - size of the pores
  - thickness of the membrane.

Low-flux dialyser

- Low-flux dialysers have relatively small pore sizes
- Provide a more conventional dialysis failing to clear large molecules, such as the potentially damaging B$_2$m
- Require less high-quality water to make dialysate
- Have a KUf of <10ml/hr/mmHg.

High-flux dialyser

- High-flux dialysers have a larger pore size
- Are able to remove molecules with molecular weights up to 40,000–50,000 Daltons (including B$_2$m, PO$_4$, PTH, and lipids)
- Have a KUf of >20ml/hr/mmHg.

High-flux dialysers are capable of removing solutes of both low and middle molecular weights whilst low flux only removes those of low molecular weight

The extra clearance of solutes is achieved not by diffusion but by solvent drag (convection) so clearance of small solutes, such as urea, is not significantly ↑ as a result of high flux.

Mass transfer coefficient (KoA)

The KoA of a dialyser is a measure of its capacity to clear solutes, specifically urea, and is a constant. KoA is determined by the membrane's surface area, pore size, and thickness. High-flux membranes (KoA 600–1200ml/min) have ↑ pore sizes compared to low-flux membranes (200–500ml/min) leading to ↑ clearance of larger molecular-weight solutes.

High-efficiency dialysis

High-efficiency dialysis utilizes dialysers which have an ↑ ability to remove urea. Highly efficient dialysers function in a similar manner to less efficient dialysers at low pump speeds, but once a threshold speed is crossed (at about 170ml/min) they start to perform more efficiently.

- Low efficiency: KoA <500ml/min
- High efficiency: KoA >600ml/min ml/min.

The extracorporeal circuit

The dialysis circuit is known as the extracorporeal circuit (EC); extra means 'outside of' and corporeal relates to 'body'. The EC begins at the point the blood leaves the patient via their dialysis access continuing along the arterial line to the blood pump (see Figure 12.5).

The blood pump is designed to minimize blood cell and platelet degradation. Blood drawn into the pump is subject to a pulling or sucking pressure which is recorded as 'arterial' pressure (arterial refers to the fact blood is coming from the patient into the EC and not because it is arterial in the physiological sense). As the arterial pressure is a negative pressure (measured in mmHg), the higher the pressure the better the flow from the patient's access.

Blood then travels into the top of the dialyser where it passes through the semipermeable membrane and out through the venous line to the 'venous' chamber. The air gap at the top of the venous chamber serves to trap any air which may have entered/been produced within the circuit preventing it being returned to the patient's circulation. The venous chamber also contains a mesh to prevent onward travel of emboli (usually blood clots). The pressure on the venous side of the circuit is positive, an ↑ in venous pressure indicates:
- Clotting in the EC
- Kinking of the venous line
- Access problems.

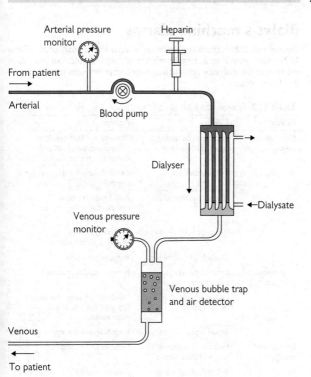

Fig. 12.5 Basic HD circuit. Reproduced with permission from Levy J, Brown E, Daley C, et al. Oxford Handbook of Dialysis, 3rd edn. Oxford: Oxford University Press; 2009.

Dialysis machine alarms

Throughout dialysis there are a number of alarms which may occur (Table 12.2). Many alarms do not cause the blood pump to stop, but may, as in the case of the dialysate conductivity alarm, interfere with the delivery of the dialysis dose.

Table 12.2 Dialysis machine alarms*

Alarm	Cause	Action
High venous pressure	Incorrect positioning of venous fistula needle	Move or readjust needle to prevent extravasation and damage to the vessel
	Venous stenosis	Avoid stenosed area. Investigate urgently
	Clot within the vessel	Avoid area. Arrange embolectomy, surgery, or thrombolysis
	Clotted circuit or dialyser	Change complete circuit and review anticoagulation
	Occluded venous lines	Remove occlusion
Low venous pressure	Error at the venous pressure sensor	Refer to operator manual
	Dislodgement of venous fistula needle	Re-cannulate with new needle Observe for bleeding or extravasation
	Blood leak in return circuit	Identify leak and correct.
Low arterial pressure	Incorrect positioning of arterial fistula needle	Remove or readjust needle
	Arterial vessel stenosis	Avoid stenosed area. Investigate urgently
	Clot within the arterial vessel	Avoid area. Arrange surgery or thrombolysis
	Occluded arterial blood lines	Remove occlusion
	Poorly developed fistula	Refer for fistula angiogram
	Hypovolaemia	Allow more time for maturation
Air and foam detector *Do not reset or over-ride alarm if air is present*	Detection of air or bubbles within the venous chamber	Ensure patient is not below dry weight. Increase the level within the chamber. If fine air bubbles within the circuit, disconnect the patient and recirculate until circuit is clear. If patient may have received an air embolus, place in Trendelenburg position, disconnect lines, attempt to withdraw the air from the fistula needle or line, and alert emergency team

Table 12.2 (Continued)

Alarm	Cause	Action
	Turbulence within the chamber caused by high blood flow	Reduce blood flow until turbulence ceases
Blood leakage	Defective or split dialyser fibres causing leakage of blood through the dialyser membrane and possible contamination of blood with dialysate. Air in the dialysate causing a false alarm	Test the effluent dialysate for the presence of blood. If blood is present discard circuit and resume dialysis
Conductivity	Incorrect concentrate, kinks in the dialysate tubing, empty concentrate cans, or a machine fault	Correct fault
H_2O failure	The flow of H_2O to the machine is at too low a pressure for the machine to adequately generate dialysate	Observe for kinking
	Kinked or compressed H_2O hose to the machine	Correct fault
	A drop in mains pressure	Correct fault
	Issues with the dialysis H_2O purification plant	Regular maintenance of dialysis H_2O plant
Power failure	Electrical supply failure	Remove venous line from air detector
	Failure of backup generator	Disconnect the patient from dialysis, hand crank the blood pump to return blood to the patient, flush dialysis access
		If power can be resumed recommence HD using new lines and dialyser
		If no power available for foreseeable future, patient's creatinine, urea and electrolytes must be checked

* Reproduced with permission from Levy J, Brown E, Daley C, et al. Oxford Handbook of Dialysis, 3rd edn. Oxford: Oxford University Press; 2009.

Anticoagulation

The interaction of blood with any foreign body will usually lead to clotting; this is true in HD where exposing the patient's blood to the EC and dialyser in the absence of an anticoagulant would lead to a marked decrease in efficiency. A lost HD circuit may be responsible for a blood loss in the region of 300ml and therefore thought needs to be given to the use of anticoagulants in the HD process in order to prevent/reduce clotting whilst not increasing the risk of bleeding.

Unfractionated heparin (UFH)

UFH is widely used for HD and may be administered either intermittently or, as a continuous infusion (e.g. 500–2000IU/hr); either approach requires an initial loading dose (e.g. 50IU/kg) to prevent clotting. As well as excess bleeding, the side effects of UFH can include:

- Abdominal pain
- Alopecia
- Dyslipidaemia
- Dyspnoea
- Excessive/occult bleeding
- Nausea
- Osteoporosis
- Pyrexia
- Thrombocytopaenia.

Activated clotting time (ACT)

As a minimum ACT measurements should be undertaken at least twice to help establish an appropriate UFH dosage for an individual patient. A small amount of the patient's blood is mixed with an assay and the time it takes the blood to congeal is measured.

The ACT of non-heparinized blood should be 90–140s. The most normal regimen is then for a bolus of 1000–2000 IU followed by maintenance of 500–2000IU/hr (raising the ACT to 170–250sec). Where a patient has a history of bleeding or has to have restricted heparin (e.g. pre or post surgery) the bolus may be omitted and the maintenance dose halved (target ACT 150–200secs).

The heparin infusion should be stopped 60–90mins prior to the end of HD for patients with AVFs or AVGs in order to avoid excessive post-HD bleeding on needle removal.

The patient's UFH heparin dose should be reassessed:

- If they develop unexplained bruising
- Clot formation noted in the EC
- They bleed excessively following needle removal
- Patient experiences other bleeding (e.g. epistaxis)
- If commence warfarin or similar anticoagulant therapy
- 3-monthly.

Low-molecular-weight heparin (LMWH)

The extended half-life of all LMWHs mean they are suitable for a single bolus injection at the start of HD, with no intra-HD infusion and are the most commonly used method of HD anticoagulation in practice.

> **Types of LMWH**
> - Bemiparin
> - Dalteparin
> - Enoxaparin
> - Tinzaparin.

▶ACT is not used to calculate LMWH dosing; doses are standardized although the measurement of factor Xa levels may be a useful when deciding dosing of UFH and LMWH which are usually renally excreted.

Nursing considerations

- There should be no visible clots in the EC at the end of HD once the circuit has been flushed through with normal saline.
- A small amount of staining in the dialyser fibres is acceptable.
- At the end of each dialysis session the EC should be observed and the length of time bleeding post AVF/AVG needle removal documented (<10mins is ideal).

Heparin-free dialysis

There are occasions when, and individuals in whom, heparin-free HD is indicated:

- ↑ Risk of, or actively, bleeding (e.g. history of cerebral bleed)
- Recent/due to have surgery with bleeding risk
- Recent liver/kidney biopsy
- Pericarditis (restricted heparin is acceptable)
- Thrombocytopaenia
- New or acute patients if abnormal clotting screens.

A HD session without anticoagulant can be achieved by:

- Giving regular bolus doses of 0.9% saline (added to total fluid to be removed)
- Maintaining BFR
- Priming EC with heparinized 0.9% saline (3000–5000 units/L) and bleeding the circuit out on connection ∴ heparin does not reach the patient
- ↓ height of blood in bubble trap (where used)
- Tight parameters of venous and arterial alarms to gain early alert to clotting.

Heparin-induced thrombocytopaenia (HIT)

Heparin-induced thrombocytopaenia type I (HITI) is observed when a small reduction in platelet count occurs at about 2–3 days after UFH use.

The platelet count will rise to normal levels within a few days even with continued use of UFH.

HITII is an uncommon immune mediated thrombocytopaenia occurring 5–10 days after starting UFH. HITII may cause serious problems with clots forming in the heart, lungs, brain, and limbs and may require pharmaceutical or surgical intervention. Patients with HITII should be changed to heparin free dialysis or another anticoagulation agent.

Alternative anticoagulants

Danaparoid is a LMW heparinoid; it contains no heparin or heparin fragments. However, similar to LMWHs, it exerts its antithrombotic effect principally through antithrombin III-mediated inhibition of factor Xa and, to a much lesser extent, thrombin.

Lepirudin is an anticoagulant that functions as a direct thrombin inhibitor. Lepirudin is a recombinant hirudin derived from yeast cells.

Fondaparinux (Arixtra®) is a synthetic, highly sulphated pentasaccharide, which has a sequence derived from the minimal antithrombin (AT) binding region of heparin.

Prostacyclin, sodium citrate, and heparin-protamine are occasionally used as anticoagulants; their use is more widespread in acute RRT.

Alteplase and urokinase are widely used (both between dialysis sessions as a lumen lock or as an infusion pre HD) to unblock all forms of dialysis catheter.

Cochrane reviews also support the use of aspirin and other antiplatelet medications (such as dipyridamole and clopidogrel) in helping maintain the patency of AVFs and AVGs especially immediately after creation, although long-term dated remains equivocal. Similar data exist on the use of warfarin to maintain AVF and AVG patency.

▶The use of oral anticoagulants is associated with ↑ morbidity and mortality in the HD population (as it is in the general population) ∴ care needs to applied when considering their use.

Reversing anticoagulation

Protamine can be given to reverse UFH-induced anticoagulation although it has only a limited impact on anticoagulation caused by LMWHs. Where protamine fails there may be a need to administer fresh frozen plasma (FFP). Nurses using alternative anticoagulant should familiarize themselves with how their effects might be reversed.

▶Infusions of protamine should be slow to avoid risk of bradycardia and shock. Protamine is not suitable for people with fish allergies.

Vascular access

Good quality VA for HD is essential to enable HD to take place, achieve an adequate dialysis and minimize infection (see Figure 12.5). Often termed the 'patient's lifeline', dialysis access creation and maintenance is one of the key aspects of the care of patients with ESKD.

Timely access creation is essential. Both NICE and the renal NSF recommend the creation of an arteriovenous fistula (AVF) at least 6–8wks before the expected date of commencement of HD.

An assessment by a VA surgeon prior to any creation of a VA allows appropriate access can be planned and agreed. Many units have a one stop access clinic where patients' vessels are assessed, relevant investigations (e.g. venogram) are carried out and an operation date is given. The patient is seen by both the VA surgeon and dialysis access nurse.

Arteriovenous fistula (Table 12.3)

AVFs are the gold standard VA for HD as they:
- Last longer than other forms of VA
- Have lower infections rates compared to other forms of VA
- Have the least mortality and morbidity of any form of VA
- Work more reliably than all other forms of VA
- Have a higher patency from creation than other VA
- Are cost-effective over time.

Formation of AVF
- AVFs are created by joining (anastomosing) an artery and a vein
- Commonly the radial artery is anastomosed to the cephalic vein in the patient's non-dominant arm.
- AVFs may also be formed using the brachial artery and cephalic vein and the brachial artery and basilic vein.
- The best patency and performance are obtained when using the radio-cephalic and brachio-cephalic to create AVFs
- Anastomoses may be made side to side, end to side, or end to end
- Where other options are not viable AVFs may be created in the leg.

▶ An AVF should not be cannulated for 6–8 wks after creation; although maturation may take up to 6 months in some patients (e.g. the elderly and those with diabetes).

⚠ AVFs should not be cannulated where there is no bruit or thrill; patients should have urgent investigation and interventions to rescue their access.

In an AVF the vein will carry arterial blood at arterial pressures. As veins are not elastic, like arteries, when they are part of an AVF they distend and become firmer. The resulting matured vein allows for the insertion of large bore dialysis cannulae. High blood flow rates within the AVF minimize recirculation of dialysed blood (see 📖 pp. 406–9).

Arteriovenous graft (Table 12.4)

- AVGs are made of polytetrafluoroethylene (PTFE), Dacron®, and occasionally grafted from the saphenous vein or from a bovine ureter
- AVG are inserted in the same sites as AVFs and may be looped or straight
- Mainly indicated in the elderly and people with diabetes who may have fragile vasculature unsuitable for AVF formation

AVGs are usually ready for cannulation after about 3–6wks when surgical swelling has subsided.

Figure 12.5 illustrates positioning of VA for HD.

Table 12.3 Advantages and disadvantages of AVF

Advantages	Disadvantages
High blood flow on HD	Can clot
Longevity of use	Aneurysms bumps and scars may disrupt patients body image
Lower infection than catheters	Problematic for those with needle-phobia
May be useable at around 6 wks	Not able to be used immediately
Easy to use	
Suitable for home HD	
Cost effective	
Reduced morbidity and mortality	

Table 12.4 Advantages and disadvantages of AVG

Advantages	Disadvantages
High blood flow on HD	Can clot
Longevity of use	Bumps and scars may disrupt patients body image
Lower infection than catheters	Problematic for those with needle-phobia
May be useable at around 2wks	Risk of infection >AVF
May be sited in patient unsuitable for an AVF	↓ access survival compared to AVF
Easy to use	
Suitable for home HD	

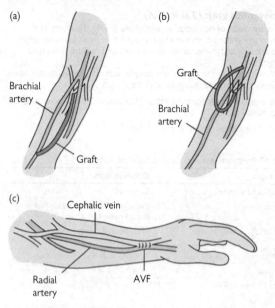

Fig. 12.6 Permanent VA for HD. (a) Forearm straight PTFE graft. (b)Forearm loop PTFE graft. (c) Radial arterio-venous fistula. Reproduced with permission from Levy J, Brown E, Daley C, et al. Oxford Handbook of Dialysis, 3rd edn. Oxford: Oxford University Press; 2009.

Care of arteriovenous fistulas and grafts

Preoperative care

Once a site for the creation/insertion of an AVF/AVG has been identified the patient should be aware it may not be used for venepuncture or measurement of BP. Preoperative preparation should include:

- What to expect of the operation (especially if under local anaesthetic)
- What to expect immediately after surgery
- Accurate marking for placement of access
- Consent
- Being adequately hydrated (helps prevent early clotting)
- If already on dialysis patient should be dialysed just prior to surgery
- Antihypertensives should be stopped
- Administer prophylactic antibiotics as per unit protocol.

Immediate postoperative care

Recover the patient safely, avoid infection, and keep them free off pain and ensure the continued patency of the access. Observe patient and their access initially at least every 30mins to ensure:

- Limited bleeding from the wound
- Wound kept clean and covered to prevent infection
- Any localized swelling is well controlled (by elevation of the limb in which the access has been created)
- The distal limb (e.g. the hand) is well perfused, i.e. warm to the touch
- BP is maintained at a reasonable level, so the AVF/AVG does not collapse
- There is an audible bruit (using a stethoscope) in the new access or a palpable thrill at or around the access site—early detection and referral of a loss of bruit/thrill may allow the surgical team to revise and ∴ save the access
- Any pain is well managed
- Signs of infection, e.g. ↑ temperature, are detected early.

Follow-up care

- Ensure patient knows how to care for their access; reinforce pre-op education and check understanding of information given
- Be aware of when the dressing should be changed, if at all, and when any stitches or clips (if appropriate) should be removed
- Know who to contact should they experience any problems.

Ongoing AVF/AVG care

- Maintain adequate hydration
- Daily hygiene and patency checking
- Do not restrict blood supply in the arm with regard to:
  - clothing
  - jewellery
  - lifting heavy objects or for prolonged periods
  - BP checking

- venepuncture
- contact sport
- Avoiding and recognizing infection
- Reporting concerns immediately
- Some patients may require help coming to terms with body image changes.

Arteriovenous fistula and graft complications

A number of complications can arise early on in the life of an AVF or AVG including: clotting; haemorrhage, and early infection (Table 12.5). These complications can be avoided by careful selection of patients, maintaining adequate hydration, use of oral anticoagulants, and good infection control procedures.

Table 12.5 Complications of AVF/AVGs

Complication	Cause	Signs and symptoms	Management	Notes
Aneurysm/ pseudoaneurysm	Repeated needling	Large swelling often around needling sites	Consider changing needle sites Surgical revision	Patient may require counselling regarding impact on body image
Bleeding	↑anticoagulation/not stopping prior to end of HD	Needle sites bleed >10mins following HD	Stop anticoagulation up to 1hr prior to the end of HD Apply directed pressure Consider pharmaceutical coagulants	Review ACT Review medications and BP
Clotting	Hypotension, dehydration, compression over AVF/AVG	Lack of thrill/bruit in the AVF/AVG	Do not needle Take blood to see if HD necessary Give thrombolytic agents Send for declotting/fistulogram/ fistuloplasty May require new access	Can occur antime following creation Educate patient regard lifestyle issues Ensure temporary access is sited
High output cardiac failure	Blood returning to the heart at arterial pressure AVF causes ↓ in peripheral resistance heart has to contract harder	Breathlessness Hypotension Oedema	May settle if mild Extreme cases may need access tying off	Very rare but potentially life threatening

(Continued)

Table 12.5 (Continued)

Complication	Cause	Signs and symptoms	Management	Notes
Infection	Poor needling technique Patient colonized with MRSA Bad personal hygiene and AVF/AVG care	Red angry exit site Purulent discharge Pain at AVF/AVG site Temperature Localized swelling	Do not cannulate Swab for cultures Treat infection AVG may need to be removed	Patient may need re educating regarding care of the AVF/AVG Patient may need admission and temporary dialysis access
Steal syndrome	Deprivation of blood distal to AVF/AVG	Cold/painful distal limb (often the hand) ↓distal pulses Necrosis	Analgesia Local applied gentle warmth Surgical revascularization	Should not be ignored Requires immediate surgical assessment
Stenosis	Hyperplasia in lumen (usually arterial side)	Difficulty cannulating; venous pressure bleeding times post HD	Angio/fistulogram Doppler US MRIof vessels Recirculation studies	May cause↑pressures AVF May cause pressure issues on HD Can ↓dialysis adequacy via recirculation

Cannulation

Cannulation of *de novo* AVFs should only be undertaken by competent HD staff. Prior to cannulation the patient should be fully appraised as to the procedure and the AVF should be checked for a bruit/thrill. When cannulating an AVF/AVG a tourniquet is now rarely used.

Local anaesthetic

The use of local anaesthetic depends on patient preference, and where possible is not used since subcutaneous lignocaine can cause scarring. Where topical anaesthesia is used (e.g. EMLA™ cream) this needs to be in place for a minimum of half an hour prior to cannulation.

AVF and AVG general cannulation guidelines

- Assess patency
- Determine direction of flow of VA (AVG use notes)
- Clean skin according to local protocol
- Administer local anaesthetic if required
- AVF:
  - cannulate >3cm from anastomosis
  - insert needle bevel upwards
  - angle needle at 25°
- AVG:
  - cannulate >5cm from anastomosis
  - insert needle bevel downwards
  - angle needle at 45°
- Avoid piercing side or back of AVF/AVG
- Site arterial needle against or with the blood flow
- Site venous needle with the blood flow
- Site arterial and venous needles >5cm apart where possible
- Flush gently with 10ml 0.9% saline
- Needle should be removed if swelling occurs or it cannot be flushed
- Secure needle as per unit policy
- Ensure access is visible during HD
- Commence HD as soon as possible.

Needle size and blood flow during HD should be appropriate to the age and maturity of the access; caution should be exercised with new access.

Following HD the needles should be removed one at a time and haemostasis attained by applying pressure to the needle site for about 10mins. The access should be checked to ensure patency prior to discharging the patient.

Cannulation techniques

There are 3 main methods for cannulating AVFs and AVGs:
- Button hole
- Rope ladder
- Area puncture.

The choice of technique relies on the age of the access (AVF), its size, and availability of site for needling as well as the competence of the individual undertaking the needling.

Buttonhole

The fistula is cannulated in the exact same spot, same angle, and depth every time. Initial cannulation is undertaken with sharp needles to develop a track over a few wks. The needles are inserted bevel upward at an angle of 40°. Once a scar tissue track develops blunt needles are used, negating the need for local anaesthetic.

Buttonhole needling is allegedly less painful, bleeds less, and fewer aneurysms form. AVFs needled in this way may be prone to increased infection as scabs form over the needle insertion sites and need to be carefully removed before each insertion. The scabs are either soaked off or picked using a sterile 'picker'.

Rope ladder

Rope ladder needling uses sharp needles inserted bevel upwards. New sites 1–2cm apart are needled on successive occasions developing the length of the AVF. It is thought rope ladder needling reduces the risk of stenosis. Buttonhole technique has superseded rope ladder as the techniques of choice for AVFs.

⚠ Area puncture needling in the same vicinity for each HD is now no longer recommended, especially for AVGs.

Complications of needling access

Complications arising from cannulation occur at one of 3 distinct times: during cannulation, during HD, and on needle removal.

Problems during cannulation

Needling an AVF which is too small, not mature enough, or very mobile can easily lead to extravasation. Extravasation or 'blowing' of the VA occurs when the needle used for cannulation inadvertently pierces through the side or back wall of the fistula of graft. Signs and symptoms include:
- Pain
- Swelling
- Bruising.

Extravasation is treated by applying pressure, ice, and administering analgesia. It is possible to commence HD using a blown arterial needle which is repositioned and from which a satisfactory flow is achieved. An extravasated venous needle should not be used for HD. Where alternative access is *in situ* the AVF/AVG should be rested for at least a week or until the swelling subsides.

Where extravasation is an ongoing problem the patients should only be needled by experienced nurses, the use of small-bore needles should be consider and referral for a surgical opinion may be appropriate.

Problems during dialysis
- Needle dislodgement:
  - may be identified by pressure alarms on the machine, bleeding from needle entry site, or excessive pain
  - observe for swelling and bruising
  - may be resolved by adjusting the needle or by removing the needle and re-cannulation
- reduced arterial pressure and mild pain or vibration at the arterial needle site may indicate the needle is sucking up against the vessel wall and the needle will need to be rotated to achieve a good flow.

⚠ Occasionally needles fall out during HD; usually the result of poorly secured needle sites, not allowing enough slack in the lines between the exit site and subsequent site of securing the EC lines or excessive patient movement.

Pressure is applied to the needle hole, the patient is taken off of HD and the EC recirculated, the remaining needle is flushed to prevent clotting. Once haemostasis is achieved the patient may be re-needled and HD recommenced.

Where the needle and dialysis line become separated during HD consideration of whether the connections have become contaminated should inform the decision as to whether to reconnect the patient using the original lines.

Problems following dialysis
Most common complication is delayed haemostasis. Associated with not turning of the heparin infusion soon enough, using too much heparin, or inadequate pressure being applied or pressure being taken off too soon following needle removal. Where over-heparinization is suspected protamine may be administered (see 📖 p. 366, Anticoagulation). Delayed bleeding from needle site after dialysis indicates manual pressure may have been taken off too soon.

Vascular access monitoring
Proactive VA monitoring is used to identify early problems such as reduced flow and stenosis. Most units have a proactive access monitoring programme which includes blood flow and venous and arterial pressure monitoring. Trends can provide evidence of changes in the quality of the blood flow through an AVF/AVG.

Common monitoring techniques used are:
- Doppler ultrasonography: converts US into an image which may be used to view fluid flow
- Transonic monitoring: US used to measure blood flow and recirculation (see 📖 p. 406, HD adequacy)
- Access recirculation monitoring: formerly done using timed blood sampling, now many devices are on the market which can do this automatically
- VA imaging and access flow studies: undertaken in a radiological setting using various imaging techniques.

Temporary haemodialysis access

When a patient requires access for dialysis in an emergency or when permanent access cannot be created, a temporary dialysis catheter is inserted; this may be tunnelled (TC) or non-tunnelled (NTC).

All patients with temporary access should be alerted to the fact that catheters are a major potential source of infection. They should be conversant with the unit's dressing regimen and exit site management policy. As with all forms of HD access the need to maintain the access purely for HD purposes to minimize infection, clotting, and loss of the access should be regularly reinforced.

Tunnelled catheter

TCs are semipermanent access and may be suitable for patients who cannot have/refuse/are awaiting the creation of an AVF/AVG.

On insertion, TCs are tunnelled under the patient's skin so there is some distance between the point of entry to the body and the blood vessel. This tunnelling, along with the presence of a Dacron® cuff around the TC, serves 2 purposes:

• Anchors the access in place
• Helps prevent the migration of infectious organisms from the skin into the blood.

TCs require priming with an anticoagulant agent at the end of dialysis in order to prevent clot formation—this 'lock', as it is termed, is then extracted and discarded prior to HD (see □ p. 381, Catheter locking).

Non-tunnelled catheter

NTCs are the least desirable form of HD access since they are associated with the highest levels of infection, morbidity, and mortality. NTCs should be replaced with more permanent access at the soonest opportunity (ideally after each dialysis when inserted femorally and at the most after 2wks for internal jugular lines). NTCs cause vascular stenosis—which affects future siting of permanent HD access. In common with TCs, NTCs are double-lumen catheters.

The key advantage of the femoral NTC is it can be used immediately after insertion. As with any catheter which penetrates the thoracic cavity, inserted into the subclavian or internal jugular vein, an x-ray is required before use to exclude pneumo/haemothorax and ensure correct placement.

Catheter complications

All catheters are subject to similar complications although those associated with NTCs are more common and often more acute in nature:

• Bruising
• Cardiac arrhythmias from poor placement of the tip (rare)
• Infection (exit site and systemic)
• Haemorrhage
• Pneumothorax
• Poor blood flow
• Stenosis of major blood vessels ↓ the chance for AVF/AVG formation
• Thrombosis.

Catheter locking

To maintain the patency of dialysis catheters they are flushed with saline after each use and an anticoagulant agent, of the right strength and amount, is instilled into each lumen. Local practice varies with many units favouring citrate-, or citrate and ethanol-containing locking solutions for their anti-coagulant and antimicrobial properties over heparin locks. Whatever form the interdialytic lock takes it must be removed prior to HD to prevent administration to the patient.

Some individuals are more prone to clotting than others and may require alteplase or urokinase to declot the catheter lumens prior to HD. Consistently poorly functioning catheters will require replacement.

Management of temporary haemodialysis access

Care of temporary dialysis access should only be undertaken by competent dialysis staff under aseptic conditions.

Non-tunnelled catheter

NTCs are prone to infections therefore temporary femoral catheters are sometimes removed after each HD session.

Prevention of infection

- Full aseptic care is needed on insertion and during connection and disconnection from HD
- Observe daily for signs of infection: redness, exudate, and odour
- Adhere to asepsis protocol when handling the catheter
- Should be removed as soon as more permanent access is established.

Infection management

- At the 1st sign of an exit infection:
  - remove catheter, send tip for culture and sensitivity
  - swab exit site and send swab for culture and sensitivity
  - peripheral and line blood cultures must be taken
  - appropriate antibiotics should be prescribed
- At the 1st sign of a systemic infection:
  - the catheter must be considered to be the most likely source of infection; there should be a low threshold for removing the catheter
  - the exit site should be inspected and swabbed for culture and sensitivity
  - peripheral and line blood cultures must be taken
  - antibiotics should be prescribed according to microbiology results.

Tunnelled catheter

TCs are less prone to infection than non-tunnelled catheters.

Prevention of infection

- Full aseptic care is needed on insertion and during connection and disconnection from HD
- Observe daily for signs of infection: redness, exudate, and odour
- Dressing should be changed at each dialysis and the exit site inspected
- Patients should be educated about the care of their catheter.

Infection management

- At the 1st sign of an exit site infection:
  - Swab exit site and send swab for culture and sensitivity
  - Peripheral and line blood cultures must be taken
  - Antibiotic requirements will be determined by the microbiology results

- At the 1st sign of an systemic infection:
  - The catheter must be consider at the most likely source of infection
  - The exit site should be inspected and swabbed for culture and sensitivity
  - Peripheral and line blood cultures must be taken
  - Antibiotic requirements will be determined by microbiology results.

▶Tunnelled catheters must be used for HD purposes only.

Assessing the patient pre dialysis

Pre-dialysis assessment of the patient is an important aspect of the dialysis process. The assessment of the ESKD patient will differ from those with AKI (see 🕮 p. 117).

Baseline assessment

Visual

- How does the patient look?
- Do they have oedema (swollen legs, ankles, periorbital oedema)?
- Are they breathless (blowing on exhaling)?
- Are they dehydrated (dry skin, dry tongue, sunken eyes)?
- Has their ability to mobilize changed between HD sessions?
- Do they have a good colour or do they look ill or anaemic?
- Does their AVF/AVG or dialysis line look clean and dry?
- Is any dressing in place where is should be?

Verbal

- How do they feel now?
- Have they been well since their last dialysis?
- Have they had cramps or felt tired?
- Have they had any problems with their VA between dialysis sessions?

Touch

- Temperature—are they hot or sweaty?
- Any signs of pitting oedema (e.g. lower legs, tested for by pressing gently) ≈fluid overload?
- Any signs of dehydration, e.g. delayed refill when applying pressure to a fingernail ≈fluid depletion or anaemia.

Clinical observations

Weight

- Each kg of excess weight gained between dialysis sessions ≈1L of additional fluid the patient is carrying
- The patient's IBW, or dry weight as it is sometimes called, represents the weight at which they are deemed to be euvolaemic—neither dehydrated nor carrying ↑ body fluid
- ↑ fluid is associated with HPT and heart disease; dehydration → ↓ BP and fainting
- Patients are weighed pre and post HD in order to determine how much fluid to remove during dialysis and to determine whether this has been achieved, respectively.

BP

- Monitoring BP pre dialysis serves 3 key purposes:
- Checks the patient is fit for dialysis
- Monitors their general state of BP health
- Allows assessment of the relationship with interdialytic fluid intake.
  A large pulse pressure (the distance between SP and DP) indicates fluid overload (the maximum range of normal being 60mmHg), while a small pulse pressure indicates dehydration.

Where dehydration is suspected, a lying (or sitting) to standing BP should be recorded. A fall in SBP of >20mmHg usually indicates dehydration (called postural or orthostatic hypotension).

▶ If BP low prior to HD, IBW may need adjusting or antihypertensive medication reviewing.

Pulse

The pulse should be assessed for both rate and rhythm. Ideally this should be done by hand as machines do not register irregular heartbeats which may result from electrolyte disturbance or disease

- A slow bounding pulse may indicate fluid overload
- A rapid weak pulse usually denotes dehydration or arrhythmia.

Temperature

Patients' temperatures are ideally checked before each HD session.

- ↑ temperature (pyrexia) may indicate infection (perhaps in the dialysis access if a line is being used). Where infection is suspected blood cultures may be indicated. If access appears infected it should not be used
- ↓ temperature may indicate dehydration or cardiovascular disease
- HD patients' normal body temperature may be lower than that of the general population and pyrexia may be present at lower absolute readings.

Respiration

The rate, rhythm, depth, and effort associated with breathing can be used to help understand the patient's condition; in some cases listening to breath sounds might be warranted.

- Shallow rapid breathing may indicate fluid overload and pulmonary oedema
- Rapid deep sighing (Kussmaul) respirations indicate severe fluid overload and/or acidosis (potentially ketoacidosis in diabetic patients). Sometime known as air hunger
- Respiratory tract infection should also be considered.

Blood glucose

- Blood glucose should be routinely checked in patients taking insulin.

Vascular access

Access should be assessed at each dialysis. AVF/AVG should be:

- Observed for signs of infection: redness, swelling or exudate
- Palpated for temperature, presence of thrill, and new stenosis.
- Distal pulses should be checked in newly formed AVF/AVGs
- Auscultated for bruit if new or small.

All dialysis catheters, whether semipermanent or temporary, should be:

- Observed for redness, swelling, or exudate at exit site
- Tested for patency prior to connection.

▶Red or swollen VA requires a medical review prior to commencing dialysis (see pp. 375–6, Infection prevention and management).

Other issues for consideration
- Recent hospitalization may have an effect on IBW:
  - poor nutrition, surgery, or reassessment
- Any problems during the previous dialysis?
  - do any blood samples taken need to be reviewed?
  - any access concerns?
  - any clotting concerns or prolonged bleeding post HD?
  - did the patient stop dialysis early?
- A fluid assessment should be undertaken each HD:
  - weight ↑↓, BP and observing for oedema
  - local policy will dictate whether re-assigning a IBW is a medical or nursing decision.

Commencing haemodialysis

All HD sessions need to be commenced following a similar pattern of activity. The aims of standardizing HD delivery are to ensure patient safety and achieve optimal dialysis dose. Universal precautions and asepsis should be observed throughout the process of preparing and connecting *all* patients to HD at *all* times.

Preparation for HD

- Undertake a thorough assessment of the patient (see 📖 pp. 384–6)
- Ensure the dialysis machine is prepared with the correct dialyser, dialysate, and anticoagulant for the patient and the EC is properly primed (see 📖 p. 360, The extracorporeal circuit)
- Ensure the correct dialysis parameters have been programmed into the dialysis machine, including any extra fluid which needs to be removed to account for intradialytic infusions
- Assess and prepare the patient's access for HD (see 📖 pp. 377–9, Cannulation and 📖 pp. 380–1, Management of temporary HD access)
- Connect the access to the dialysis lines (the EC) following local protocol either bleed out the priming saline or straight connect the patient
- Administer anticoagulation as prescribed (see 📖 pp. 364–6, Anticoagulation)
- Ensure the access is securely fastened according to local protocol and that if an AVF or AVG are in use they are visible
- Observe and record the various machine pressures ensuring they are within safe limits and any guards which need to be set have been set correctly.

Patients undergoing dialysis for the 1st time

Preparation for the 1st HD will depend on whether the patient has presented acutely (see 📖 pp. 116–19) or whether they have been referred via the advanced kidney care clinic (see 📖 pp. 154–7).

The aims of the 1st HD session for the new ESKD patient are to:
• Ensure patient receives a safe HD
• Assess the patient's dialysis needs
• Set initial treatment parameters
• Ensure the safety of other patients and staff.

The initial HD sessions will be very different from subsequent HD sessions. Of concern is the potential for dialysis disequilibrium syndrome (DDS; see 📖 p. 118) arising from the rapid reduction in plasma urea as well as the potential for haemorrhage due to high urea levels. Cardiovascular tolerability toward fluid removal also needs to be assessed; therefore the 1st HD should:
• Be ~2hrs ↑ to 3hrs for the 2nd session and 3.5/4h subsequently
• Use a low efficiency dialyser
• Achieve a URR of ~30%
• Run ↓ BFR ~200ml/min
• DFR ≤500ml/min
• Anticoagulated as per unit protocol (possibly heparin free)
• Remove ≤2L fluid.

▶ All new patients should be treated as an infection risk until their viral screen/MRSA swabs have been returned.

Of particular nursing concern is ensuring the patient understands what HD is, how often it occurs, their fluid and lifestyle restrictions including access monitoring and care.

New patient dialysis prescription
• Setting the dialysis prescription for new patients needs to take account of:
• Residual kidney function
• Nutritional status
• Patient size (weight/height)
• Age
• Cardiovascular stability and general health.

▶The dialysis prescription will need to be reviewed frequently in the 1st few wks of HD.

Dialysate for patients undergoing dialysis for the 1st time
Blood chemistry which is <24hrs old is a requisite for planning HD for all new patients. This will aid in setting dialysate levels which help avoid complications arising. Rapid correction of longstanding abnormal blood chemistry may give rise to potentially life-threatening complications and should be avoided.

Alkalotic and acidotic patients may require reduced HCO_3 in order to avoid overcorrection.

▶ Hyponatraemia should not be corrected too quickly (dialysate <20mmol higher than plasma level) while hypernatraemia should not be corrected too early as risk of IDH (see 📖 p. 404).

⚠ Fluid shifts due to rapidly ↓ plasma Na^+ concentration may give rise to severe IDH, loss of consciousness, and cardiac arrest.

▶ Rapid ↓ in Ca^{2+} may also contribute to IDH and ↓ Ca^{2+} dialysate should therefore not be used.

▶ Patients with CKD are more tolerant of and adapt to recurring hyperkalaemia. A rapid ↓ in K^+ during 1st HD may predispose to cardiac arrhythmias. The use of 0mmol/L dialysate K^+ for hyperkalaemic patients should be resisted.

The dialysis prescription

Individual patients require individual dialysis prescriptions. A HD prescription needs to take into account patient-specific variables:
• Individual total body water (size, and disease dependent)
• Urea generation rate (affected by diet and liver function)
• Residual kidney function
• Interdialytic fluid intake.

There are a number of dialysis variables which may be altered in order to achieve a good dialysis:
• Dialyser size
• Dialyser type
• Dialysis length
• Dialysis frequency
• Type of dialysis (high flux/low flux)
• Change to HDF (see 📖 p. 416, Therapies derived from HD)
• Access type
• BFR.

Decisions about an individual's dialysis prescription should include:
• Anticoagulation
• Dialysate prescription
• IBW changes
• Dietary advice.

The dialysis prescription should be regarded as a holistic, rather than mechanical, decision making process (see 📖 p. 388, Patients undergoing dialysis for the 1st time).

Dialyser

The choice of dialyser size will depend on:
• Patient size
• Tolerance of HD.

Use of high flux will depend on patient need and local protocol.

BFR

BFR directly affects solute clearance; each dialyser has a set clearance of urea (KoA) in relation to BFR (see 📖 pp. 358–9, The dialyser). This information is found in the manufacturer's information leaflet. This will depend on the patient's dialysis requirements and the quality of the access they have.

Fluid removal

Will depend on the patient's need, and ability, to tolerate UF. In new patients this should be undertaken cautiously to avoid complications (see 📖 pp. 394–6, Methods of fluid removal).

Adequacy

The main purpose of any dialysis prescription is to attain a dialysis which is better than adequate for the individual patient's needs (URR >70% or Kt/V >1.3)

Nursing considerations during dialysis

- Carry out a full pre-dialysis assessment
- Discuss fluid/weight gain with patient, offer support and education about fluid management
- Check patient aware of fluid and dietary parameters/restrictions—refer to dietitian if required for further support
- Take any blood samples requested pre, post, or during dialysis
- Ensure patient receives correct dialysis prescription
- Ensure quality of dialysis: observations, BFR, complete prescribed hrs
- Ensure safe dialysis: prevent needle dislodgement, reduce risk of complications during treatment
- Document and report any deviations from prescribed dialysis to senior staff/medical staff
- Check patient is taking medication as prescribed
- Administer any drugs prescribed to be given during dialysis, e.g. ESA, IV iron, IV alfacalcidol
- Be aware of patient's psychological and social needs
- Promote self-care and encourage patient to participate in aspects of dialysis, e.g. weighing, BP, care of VA
- Ensure infection prevention and management procedures are followed.

Routine tests

Blood tests

It is recommended that routine blood tests be taken before a mid-week HD session using a dry needle/syringe (access dependent).

Monthly blood testing includes:
- Dialysis adequacy (Kt/V, URR)
- Cr
- U&Es
- HCO_3
- Renal bone profile (Ca^{2+}, PO_4, Alb)
- FBC
- Glucose/HbA1c (if diabetic and if not checked in 1° care).

3-monthly blood testing include:
- Iron studies (ferritin, % TSAT, % HRC)
- CRP
- Aluminium (if taking Alucaps®)
- Hepatitis B and C.

6-monthly blood testing includes:
- PTH
- Chol
- B12 and folate.

Testing for conditions such as HIV is undertaken with consent when a patient commences HD for the 1st time and then again only as indicated, e.g. after HD abroad in an 'at-risk' environment.

Additional testing
Further tests, such as MRSA swabs, may be required if the patient
- Has any health concerns
- Has been unwell
- Has been an inpatient
- Has undertaken HD in a different unit.

Methods of fluid removal

Management of fluid removal starts outside of the HD unit and the patient's ability to tolerate large volumes of fluid removal should not preclude attempts at reducing fluid intake. Proactive strategies include:
- Frequent dietetic input regarding salt and fluid intake
- Psychological support/referral where adjustment is proving hard
- Not taking antihypertensive pre HD
- Use of BP supporting medications, e.g. midodrine and carnitine (in deficient patients).

Intradialysis there are a number of potential strategies which help maintain BP and hence enable fluid removal.

Sodium profiling

This remains a controversial choice. Profiling refers to dialysis which is delivered using a ↑ Na^+ concentration in the dialysate at the start of dialysis and a ↓ concentration at the end. The ↑ Na^+ will dialyse *into* the patient's blood via the dialyser, ↑ their plasma Na^+. The ↑ Na content of the blood generates an osmotic gradient which attracts fluid from the interstitium into the circulation supporting the patient's BP.

The level of Na^+ in the dialysate ↓ throughout dialysis (either as programmed, stepwise, or linearly, or manually at set times). Simultaneous to the ↓ in dialysate Na^+ the UFR also ↓. The ↓ Na^+ level at the end of HD is thought to help reduce intradialytic thirst.

The role of calcium

↓ plasma Ca^{2+} levels reduce cardiac contractility and hence BP. ↑ Ca^{2+} calcium dialysate (1.5–1.75mmol/L) helps maintain contractility but may ↑ Ca^{2+} load.

Isolated ultrafiltration

Isolated UF is gentler than simultaneous HD and UF and is performed in the 1st hour of HD when plasma urea and sodium are at their highest (encouraging plasma refill from the extravascular fluid compartment). Dialysis is then performed in the usual manner at a low UFR.

Low temperature dialysis

There are many studies which support low dialysate temperatures (35–36°C) as a means of promoting vasoconstriction/preventing vasodilation and therefore supporting BP. Some patients may find low dialysate temperatures uncomfortable.

Increased dialysis time

Will increase the amount of time available over which to remove fluid thereby reducing UFR. Some patients will find this unacceptable and may refuse to allow it.

Nursing considerations for fluid removal

All strategies to enable ↑ fluid removal risk encouraging ↑ fluid intake.
↑ fluid intake, is associated with:
- HPT
- LVH
- Peripheral and pulmonary oedema
- Morbidity
- Death.

The role of the nurse is to assess the patient and make appropriate referrals to other professionals whose input may be of benefit:
- Dietitian
- Pharmacist
- Psychotherapist
- Counsellor
- Social worker
- Occupational therapist.

Case study

David is 67yrs old, has type II diabetes and hypertension, and has been on dialysis for 3 months. David is dialysed for 4hrs three times a week on a low-flux dialyser and usually needs 3.5L of fluid removing plus washback.

David takes 3 antihypertensive agents, although he is always hypertensive (180/110mm/Hg) pre dialysis. At about 2½hrs into each dialysis session David experiences severe IDH and vomits before losing consciousness.

The nurses in the team decide to devise a strategy to help manage David's IDH. Since David takes on too much fluid between dialyses, he is referred to the dietitian regarding his salt and fluid intake.

On discussion David is struggling to come to terms with being on HD and as he lives alone, and he is tired all the time, he lives on ready meals. Since he is not anaemic and his URR is 73% David is referred to the renal counsellor. The renal social worker also visits David and arranges dialysis appropriate meals on non-dialysis days.

David is requested not to take his antihypertensive prior to HD and not to eat or drink in the 2hrs prior to dialysis. The team decide to alter David's dialysate temperature to 35.5°C.

The case study illustrates the importance of joined up thinking and the use of the full multidisciplinary team in the management of IDH. The strategy focuses on David as an individual and recognizes how the social and psychological influence on him are potentially contributing to his IDH. The emphasis is on a number of small, subtle interventions which collectively could have a large impact on David's HD experience.

Observations during dialysis

For the majority of patients, checking vital signs just once during HD is sufficient. The frequency of observations should be ↑ for patients who are:
- New to HD
- Suffer frequent IDH
- Are systemically unwell
- Elderly.

For patients who are particularly unstable on HD the use of automated monitors may be useful. However visual assessment of the patient is essential and less stable patients are best dialysed close to the nursing station. At a minimum, intradialytic observations should include BP and pulse. Some HD machines have in-line haematocrit monitors which detect changes in the fluid status of an individual patient which may pre-empt an episode of IDH.

It is worth noting in individual patient's notes their usual signs and symptoms for going flat (IDH) since these can provide useful early warning of what might become a more serious episode.

Ending dialysis

The routine followed at the end of HD has 2 purposes:
• To ensure the goals for the session have been achieved (e.g. patient has attained their IBW)
• To ensure they are fit to be discharged (e.g. BP is adequate).

Prior to disconnecting the patient from HD it is important to check the machine has removed the correct amount of fluid and any HD drugs have been administered. The amount of blood dialysed (recorded as litres processed) should be recorded.

The blood pump should be stopped and the arterial access flushed and clamped. The arterial EC line should be clamped and attached to the 'washback' saline. The blood pump should be restarted at 150ml/min and should run until the EC is almost clear of blood; usually at about 2mins.

At this stage the patient's vital signs should be checked to ensure no further fluid is needed to support their BP and then the HD needles may be removed/the HD catheter flushed and locked with anticoagulant.

Any excess clotting on the EC or the dialyser should be documented and a recommendation for increasing anticoagulation documented.

Once the access is removed/locked the HD machine may be stripped and disinfected. The patient should be weighed to ensure they have reached their IBW (see p. 384, Assessing the patient pre-dialysis). Once the patient has been discharged the bed/chair and table at the HD station should be cleaned and disinfected.

Assessing the patient post dialysis

Post-dialysis assessment of the patient serves 2 key purposes:
- Assessing and documenting the quality of the dialysis delivered
- Assesses whether the patient is safe to be discharged home.

Baseline assessment

Visual
- How does the patient look?
- Does their AVF/AVG or dialysis catheter look clean and dry?
- Is any dressing in place where is should be?

Verbal
- How does the patient feel?
- Have they remained well during dialysis?
- Have they had cramps during the session?

Touch
- Are they hot or sweaty or cold and clammy (i.e. have they become septic or are they hypovolaemic?).

Clinical observations

BP
- Post HD the patient's BP should be taken to ensure it is safe for them to stand
- ▶Where dehydration is suspected, a lying/sitting BP should be undertaken with some caution
- Recommended post-HD BP ≤130/80mm/Hg
- Where a patient's post-HD BP is >130/80mm/Hg they should take their antihypertensives as soon as possible
- If the patient has a large ↓ in pulse pressure post HD, their IBW may need reassessing.

Weight
- Has the patient achieved their IBW during dialysis?
- If ↑ IBW why is this? Consider reinforcing education about the need for salt and fluid restriction
- If they are very much over their IBW consider the need for further dialysis/UF especially prior to the weekend inter dialysis break
- If they are under their IBW why is this? Are they safe to go (check BP sitting/lying and standing). Consider the need to give extra fluid.

Pulse
- The post HD pulse is best taken by hand to assess rate and rhythm
- Cardiac arrhythmias, which are not normal for the patient, may be indicative of an electrolyte disturbance and should be investigated.

Temperature
- Generally it is not necessary to take the patient's temperature after dialysis unless they have signs or symptoms of fever
- Ideally if this is the case the temperature should be taken before removing needles or heparinizing and capping the dialysis catheter as blood cultures may be needed.

Respiration
- Post-HD breathlessness in patients without a history of respiratory or cardiac disease may indicate continued fluid overload, the presence of a respiratory tract infection, or the development of congestive cardiac failure and should be documented and investigated.

Blood glucose
- Blood glucose measures post dialysis are only needed if the insulin-dependent diabetic patient is complaining of light-headedness

The documentation of the post-HD condition of the patient is important as it forms the basis of the assessment at the start of the next HD session.

Patient involvement in dialysis

The last 10yrs have seen an ↑ interest in promoting self-care, underpinned by the first renal NSF (2004) and NICE (2002) guidelines.

Patient ability to become involved in self-care will depend on:
- Age
- Physical and mental ability
- Willingness to participate
- Cultural factors
- Availability of support.

The ability of staff to train patients to partake in aspects of their own care is driven by staff training, willingness, time, and resources. Patient involvement requires the input of the whole MPT. Individual targets for participation need to be agreed, according to need and ability. Patient involvement with HD can range from contributing to their own preparation for HD (i.e. weighing themself) right through to taking ownership of the whole HD process and finally home HD.

Methods of delivering education need to be individualized (see 📖 pp. 604–5).

Suggested content of HD patient training programme
- The nature of HD
- Understanding and doing observations
- IBW, weighing, and setting fluid removal
- VA care
- Lining and priming
- Commencing HD
- Troubleshooting alarms, machine issues, and access problems
- Ending HD
- Documentation
- Universal precautions and waste disposal
- Diet and fluid restrictions
- Understanding medications
- Where to get support.

Other topics which patients may benefit from information about include:
- Diet
- Fluid management
- Body image
- Sexual health
- Understanding symptoms
- Medication management
- Financial support.

For further information see 📖 pp. 531–63.

Supporting the haemodialysis patient

There are a number of ways in which support can be given to HD patients and a number of professionals who can be involved. Proactive support from the MPT and education of HD patients can help avoid potential problems arising as well as enabling patients to deal with problems which do arise during care.

HD clinics

Ideally all HD patients should be seen outside of the dialysis setting on a regular basis (at least bi-annually), medication reviewed, problems pre-empted, education provided, and the dialysis prescription and IBW reviewed. HD clinics are an opportunity for the patient to raise any concerns they may have and for appropriate referrals to be made. Alternatively patients may be seen regularly by a nephrologist whilst dialysing.

Dietetic review

This should happen at least bi-annually. Information regarding all aspects of diet and fluid intake should be covered and levels of understanding assessed and dietetic plans reinforced. Ideally this should be undertaken away from the dialysis setting. Advice given should be age and culturally appropriate.

Psychological and social support

Where possible this should be undertaken in a proactive manner. Referrals for support should be made in response to specific life events and/or concerns raised by the patient. Significant events might include body image issues relating to the formation of access and scarring, fear regarding life chances and observing the death of fellow dialysis patients. Counselling and psychological referral should be made to a professional who is conversant with the issues pertinent to HD patients. Named nurses or nursing teams should recognize signs of anxiety, stress, and acopia.

Other specialities

The presence of concomitant disease and illness should never be forgotten. For example, patients with diabetes need the input of the diabetes as well as the nephrology team. The HD nurse should ensure patients are referred to and reviewed regularly by appropriate specialists.

Intradialytic complications

There are a large number of issues which may affect any patient on HD. Recognizing and responding to intradialytic problems quickly and appropriately may help avoid ↑ morbidity and mortality.

Fever and chills
Due to:
- Exit site infection
- Systemic infection from access
- Other infection (e.g. respiratory tract)
- Dialysate temperature
- Blood transfusions.

Recognition and removal/treatment of the cause, administration of antibiotics and paracetamol, blood cultures/exit site swabs is essential.

Headache
Due to:
- Anxiety
- Caffeine/nicotine withdrawal
- Dialyser reaction
- DDS (see 🕮 p. 118)
- Excessive/inaccurate fluid removal
- Inaccurate IBW
- Hypertension/hypotension.

Management includes identifying and rectifying the cause, proving support and reassurance, and the administration of analgesia.

Chest pain
Causes include:
- Air embolism
- Anaemia
- Anxiety
- Cardiac event (e.g. angina, MI, arrhythmia)
- Electrolyte imbalance
- Gastric reflux
- Hypotension.

Management
- Obtain baseline observations immediately and alert other staff.
- Set UFR on the machine to zero and ↓ BFR. Identify cause, treat if possible or refer as required.

Cardiac arrest
May be precipitated by:
- Anaphylaxis (e.g. ethylene oxide, protamine)
- Cardiac event (e.g. myocardial infarction)
- Cerebral event (e.g. haemorrhage)
- Hyper/hypokalaemia

- Hypocalcaemia
- IDH (excessive fluid removal)
- Pericarditis.

Management
Commence CPR immediately whilst a cause is identified and if possible reversed. Wash back the patient if possible and stop HD, preserve access to enable taking of blood samples/drugs administration.

Air embolism
Signs and symptoms
- Confusion and dizziness
- Coughing and dyspnoea
- Double vision
- Death
- Fitting
- Pain/tingling in chest
- Roaring sound in ears
- Slurred speech.

Causes
- Inadvertent removal of central venous access (falling out)
- Separation of venous line and dialysis catheter
- Malfunctioning air detector
- Cracked/split dialysis catheter
- Turbulence in the venous chamber due to ↑ BFR.

Management
▶ Treatment needs to be rapid and decisive in order to preserve life:
- ↑ level of blood in venous chamber and ↓ BFR
- Turn BFR off and clamp all lines
- Place patient in Trendelenburg position—head down and on their left side (keeps air trapped in right ventricle)
- Try to withdraw air from venous access
- Administer O_2.

Convulsions
Causes
- Anaphylaxis (e.g. ethylene oxide, protamine, endotoxins)
- Arrhythmias
- DDS (see 📖 p. 118)
- Electrolyte disturbance
- Hypoglycaemia
- IDH
- Epilepsy.

Management
The BFR and UFR should be stopped and washback considered. Airway maintenance is the priority. The cause should be removed/treated.

Intradialytic hypotension (going flat)

This is the most common intradialytic complication and is usually the result of intolerance of/excessive fluid removal. Other causes include:
- Air embolism
- Anaemia
- Anaphylaxis
- Antihypertensives: incorrect dosage/taken pre HD
- Arrhythmia, ► check pulse manually
- Dialysate temperature too ↑
- Dialyser membrane reaction
- Disconnection of blood lines/haemorrhage
- Eating or drinking on HD
- Haemolysis
- Myocardial infarction
- Septicaemia.

Management

Individual patients display different signs and symptoms of IDH which should be documented. IDH may progress to cardiac arrest ∴ treatment needs to be rapid and includes airway maintenance, cardiovascular refilling, ensuring blood flow to the brain. On recovery reassessment of IBW and HD fluid removal target should be undertaken. An ECG may be needed to exclude a cardiac event. Education may be required regarding use of antihypertensive pre HD, and eating and drinking on and off HD. Onward referral (e.g. to the dietitian) may be advisable. See 📖 pp. 394–5.

Cramps

May occur either in peripheral muscles or abdominally. Cramps may be a complication on their own or a sign of something else (e.g. IDH).

Causes include:
- DDS
- Excessive/inaccurate fluid removal/hypovolaemia
- Na⁺ imbalance
- ↓ K⁺ level.

Management

The immediate response includes ↓ both UFR and BFR, replacement fluids may be needed. Heat and massage may help. The IBW may need reviewing. Education and support regarding fluid intake should be given.

Nausea and vomiting

Causes include:
- Contaminated dialysate
- DDS (see 📖 p. 118)
- Gastroenteritis
- Hypo/hyperglycaemia
- Hypotension/hypertension
- Infection
- Uraemia.

Management

Consider ↓ fluid removal, in severe cases slow down or stop dialysis. Remove/treat cause and administer antiemetic medication.

Pyrogenic reactions

These manifest with a variety of symptoms including:
• Anaphylactic type reaction
• Chest pain
• Chills
• Clamminess
• Hives
• Hypotension
• Pyrexia
• Rigors.

Causes

Bacteria or bacterial endotoxins entering the body rapidly as the result of contaminated dialysate.

Management

Stop dialysis with no wash-back. Water and blood samples should be sent for microbiological testing. Consider admitting the patient for observation.

Nursing considerations

With HD units being such public places the need to protect the patient's dignity in all scenarios is important. In some instances the need to provide support and reassurance to patients who witness potentially distressing events should be considered.

All complications of dialysis give rise to the need for support, education, and potentially referral of the person affected. The nurse should consider who is the best person to address the patient's needs and ensure the appropriate referral is made. Patients who experience recurrent events may require preventative strategies to be put in place.

Adequacy

Adequate, and better than adequate, dialysis improves the quality and longevity of HD patients' lives. Good quality dialysis is about more than merely reducing levels of circulating toxins and waste products of dialysis. In order to minimize morbidity and mortality associated with ESKD the dialysis nurse needs to be concerned about the management of:

- Ca^{2+}/PO_4 product
- Exercise capacity
- Hb
- Infection
- Nutritional intake.

Urea is a small, water-soluble waste product of protein metabolism, and often used as a cheap and easy to process means of measuring both renal function and dialysis efficiency.

If sufficient urea, and, by association, other important toxins (both known and unknown), are removed by HD, then patient survival improves as do other markers of morbidity and QOL. The amount of urea removed during dialysis is calculated using the urea reduction ratio (URR). Most guidelines suggest a target URR of > 70%/Kt/V > 1.3/1.4.

Exceeding the targets is ideal, while failure to meet these target figures requires prompt intervention to improve adequacy.

- Pre-HD urea 20–30mmol/L is a good indicator of patient health
- Plasma urea <20mmol/L is indicative of malnutrition, vegetarianism, or partial residual renal function
- Pre-HD urea >30mmol/L is indicative of poor HD adequacy; often the result of inadequate access.

Urea reduction rate

The URR is a real measure of the drop in urea levels during a single dialysis session and may be calculated as:

$$\frac{\text{Pre urea - post urea}}{\text{Pre urea}} \times 100 = \text{URR (\%)}$$

$$\text{Example}: \frac{25 - 7}{25} \times 100 = 72\% \rightarrow \text{adequately dialysed}$$

Being a measure of the change in urea in one dialysis session means URR needs to be interpreted against other measures of well-being and dialysis efficiency for each individual patient. The quality of an individual HD session may not reflect all HD sessions, for example, if the dialysis access is intermittently good affecting the amount of blood processed during HD.

Variables which will affects dialysis adequacy include:

- Access quality
- Access type
- BFR
- DFR
- Dialyser size

- Recirculation of dialysed blood
- Time on the machine.

Other markers of adequacy such as Cr levels and anaemia are useful at indicating whether the URR is representative of the true adequacy of HD a patient is receiving.

Sampling for URR

It is important the initial sample pre dialysis is not contaminated with 0.9% saline or line lock. It is usual practice to obtain samples using dialysis needles which have not been primed and from dialysis catheters after the removal of the locking solution, before flushing.

The post HD sample is taken according to unit policy where consistency is key, with the same collection method used at all times. Therefore any changes in patient results are attributable to clinical, rather than sampling issues. Commonly units either stop the dialysate flow for about 5mins and/ or reduced the BFR to 150–200ml/min for 2–3mins before sampling from the arterial line.

Kt/V

Kt/V is essentially a theoretical measure of the adequacy of dialysis calculated using 3 variables:

- K = urea clearance of the dialyser in ml/min (obtained from manufacturer)
- t = session time in mins
- V = is an estimation of the patients total body water (in ml).

K is a constant for a given dialyser and therefore can only be altered by altering the dialyser. Time on dialysis can be lengthened or shortened thereby changing t. The patient's body volume of water is not alterable therefore little can be done about V.

The most straightforward method of estimating V is to presuppose V is 55% of the total body weight for ♀ and 58% for ♂ (remembering each kilo of weight equates to 1L of water).

- A 58kg female patient would have a urea distribution volume (V) of 55% × 58 = 31.9L = 31900ml
- If the patient were given a treatment with a dialyser clearance of 180ml/min lasting 3.5hrs (210mins) then the prescribed Kt would be
- 37,800; 37,800/31,900 = Kt/V 1.2.

▶The calculated Kt/V and adequacy of dialysis may not be synonymous perhaps because of poor access.

Kt/V calculations may be modified to represent a more correct measure of dialysis adequacy; however, true measures of adequacy do require the measurement of blood samples pre and post HD which may be used to calculate Kt/V using natural logarithms.

More accurate methods of calculating Kt/V (e.g. urea kinetic modelling) involve intricate patterns of blood sampling and other physiological measures (e.g. RRF and diet) as well as complex computer programs which make them impractical for large-scale use.

Online clearance monitors (OCM)
OCMs may be used to monitor the removal of urea during HD in real-time

Signs of a well-dialysed patient include:
- Acceptable libido
- Adequate Hb
- Being infection free
- Good QOL
- Limited access recirculation <10%
- ↓ morbidity
- ↓ mortality
- Reasonable exercise tolerance
- Reasonable nutritional status
- URR >70%/Kt/V >1.3
- Ca^{2+}/PO_4 product <4.5.

Ways to improve HD adequacy
- Ensure patient completes each HD session in full
- Good quality access
- ↑ needle gauge
- Reduce/prevent access recirculation
- Use AVF/AVG for HD
- Ensure adequate anticoagulation
- Change type/frequency of dialysis:
  - high flux
  - HDF
  - daily
- ↑ BFR
- ↑ dialysis time
- ↑ DFR (to a point)
- ↑ dialyser size.

Recirculation
Recirculation occurs when blood which has already been dialysed passes back into the arterial side of the patient's access. This phenomenon affects AVGs and AVFs more than dialysis catheters. Recirculated blood is already low in waste products and therefore the diffusion gradient is diminished and the adequacy of dialysis affected.

Causes
In AVFs and AVGs, includes reduced or retrograde blood flow through the access (perhaps as the result of a distal stenosis) and dialysis needles which are sited too close together. The suggested target for recirculation is <10%.

2 common ways to measure recirculation include a 2-needle technique and US dilution technique.

2-needle measurement of recirculation*

- Perform test after 30mins of dialysis with UF switched off
- Take arterial (A) and venous (V) blood samples from the access lines
- Reduce blood flow rate to 120ml/min for 10secs then switch off pump
- Clamp arterial line above sampling port and take systemic arterial sample (S) from arterial line
- Resume dialysis.
- Measure urea in arterial, venous, and systemic sample (A, V, and S).

$$\text{Recirculation} = \frac{S - A}{S - V} \times 100$$

This method is less accurate than dilution techniques, but easy to perform and reliable. Dilution methods are increasingly used though as more dialysis machines come equipped with appropriate technology.

US dilution techniques for measurement of recirculation*

Recirculation can be measured using US measurement of the dilution of saline (e.g. transonic device) or by temperature change, as for measuring flow but with blood lines not reversed. A bolus of saline injected into the V line will be detected at the A line if there is significant recirculation.

* Reproduced with permission from Levy J, Brown E, Daley C, et al. Oxford Handbook of Dialysis, 3rd edn. Oxford: Oxford University Press; 2009.

Long-term complications

As people are surviving longer on HD the management of the long-term complications of dialysis become an ever more pressing issue for the nephrology team. Long-term complications can have a serious impact on:

• QOL
• General morbidity (often measured as hospitalization)
• Longevity of life.

Cardiovascular disease

CVD in HD patients is often a result of their initial presenting disease (e.g. hypertension or diabetes) or as a co-morbidity of the ESKD itself (e.g. poor BP control, poor fluid management, anaemia, electrolyte disturbance, and dyslipidaemia). CVD is the leading cause of death in patients at all stages of CKD. Key manifestations of CVD include:

• Angina
• Arrhythmia
• Coronary ischaemia
• LVH
• PVD.

Management of CVD complications ∴ include adequate dialysis and the management of potential causes through pharmacological, dietetic, and educational means (see 📖 p. 79).

Gastrointestinal problems

GI disturbances play a leading role in the malnutrition which is so often associated with ESKD and which is associated with ↑ morbidity and mortality. The probable causes of GI disturbances in patients with ESKD include:

• Age
• Inadequate dialysis
• Medications
• Metabolic acidosis
• Metabolic disturbance (e.g. diabetes)
• Psychosocial factors
• Uraemic toxins.

Key manifestations of GI disturbance in CKD/ESKD include:

• Constipation/diarrhoea
• Dyspepsia
• Gastroduodenal inflammation
• Malnutrition
• Nausea/vomiting.

Management of GI disturbance ∴ requires adequate dialysis, the use of medications, education, and dietetic input and perhaps onward referral.

Immune dysfunction

Immune dysfunction in ESKD arises as a result of many factors including the presence of uraemic toxins. Good infection control practices, immunization, and dietetic input all help prevent the onset of sepsis. The presence of immune dysfunction may in characterized by increased risk of infection and tissue degeneration.

Neurological issues

Neurological problems arise as the result of pre-existing disease (e.g. diabetes) and the impact of ESKD, especially the build-up of uraemic toxins. The signs and symptoms of neurological dysfunction include:

- Confusion
- Fatigue
- Headache
- Hiccups
- Insomnia
- Irritability
- Peripheral neuropathy
- Restless leg syndrome
- Sensory impairment.

Issues with vision

Visual problems are common in HD patients and include retinopathy, cataracts, and glaucoma. The presence of these in HD patients is attributable in large part to the increased prevalence of diabetes and hypertension. Signs and symptoms include:

- Blurred vision
- Conjunctival haemorrhages
- Loss of vision (including peripheral)
- Pain.

Renal osteodystrophy

Renal bone disease is a pressing problem in HD patients and results from disturbed Ca^{2+}/PO_4 metabolism. Signs and symptoms include bone and joint pain as well as deformation and propensity to fracture. As ever, good management includes adequate dialysis, pharmaceutical intervention, and dietetic management (see 📖 pp. 192–6).

Amyloid

Dialysis-related amyloidosis (DRA) is unique to patients undergoing long-term HD. It is caused by the deposition of B_2m. The pathogenesis and pathophysiology of DRA is not fully understood, but is probably affected by patient age, length of time with CKD/on HD, and biocompatibility of HD membranes. DRA affects bones and joints; predominantly hips, wrists, shoulders, spine, and knees. DRA is manifested as osteoarthropathies and erosive joint and bone disease. Improved biocompatibility and the use of HDF both contribute to preventing the genesis and progression of DRA

Infection prevention and management

After sudden cardiovascular death, and possibly withdrawal from dialysis, the leading cause of mortality amongst ESKD patients undertaking HD is infection. Infection is preventable.

Factors increasing risk of infection in HD patients include:

- DM
- Older age
- Malnutrition
- Temporary or semipermanent vascular catheters
- Regular hospital attendance
- Immunosuppression 2° to uraemia
- Poor skin integrity
- Exposure of blood to dialysis.

▶ Universal precautions are a fundamental part of infection control and be considered as protective to both staff and patients.

Standard infection control measures

- The most important universal precaution is good hand hygiene, i.e. hand washing before and after patient contact regardless of whether gloves are worn. The appropriate use of alcohol gel
- The use of personal protective equipment: gloves, aprons, goggles/face shield, changed (where appropriate) between patients Where items for HD use are not single use they should be thoroughly cleaned according to a local protocol between HD sessions
- Dialysate containers should be discarded/recycled after single use
- Dialysis lines and dialysers should be double bagged and removed to the bin immediately after use
- Sharps bins should be available within reach every time a medical sharp is used
- Visitors and visiting professionals should clean their hands on entering and leaving a dialysis unit.

Infections affecting dialysis units

The nature of HD means BBV and other infections are of special importance:

- *Clostridium difficile*
- HBV
- HCV
- HIV
- MRSA
- *Staphylococcus aureus*
- VRE.

Management of patients with BBV

Patients with BBV are an infection risk to both other patients and staff. National and local policies determine what intervention is needed. Alongside good clinical practice, universal precautions, immunization, and procedures outlined in the rest of this section, the following issues apply to the management of BBV in the dialysis unit:

- The machine's exterior should always be cleaned between each use as per unit protocol. If there is any suspected blood seepage into the machine through panels sensors or transducers the machine must be removed from use immediately and decontaminated as per manufacturer's instructions
- Heat disinfection of machines should always follow each patient use.

▶ If a patient dialyses away from their unit in an area where there is potential risk of exposure to BBV, they should be segregated until known to HbsAg negative. This is not required if they have known HBV immunity.

HBV

The increased use of universal precautions and routine vaccination has reduced the prevalence of HBV in HD units.

Patients commencing HD or returning to HD from another RRT modality need to be tested for HbsAg and be proven to be negative before having dialysis on the main dialysis unit. Alternatively they should be isolated until the results are known.

Separate dialysis machines are recommended for patients who have HBV and those with HBV should be segregated. Only HBV immune renal staff should care for HBV +ve patients. A machine that has been used for HBV patients can be used again for non-infected patients only after it has been thoroughly decontaminated.

HBV vaccination

Nephrology services need to ensure patients are vaccinated prior to commencing HD. Those who have responded to HBV vaccination should have annual HBsAg titres (>10m units/ml). Those who have not responded should be tested for HBsAg every 3 months.

HCV

HCV is the major liver disease affecting HD patients despite its prevalence being on the decline. Isolated machines are not required provided disinfection processes are properly carried out as per local protocol.

HIV

Isolated machines are not required, provided that that the disinfection processes are properly carried out as per local protocol.

6-monthly screening is recommended for high-risks groups, including patients returning from holiday dialysis in a high-risk area.

See 📖 Pathophysiology for further information.

Management of other common infections in the HD unit

Due to the large numbers of people who visit the HD unit, the widespread use of antibiotics, and the immunocompromised nature of HD patients, the incidence and prevalence of infections in the HD population are high. As well as managing the risk of infection from BBVs, HD staff need to be alert to the risk of other infections which may impact the QOL of patients and which, in some cases, may prove fatal.

Meticillin-resistant Staphylococcus aureus (MRSA)

MRSA is derived from antibiotic resistance which came about as a result of the widespread, often indiscriminate use of antibiotics, usually in the hospital setting. While no more virulent than other infections MRSA is becoming more difficult to treat.

The majority of HD units isolate MRSA positive patients, until they have had 3 sets of MRSA negative swabs on consecutive wks whilst not on MRSA treatment.

All HD patients should be screened for MRSA:
• 3-monthly
• After dialysing in another unit
• Following hospitalization.

The management of MRSA infection should be thorough and directed by the local infection control team. For HD patients this may include the removal of dialysis catheters.

Alongside MRSA, some units test for *S. aureus* and subject +ve individuals to decolonization treatment in order to ↓ morbidity.

Vancomycin-resistant enterococci (VRE)

VRE appears able to transfer vancomycin resistance to other bacteria such as MRSA. Despite the low incidence of VRE it is good practice to avoid the use of vancomycin, cephalosporins, and quinolones in order to prevent its development.

Clostridium difficile (C. diff)

C. diff is quiescent until a person carrying it takes antibiotics. At this point it is activated and causes diarrhoea as a result of the toxins it produces. In the HD population, because of the widespread use of antibiotics, any patient who presents with diarrhoea may have C. diff as the causative agent; therefore a stool sample needs to be sent for culture and C. diff toxicity screening.

Patients with C. diff colonization of the GI tract do not need to be isolated unless they have diarrhoea. Symptomatic C. diff is usually treated with oral or IV metronidazole, or sometimes oral vancomycin.

Therapies derived from haemodialysis

Haemodiafiltration (HDF)

HDF combines diffusion, UFR, and convection using a high-flux membrane. HDF provides a more haemodynamically stable RRT than HD as ultrafiltrated fluid is replaced, by substitution fluid, in real-time, decreasing treatment-induced osmotic gradients in the body and hence slowing down the movement of water between body compartments. The haemodynamically stable nature of HDF makes it very suitable for the elderly, those with cardiovascular disease, and patients who experience regular IDH.

The benefits of convection, e.g. the removal of 'middle molecules (B₂m) are balanced by the requirement for ultrapurified water with which to make the substitution fluid. This substitution fluid is produced 'online' by the HD machine (similar to dialysate production) and introduced into the HDF circuit either before or after the dialyser (pre or post dilution).

Plasmapheresis

Plasmapheresis, also known as plasma exchange, entails the subtraction of plasma from whole blood using a semipermeable membrane and hydrostatic pressure. The resulting filtrate contains not only water but also some large molecular compounds, such as pathogenic antibodies, immune complexes, and lipoproteins. A replacement fluid of equal volume to the amount of plasma removed is infused to maintain the patient's circulating volume. A single treatment of plasmapheresis will replace about 75% of the patient's plasma, whilst a course of 3 sessions over 3 days will replace about 95%.

Indications for treatment

Plasma exchange is a cornerstone of the treatment of any number of renal, immunological, haematological, and neurological disorders (see 📖 pp. 1–36) such as:

• Goodpasture's syndrome (antiglomerular basement membrane (anti-GBM) antibody disease)
• Rapidly progressive glomerulonephritis (RPGN)
• ANCA (antineutrophil cytoplasmic antibodies) +ve nephritis
• Thrombotic thrombocytopenia purpura (TTP)
• Haemolytic uraemic syndrome (HUS).

Replacement fluids

Options for fluid replacement include: Alb (which does not replenish some electrolytes and clotting factors); a mix of Alb and saline (in the ratio 2:1) and FFP in patients with clotting deficiencies or bleeding disorders.

▶When using FFP precautions against clotting need to be taken, including the use of graduated elastic compressions stockings and the use of LMWH once the platelet count starts to rise.

Complications

Plasmapheresis is associated with all of the same potential complications as HD with respect to fluid and electrolyte depletion; and the same complications which can arise as the result of using an EC. In addition the removal of clotting factors ↑ risks associated with haemorrhage.

Blood sampling

Serum Cr, U&Es, bone profile, are taken pre and post plasmapheresis to ensure appropriate amounts of Ca^{2+}, Mg^{2+}, K^+ are given in the replacement fluid.

Anticoagulation

Although the process of plasmapheresis removes coagulation factors from the blood, patients on plasmapheresis will still require anticoagulation to ensure the EC does not clot. Heparin is the anticoagulant of choice and is titrated to patient need.

Immunoadsorption (IA)

Plasma is collected from the patient in a procedure like plasmapheresis. The plasma is subsequently passed over a protein column (containing protein A; isolated from *S. aureus*). Circulating immune complexes and IgG selectively bind to protein A and are ∴ removed from plasma. The adsorped plasma is then returned to the patient removing the need for plasma exchange.

IA removes ~80% of immunoglobulins from plasma without the need for replacement fluids.

Indications for IA

- ABO incompatible transplantation
- Goodpasture's syndrome (anti-GBM antibody disease)
- Cryoglobulinaemia
- FSGS
- Guillain–Barré syndrome
- SLE
- High levels of HLA antibodies.

Double filtration plasmapheresis

Plasma is separated from whole blood and then filtered through an additional filter of smaller pore size; large molecular-weight solutes are then dispensed with and smaller ones being returned to the patient. This negates the need for replacement fluid.

Delivering haemodialysis

Modes of delivery

Conventional HD
Most widely used in patients with ESKD. Usually 3–4hrs, 3 × /wk.

Daily HD
Daily HD is most often undertaken in patient's home. Length of HD will depend on need. Daily HD indicated in: severe heart disease, resistant anaemia, osteodystrophy, and peripheral neuropathy.

Nocturnal HD
Nocturnal HD is usually undertaken 6 nights a week for 6–10hrs a night at slow pump speeds. May occur in the patient's home or a hospital unit.

Benefits of daily and nocturnal HD
- Maintaining near normal fluid, electrolyte, and waste product levels in the patient's blood
- Less rigorous dietary and fluid restrictions
- Improved management of anaemia and hypertension
- ↓ morbidity
- ↓ mortality.

Acute HD
Used to treat severe presentations of acute kidney injury (see 🕮 p. 116).

Venues of delivery

Hospital HD
Both long-term and acute HD is provided in the hospital setting. HD for ESKD is almost exclusively provided 3 days a week (Monday, Wednesday, and Friday or Tuesday, Thursday, and Saturday) in a dedicated facility. Hospital HD is usually recommended for patients who are:
- Highly dependent (e.g. very elderly, immobile)
- Prone to intradialytic complications
- Unable to dialyse themselves at home
- Temporarily resting from PD
- New to HD
- Live close to the facility.

Acute HD is usually provided on the nephrology ward by a dedicated team of experienced dialysis nurses (see 🕮 p. 116). Patients cared for by the acute dialysis team include:
- Patients with AKI
- Patients admitted with previously undiagnosed ESKD
- ESKD, HD patients who are unwell
- PD patients who are unwell
- Patients recovering from transplantation
- HD patients recovering from surgery
- Patients for whom a regular HD space in unavailable.

Satellite HD

Satellite HD units often operate on a 'hub and spoke' model (where the main unit is the hub and satellite units are spokes). Satellite units may be based in hospitals which do not have nephrology services or may be free standing. Dialysis staff working in satellite units have a lot of autonomy and need to be trained in resuscitation and emergency care as well as being dialysis proficient. Satellite units are usually of a modest size. Patients suited to satellite HD include those who:

• Live close to the unit
• Are relatively self-caring/have low levels of dependency
• Are stable on dialysis.

Services offered at satellite dialysis units may be limited by the skills of the staff available.

Home HD

Home HD (HHD) is usually offered to patients with a high capacity for self-care, or those with a carer at home. Patients having HHD may undertake HD 3 times a week, daily and/or nocturnally. Benefits for the patient include not having to travel to and from a dialysis unit, being flexible with dialysis times, maintaining lifestyle/independence, and the potential for lower infection rates.

Despite NICE recommendations advocating choice around place of HD, only about 2.5% of all HD patients undertake HHD.

In part, this is the result of their need to be well established and stable on HD with good VA as well as having the physical, social, and psychological capacity to perform HHD and the room at home to do so.

The timing and frequency of HD may be varied in the home setting with opportunities for nocturnal and daily dialysis which may not exist in the hospital setting. Taking on HHD places control back with the patient and can have a positive impact on all aspects of their personal life as well as their medical well-being.

Patients with concomitant illness, those unstable on HD or those unable to concord with various aspects of their treatment regimen may be unsuitable for this type of dialysis. The social set up at home and psychological issues may mean HHD is not a good choice for some patients.

Training and support

Patients being considered for HHD need to undertake a training programme, usually in a specific HHD training or satellite unit. As well as the basic aspects and understanding of HD, training for HHD should cover:

• All aspect of HD session management
• Intra- and interdialytic complications and their management
• Interpretation and response to basic blood tests
• HD adequacy
• The principles of universal precautions
• The maintenance of HD and associated equipment
• When to ask for and where to go for help and advice.

Haemodialysis: the future

Despite NICE and Department of Health aspirations to dramatically increase the amount of HD undertaken at home, the demographics and age of the HD population tend to suggest this will not be realized to any great extent using present methods and modes of delivery.

Access issues have bedevilled HD since its inception. The new dialysis access of the future will have none of the issues with infection seen with dialysis catheters and will not cause scarring and be susceptible to clotting and bleeding. The increased use of SC VA devices, especially in the USA, shows some promise for the future. These small metallic devices, which are needled in a manner similar to AVF/AVGs, give rise to much lower infection rates than temporary dialysis access and can be sited in patients who might usually have a catheter.

The ideal access of the future would be very biocompatible, have low infection rates, be easily sited and accessed for dialysis, and have a good blood flow. From the patient point of view, they should not be unsightly and should cause minimal interference with day-to-day life.

Frequency of HD has long been known to correlate well with survival. Long slow HD may yet prove to be the best solution for patients who need HD. One of the most promising features of long slow daily dialysis is its focus on achieving optimum rather than merely 'adequate'. This refocusing of the objective of HD should set a precedent for the future whereby the quality of dialysis is not measured against a minimal standard. Alongside achieving good blood chemistry the dialysis of the future will focus on the drug-free management of hypertension, improving anaemia control, and attaining a patient defined improvement in QOL.

The portable (wearable) HD has been promised for some years. The human nephron filter uses 2 filters to replace the function of the kidney, while the wearable artificial kidney uses a HD-like system in which the dialysate is regenerated and HCO_3 added to make HD as close to portable as possible. The minimization and portability of such devices makes them potential candidates for a life on HD which is less restricted and where the dialysis is undertaken with increased frequency promoting improved survivability and QOL.

Further reading

Daugirdas J, Blake P, Ing T. *Handbook of Dialysis*, 4th edn. Philadelphia, PA: Lippincott, Williams & Wilkins; 2007.

EDTNA-ERCA. Guidelines for the control and monitoring of microbiological contamination in water for dialysis. *EDTNA-ERCA Journal* 2002; **28**:107–15.

European Best Practice Guidelines for HD. (Part 1 Section IV) Dialysis fluid purity. *Nephrol Dial Transplant* 2002; **17**(Supplement 7): S45–S46.

Department of Health. *Good practice guidelines for renal dialysis/transplantation units: prevention and control of blood-borne virus infection*. London: Stationery Office; 2002.

Department of Health. *National Service Framework for renal services: Part1—Dialysis and Transplantation*. London: Department of Health; 2004.

International Organization for Standardization/British Standards. *Quality of dialysis fluid for HD and related therapies*. BS ISO 11663. 2009.

International Organization for Standardization/British Standards. *Concentrates for HD and related therapies*. BS ISO 13958. 2009.

International Organization for Standardization/British Standards. *Water for HD and related therapies*. BS ISO 13959. 2009.

International Organization for Standardization/British Standards. *Water treatment equipment for HD and related therapies*. BS ISO 26722. 2009.

International Organization for Standardization/British Standards. *Guidance for the preparation and quality management of fluids for HD*. BS ISO 23500. 2009

Levy J, Brown E, Daley C, et al. (eds). *Oxford Handbook of Dialysis*, 3rd edn. Oxford: Oxford University Press; 2009.

Pauly R. Nocturnal home HD and short daily HD compared with kidney transplantation: emerging date in a new era. *Adv Chronic Kidney Dis* 2009; **16**(3):169–72.

Misra M, Phadke G. HD adequacy, dialysate composition in HD and HD access—a compendium. *US Nephrology* 2011; **5**(2):65–70.

National Kidney Foundation Kidney Disease Quality Outcomes Initiative. *NKF-KDOQI Clinical Practice Guideline for VA*, 2006. Available at: <http://www.kidney.org/professionals/kdoqi>

Osborn, G. Escofet, X, Da Silva, A. Medical adjuvant treatment to increase patency of arteriovenous fistulae and grafts. *Cochrane Database Syst Rev* 2008; **8**(4):CD 002786

Rahman T, Harper L. Plasmapheresis in nephrology: an update. *Curr Opin Nephrol Hypertens* 2006; **15**:603–9.

Raimann JG, Kruse A, Thijssen S, et al. Metabolic effects of dialysate glucose in chronic hemodialysis: results from a prospective, randomized crossover trial. *Nephrol Dial Transplant* 2011; **25**(5):597–602.

Thomas N. *Renal Nursing*, 3rd edn. Edinburgh: Bailliere Tindall; 2008.

Willms L, Vercaighe LM. Does warfarin safely prevent clotting of hemodialysis catheters? *Semin Dial* 2008; **21**(1):71–7.

Useful websites

<http://www.cari.org.au/dialysis_adequacy_published.php>

<http://www.kidney.org/professionals/kdoqi/guideline_uphd_pd_va/index.htm>

<http://www.kidneycare.nhs.uk>

<http://www.nice.org.uk/TA48>

<http://www.nocturnaldialysis.org/>

<http://www.renal.org/clinical/GuidelinesSection/HD>

<http://www.renal.org/clinical/GuidelinesSection/BloodBornevirusInfection>

<http://www.renalweb.com/topics/infection/infection.htm>

Transplantation: supply and demand

Introduction

Transplantation (Tx) is the treatment of choice for suitable patients with end stage kidney disease (ESKD) and the only option for renal replacement therapy (RRT) that avoids dialysis. The first successful kidney transplant was performed in Boston, USA in 1954 between identical twins and the first deceased donor (DD) transplant in the UK was in 1960. Since then, advances in clinical practice have improved outcomes, benefiting thousands of patients. Activity is limited by the availability of suitable organs. All UK transplant activity is monitored and recorded by the Directorate of Organ Donation and Transplantation (ODT) at NHS Blood and Transplant (NHSBT). The National Transplant Database provides up-to-date statistics on all aspects of organ donation and Tx.

Organ Donation Taskforce

In January 2008, the Organ Donation Taskforce (ODTF) published 14 recommendations, based upon global expertise, to achieve a 50% increase in deceased organ donation in the UK in 5 years (by 2013). Services were re-organized to include:
- New systems of organ retrieval
- Donor and recipient management
- In-house co-ordination embedded in ICUs
- Clinical leadership to improve the interface between transplant and intensive care teams.

In a supplementary report, the ODTF examined the option of presumed consent (opt-out system) and concluded that this should only be revisited if the listed initiatives did not meet expectations.

UK facts and figures

- Since 2002, there has been a 38% ↑ in patients registered on the national transplant list (NTL) to receive a kidney or a combined kidney and pancreas transplant. In 2010–2011, the NTL ↓ < 7000 for the first time in 3 years (Figure 13.1)*
- In 2010–2011, there was a 5% ↑ in solid organ DDs (n=1010), with an 11% ↑ in donors after circulatory death (DCD) and a 2% ↑ in donors after brain death (DBD)
- 95% of DDs donate their kidneys and kidney transplants ↑ to 1667 in 2010–2011 (Figure 13.2)*
- Living donor (LD) transplants comprise 38% (n=1020) of UK kidney transplant activity and has trebled in 10yrs, despite a 2% ↓ in 2010–2011 (Figure 13.3)*
- A new pancreas allocation scheme for DD was introduced in December 2010. In 2010–2011, there was a 5% ↑ in pancreas donors and transplants performed (n=210) with a 4% ↓ in patients waiting. 13 pancreatic islet transplants were performed in year (Figure 13.4).*

* Data courtesy of NHS Blood and Transplant, ✆ <http://www.nhsbt.nhs.uk>.

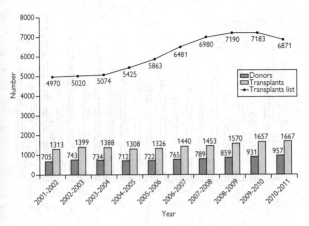

Fig. 13.1 Deceased donor kidney programme in the UK, 1 April 2001–31 March 2011. Numbers of donors, transplants, and patients on the active transplant list at 31 March 2011.

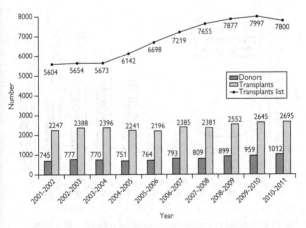

Fig. 13.2 Number of deceased donors and transplants in the UK, 1 April 2001–31 March 2011, and patients on the active transplant list at 31 March 2011.

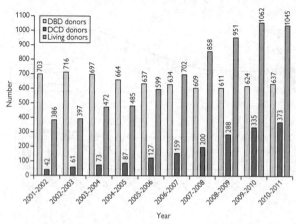

Figure 13.3 Number of deceased and living donors in the UK, 1 April 2001–31 March 2011.

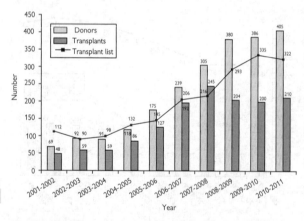

Fig. 13.4 Deceased pancreas and islet programme in the UK, 1 April 2001–31 March 2011. Numbers of donors, transplants, and patients on the active transplant list at 31 March 2011.

The NHS Organ Donor Register

The Organ Donor Register (ODR) was established in 1994 and is a national register of everyone who wishes to donate their organs after death. It is administered by NHS Blood and Transplant (NHSBT). Under the Human Tissue Acts (HT Acts) and the guidance set out by the Human Tissue Authority (HTA), the ODR is the first point of contact for healthcare professionals in establishing the wishes of potential DD (see 📖 p. 428, Legal framework (UK)). 90% of the general population claim to be supportive of organ donation and Tx but, although ODR registrations have ↑, only 33% of people have actually signed up to the ODR.

See 📖 p. 442, Further reading.

Legal framework (UK)

Organ donation and Tx in the UK are governed by the Human Tissue Act 2004 (England, Wales, Northern Ireland) and the Human Tissue (Scotland) Act 2006 (HT Acts) which came into force in September 2006. The HTA is the regulatory authority under the Acts and it is responsible for licensing the use and storage of human tissues and organs for Tx. The HTA Codes of Practice that specify expected standards of practice for both living and deceased donation are
• Code 1: Consent
• Code 2: Donation of solid organs for Tx.

Both Codes are available on the HTA website at ℘ <http://www.hta.gov.uk>.

Donation from deceased donors

To facilitate donation from DDs, the HTA makes it explicit that the decision of an adult in life to consent to donation after death takes legal precedence, i.e. shifts emphasis away from the wishes of the family to the wishes of the deceased. The ODR is central to establishing if a person has registered a preference for organ donation during his/her lifetime but it is not foolproof. In practice, if the person has not shared his/her wishes with loved ones and they are against organ donation, it is difficult to proceed. Where the wishes of the deceased are not known, the Codes allow for a nominated representative within a hierarchy of qualifying relationships to give consent on behalf of the person who has died.

Donation from living donors

The HTA is responsible for the approval of all LD transplants following independent assessment of each donor/recipient pair or, in the case of non-directed altruistic donation (NDAD), the donor alone (see 🕮 p. 434, Sources of organs). An approval notice is issued by the HTA which is valid for 6 months and allows donation to legally proceed. The purpose of the independent assessment is to establish:
• That there is evidence to support the claimed relationship between donor and recipient
• That the donor is able to give free and voluntary consent to donation, having been fully appraised of the benefits, risks, and possible complications of the procedure.

The independent assessment takes place when both donor and recipient have been through full clinical evaluation for donation/Tx. Independent assessors (IAs) are senior colleagues working within the healthcare system and have no direct or vested interest in the transplant programme. They are trained, accredited, and monitored by the HTA and usually provide an IA service within their own hospital/Trust. The HTA provides guidance for transplant teams and independent assessors.

The HTA Acts allowed LD kidneys to be 'shared' to ↑ the donor pool. The National Living Donor Kidney Sharing Schemes (NLDKSS) (see 📖 p. 434, Sources of organs) include:

- Paired/pooled donation (PPD) between 2 donor and recipient pairs (paired) or more (pooled)
- NDAD to a recipient who is unknown to the donor
- Altruistic donor chains (ADCs) where a NDAD donates into the PPD scheme to initiate a chain of transplants.

See 📖 p. 442, Further reading.

Ethics of organ donation and transplantation

Public confidence in organ donation and Tx are essential to the survival of the national transplant programme. The UK legal framework underpins these principles (see 📖 pp. 428–9, Legal framework). Moral dilemmas are inevitable in such a rapidly growing and pioneering area of clinical practice and a framework, based upon the following ethical principles, may be helpful in decision-making:

- Altruism—selfless act of giving/acting in the interests of others
- Autonomy—right to self-determination
- Non-maleficence—'do no harm'
- Beneficence—promoting well-being, balancing benefit vs harm, duty of care
- Justice—right to fair treatment and equity
- Dignity—protection from human degradation
- Reciprocity—mutual exchange of benefits
- Utility—the greatest good/happiness for the greatest number

Several perspectives interplay in moral decision-making. These can be considered from the:

- Donor perspective
- Recipient perspective
- Healthcare perspective—individual rights, professional responsibilities.

Donor perspective

Deceased donors

Key moral dilemmas:

- The definition of death; when does a 'patient' become a 'donor' in both the DBD and DCD situation?
- Rights of the donor before and after death; donor management/ optimization; how far should the wishes of the deceased to donate influence decisions about donor management/interventions to maximize use of donated organs?
- Consent to organ donation; is the ODR fit for purpose as an expression of consent to 'opt-in' to organ donation? Is presumed consent ('opt-out' system) really 'no' consent and/or what are the alternatives?
- Law vs ethics: the role of the family in facilitating/creating barriers to donation. Legally, the wish of a competent adult who has expressed a wish to donate after death takes precedence; morally it is complicated in the face of family objection at the point of donation.

Living donors

LDs may donate directly to family or loved ones, indirectly via the PPD scheme or as a NDAD (see 📖 pp. 434–7, Sources of organs). Generic and specific considerations will apply to each, according to the donor– recipient relationship.

- Valid consent and voluntariness

- Donor autonomy vs medical paternalism: donor safety and well-being; physical and psychological harm
- Risks to the donor vs benefits for the recipient; particularly when donor and recipient case-mix are more complex and co-morbidity is higher
- Anxiety about coercion and reward; upholding the best interests of the donor; expanding the LD pool e.g. 'directed' altruism
- Complex motivation; the spectrum from egoism (selfishness) to altruism (selflessness), depending upon the donor–recipient relationship
- Privacy and information sharing between donor and recipient in the context of the NLDKSS.

Recipient perspective

Key considerations:
- A patient hopes to achieve the best possible outcome from his/her transplant, i.e. improved QOL for as long as possible. Outcomes are influenced by both donor and recipient factors (see 📖 p. 447)
- Innovation and practice mean that more recipients are now considered for Tx than ever before (see 📖 pp. 446–7)
- Sources of donated organs have expanded the donor pool (see 📖 pp. 434–5, Sources of organs)
- Not all recipients will benefit equally from Tx and potential transplant recipients must be as informed as soon as possible about their best options and the implications of their choices when consenting to Tx (see 📖 pp. 446–7). The NHSBT and BTS *Guidelines for Consent for Solid Organ Transplantation* support a 2-stage consent process:
  1) prior to listing on the NTL
  2) on admission for transplant surgery, with annual confirmation of consent to ensure that the decision is still valid (see also 📖 pp. 454–5)
- National allocation of organs relies upon agreed selection criteria to ensure equity of access for patients to DDs and LDs from the NTL and/or NLDKSS. It may not be appropriate for some patients to be considered for DD transplantation (DDKT) if the likelihood of success is very low. LD kidney transplantation (LDKT) may be considered instead if both donor and recipient fully understand the implications and the transplant team are willing to proceed. In this situation, another recipient on the NTL is also not deprived of an organ
- Equity of access for patients to the DD pool is directly influenced by listing practices and the duration of preparation prior to transplant listing.

Healthcare perspective

Deceased donor transplantation

DD organs are a scarce resource and demand outstrips supply. In the procurement, allocation and distribution of organs, there are many competing moral obligations:
- To do what is best for the donor/recipient/patient in front of them—duty of care, dignity

- To consider all the patients who may benefit from a transplant—utility, greater good, equity of access
- To consider the impact on the health economy
- To safeguard the reputation of donation and Tx practice and inspire public confidence.

Ethical donation

There is not always agreement between intensive care teams and transplant teams about when it is morally acceptable to approach a family about donation and who should be involved in the discussion. The UK Donation Ethics Committee (UKDEC) has developed guidance to help in this area (see 📖 p. 442, Further reading).

Ethical allocation

The scarcity of organs for Tx complicates the process of distribution because supply does not meet demand (see 📖 p. 440, Allocation of organs). The national allocation scheme for DD organs, administered by NHSBT is regularly reviewed and aims to achieve equal distribution of kidneys. The criteria attempt to balance 'utility' (greatest good for the greatest number) and 'deontology' (duty-based) by:

- Respecting the wishes of the DD
- Utilizing donated organs most effectively on the basis of need
- Selecting recipients fairly and without bias
- Offering equity of access to DD Tx.

Healthcare professionals are responsible for selecting suitable recipients for Tx to ensure that the best outcomes are achieved for individual patients and for all potential recipients on the NTL (see 📖 pp. 454–5, recipient selection).

Living donor kidney transplantation

98% of LD Tx in the UK is in kidney Tx, which has become the treatment of choice for many patients because of superior outcomes and the opportunity to plan the date of donation and Tx (see 📖 p. 468, Choices). It is one of the most progressive areas of Tx and activity has trebled in 10yrs. This creates some unique moral challenges:

- The proximity of donor and recipient—boundaries of confidentiality must be clearly defined and respected. Separate clinical teams for donor and recipient are advised
- Sharing LD kidneys through the NLDKSS—respect for privacy and anonymity between all parties
- Recipient and donor preparedness to take on risk—challenges professional responsibilities if the transplant team considers the risks to be unacceptable for either donor or recipient
- Second opinion may be appropriate
- Evidence-based British Transplantation Society/Renal Association *UK Guidelines for living Donor Kidney Transplantation*, offer professional guidance re: complex choices in LDKT.

Organ sales and 'transplant tourism'

Regulated or unregulated organ trafficking is illegal in the UK. Prohibition is controversial. Proponents of a regulated payment system suggest that it would:

- Supply sufficient organs to meet demand
- Stop the 'black market' in organ sales
- Allow would-be donors to express individual autonomy and choice.
  Opponents argue that there would be a negative impact upon:
- The principle of 'gifting'
- The altruistic motivation to donate with ↑ financial incentives
- Exploitation of the poor.

'Transplant tourism' (TT), in which people travel overseas to pay for an organ, is associated with poorer outcomes, exploitation, and inequality. Healthcare professionals have a duty of care to all transplant recipients, regardless of the source of the organ. TT increases when the supply of organs is limited, so all options for Tx within the UK for eligible patients should be fully explored to minimize the risks associated with TT.

See 📖 p. 466, Further reading.

Sources of organs

There are 2 sources of organs for Tx:
- Deceased donors (DDs)
- Living donors (LDs).

Deceased donors

Donors after brain death (DBDs)

DBD are donors who are brainstem dead; requiring full respiratory support in the ICU. The vital organs are perfused and oxygenated until ventilator support is withdrawn. DBDs offer the best organs for Tx but the numbers are static in the UK in comparison with DCD donors.

Donors after circulatory death (DCDs)

DCDs are categorized as 'controlled' and 'uncontrolled' according to the Maastricht Criteria (Table 13.1). Donation from 'controlled' DCDs has ↑ in the UK and accounts for the overall rise in DDs.

Table 13.1 Categorization of DCD donors

I	Brought in dead	Uncontrolled
II	Unsuccessful resuscitation	
III	Awaiting cardiac arrest	Controlled
IV	Cardiac arrest after brainstem death	
V	Cardiac arrest in a hospital inpatient	Uncontrolled

Kidneys from DBDs and DCDs can be used for Tx. Outcomes from DBD and controlled DCD kidney transplants are comparable.

Pancreata for Tx are ideally retrieved from young, slim DBDs without a FH of DM but suitable organs can also be retrieved from DBDs and DCDs up to 60yrs of age. ~60% of retrievals result in a pancreas transplant.

Living donors

Kidneys from LDs account for 38% of all kidney transplants performed in the UK, offering more opportunity and choice to patients and excellent results (see 📖 p. 447).

Directed donors

Most LDKTs in the UK are directed donations, i.e. the donor and recipient are either genetically related (blood relatives) or emotionally related (spouse, partner, friend).

National living donor kidney sharing schemes

This is a UK-wide scheme in which kidneys from LDs are shared to increase the donor pool and maximize the opportunity for Tx for patients waiting for a kidney. The NLDKSS include:
- PPD
- NDAD
- ADCs.

Paired/pooled donation

Donor-recipient LDKT pairs may register in the PPD scheme rather than donate directly to one another (see 🕮 p. 450) because:

- They are incompatible due to ABO blood group antibodies (ABOi)
- They are incompatible due to human leucocyte antigen (HLA) antibodies (HLAi)
- They are both ABOi and HLAi
- They are ABO and/or HLA *compatible* but prefer a better HLA or age match
- Process for PPD:
- Fully assessed donor-recipient pairs (see 🕮 pp. 476–7, Living donor kidney transplantation) register into a national scheme
- A computerized kidney donor matching run (KDMR) is performed 4 times per year by NHSBT to identify 2-way (paired) or 3-way (pooled) compatible 'exchange' transplants (Figure 13.5)
- A scoring system optimizes the number of transplants that can be achieved from each KDMR; benefiting recipients who have waited longest in the scheme and are most difficult to match to a donor
- Once compatibility between all 'matched' pairs has been confirmed, independent assessment and HTA approval are obtained
- Dates for surgery are scheduled with same-day, synchronous donor operations in each transplant centre. Donor–recipient pairs usually stay in their local transplant centres and kidneys travel from the donor to recipient centres.

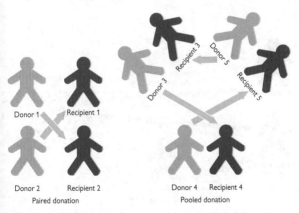

Fig. 13.5 Paired (2-way) pooled (3-way) exchanges. Reproduced courtesy of NHS Blood and Transplant.

Non-directed altruistic donation

Altruistic donation in the UK is typically 'non-directed', i.e. to a recipient who is unknown to the donor, although 'directed donation' to a recipient with whom the donor has no prior relationship is not precluded under the HT Act. There is an increasing trend in NDAD. Donors are fully assessed to ensure suitability to donate, including mandatory mental health assessment and independent assessment for the HTA (see 📖 p. 476, Living donor kidney transplantation) prior to registration with NHSBT. Kidneys are allocated to potential recipients who are on the NTL as per DD allocation criteria (see 📖 p. 440, Allocation of organs).

Altruistic donor chains

ADCs were introduced into the NLDKSS in January 2012. A 'chain' of transplants can be initiated when a NDAD donates to a recipient in the PPD scheme and the donor for that recipient donates to someone else. The final transplant goes to a recipient on the NTL. Short chains (involving 1 donor-recipient pair) and long chains (involving several donor-recipient pairs) are possible (Figure 13.6). Simultaneous dates for surgery are scheduled for all donors and recipients in the chain so that all the donor operations start at the same time, as for PPD. NDADs are offered a choice to 'opt-in' or 'opt-out' of the ADC scheme at the time of registration with NHSBT. If they 'opt-out' kidneys are allocated directly to the NTL; if they 'opt-in', high priority recipients on the NTL will still be offered kidneys first, before an ADC is considered (see 📖 p. 440, Allocation of organs).

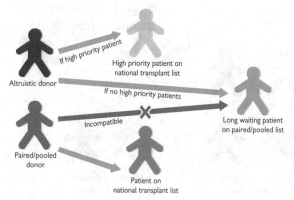

Fig. 13.6 Altruistic donor chain.

Domino kidney donation (DKD)

DKD can be confused with *domino-paired donation* which is used in many other countries to describe ADCs. In the UK, DKD is when a kidney is donated following nephrectomy as a *therapeutic procedure* and re-implantation of the kidney in the same patient is not appropriate (e.g. haematuria-loin pain syndrome). Key points:

• Nephrectomy is only considered if it is the best treatment option for the patient and then he/she should be given the choice to donate the kidney
• HTA approval is not required because the donation occurs as a consequence of treatment
• Donated kidneys are allocated locally via NHSBT rather than nationally (see 📖 p. 440, Allocation of organs) to promote the best outcome by minimizing cold ischaemic time (CIT). The recipient can also be counselled in advance about the risk of the transplant not proceeding if the kidney is not viable on retrieval
• Transplants from DKDs should be recorded differently from other LDKTs as the outcomes for both donor and recipient may be influenced by the unique clinical circumstances.
  See 📖 p. 442, Further reading.

Procurement

The National Organ Retrieval Service (NORS) was established in April 2010 in response to ODTF recommendations to:
- ↑ efficiency of organ retrieval arrangements via a UK-wide network of dedicated, self-sufficient Organ Retrieval Teams
- Optimize procurement of organs from multi-organ DBDs and DCDs
- ↑ the number of transplantable organs.
  Arrangements to support NORS were put in place, as follows:
- NHSBT to commission and performance manage NORS
- Published 'National Standards for Organ Retrieval from Deceased Donors', setting out roles and responsibilities of the MPT, donor hospital and transplant centre
- Dedicated abdominal (kidneys, liver, pancreas) and cardiothoracic (heart, lungs) retrieval teams
- Retrieval zones based upon proximity of team closest to donor hospital with 1st and 2nd on-call team structure
- Local procurement agreed for 'kidney-only' donors
- Local retrieval for uncontrolled DCDs due to time constraints
- All potential donor organs to be offered unless subject to absolute contraindication (e.g. disseminated malignancy)
- Dedicated MPT in each retrieval team; minimum dependence on staff in the donor hospital; 24hr, 7-day/wk service
- Training opportunities within teams to ensure safety and sustainability
- Donor hospital to provide donor care, together with the specialist nurse for organ donation (SN-OD) up to the time of donation; safe transfer to an appropriately equipped and staffed operating theatre
- Recipient transplant centre MPT to be responsible for ensuring that the transplant process progresses to plan with consultant transplant surgeon ultimately responsible for safe implantation of donated organs.

SN-OD provides key role in:
- Liaising with and supporting staff in the donor hospital
- Facilitating optimal donor management and family support
- Communication with retrieval teams
- Offering organs for Tx to recipient centres.

Recipient co-ordinator/transplant nurse provides key role in:
- Co-ordinating recipient admission and surgery
- Communication with transplant teams re: organ offers
- Facilitating timely implantation of donated organs.

See 📘 p. 442, Further reading.

Allocation of organs

Deceased donors

Kidneys are the most commonly transplanted organ and the number of people requiring a kidney transplant exceeds the supply of available organs. The National Kidney Allocation Scheme was initially revised in April 2006 and has subsequently been reviewed to ensure that:

• There is equity of access to Tx for all patients
• Every donated kidney is used to the best possible advantage and is allocated to the person who needs it most
• There are agreed criteria for the allocation of kidneys which include waiting time on dialysis, HLA type, blood group, age, and body size (children).

DBD kidney allocation

All patients waiting for an organ transplant are registered on the NTL and all DBD kidneys are allocated on a national basis. Kidney matching runs (KMRs) are performed by the Duty Office at the Directorate of Organ Donation and Transplantation (ODT) within NHSBT. There are 5 tiers (A to E) (Table 13.2). Key points:

• Tier A has priority
• Within tiers A and B, children are prioritized according to their waiting time
• In April 2011, an additional 'clinically urgent' category for children was introduced, which gives priority above tiers A to C
• In tiers D and E, patients are prioritized using a points system according to agreed criteria. Organs are allocated to patients with the highest number of points.

Table 13.2 Tiers for DBD kidney allocation

Tier	
A	HLA identical for highly-sensitized children (<18yrs)
B	HLA identical for other children
C	HLA identical for highly-sensitized adults
D	HLA identical for other adults + well-matched children
E	All other eligible patients (adults and children)

DCD kidney allocation

Historically, local allocation of DCD kidneys was agreed to minimize CIT and to promote the best outcomes. As the number of DCD kidneys increases in comparison with DBDs and transplant outcomes are similar, allocation of DCD kidneys is under review to improve equity of access across the UK.

Pancreas allocation

Recipients of combined/simultaneous pancreas and kidney transplants (SPKs) benefit from the national allocation system because donors are typically younger and waiting times for a combined transplant tend to be shorter. It is argued that this is appropriate, given that these patients have limited opportunity to be successfully transplanted because of the combined co-morbidity and mortality associated with diabetes and kidney failure.

Living donors

Directed donations

LDKT practice influences how patients are listed for Tx and hence the overall distribution of kidneys. Recipients who have willing donors may choose not to be listed for DD Tx whilst evaluation for LDKT is ongoing if this is likely to offer them the best transplant outcome. Others may choose or be advised to remain on the NTL, depending upon individual circumstances for both donor and recipient. As a general rule, DD listing should reflect best practice; a transplant from a DD for a recipient with a fully assessed, suitable, and willing LD, may not be in the interests of the donor, recipient, or the wider transplant community.

National living donor kidney sharing schemes

See 📖 p. 434, Sources of organs, for the allocation of LD kidneys through the NLDKSS. In both the PPD and ADC schemes, recipients can also be listed on the NTL for DD Tx. If a potential match is identified through the NLDKSS, NHSBT suspend all recipients involved in the potential kidney exchange from the NTL. If the immunological crossmatches between the matched donor–recipient pairs are all negative, the recipients remain suspended from the NTL until the transplants proceed. If any of the 'exchanges' cannot go ahead, recipients can be reinstated on both the NTL and in the NLDKSS if they wish.

Domino kidney donation

Kidneys donated through DKD are allocated locally. A KMR is performed by NHSBT at the request of the transplant centre to identify a local recipient on the NTL (see 📖 p. 434, Sources of organs).

See 📖 p. 442, Further reading.

Further reading

Danovitch GM (ed). *Handbook of Kidney Transplantation*, 5th edn. Philadelphia, PA: Lippincott Williams & Wilkins; 2010.

Ohler L, Cupples S, International Transplant Nurses Society (eds). *Core Curriculum for Transplant Nurses*. St Louis, MO: Mosby Elsevier; 2008.

Torpey N, Moghal NE, Watson E, *et al.* (eds). *Oxford Handbook of Renal Transplantation*. Oxford: Oxford University Press; 2010.

Useful websites

British Transplantation Society (BTS) website. Available at: ℞ <http://www.bts.org.uk>
Access 'Active Standards and Guidelines' for:

- NHSBT/BTS: *Guidelines for Consent to Solid Organ Transplantation in Adults*, March 2011
- BTS/RA: *UK Guidelines for Living Donor Kidney Transplantation*, 3rd edn, May 2011
- BTS: *Antibody Incompatible Guidelines*, 2nd edn, January 2011
- Renal Association (RA): *Guidelines for Assessment for Renal Transplantation*, 4th edn, 2008
- BTS/ICS: *Consensus Guidelines on Organ Donation after Circulatory Death*, December 2010
- BTS: *Guidelines for Donation after Circulatory Death*, 2nd edn, 2012.

Department of Health website. Available at: ℞ <http://www.dh.gov.uk>
Access 'Publications' for:

- *National Service Framework for Renal Services, Part 1, Dialysis and Transplantation*, 2004
- *National Service Framework for Renal Services, Part 2, Chronic Kidney Disease, Acute Renal Failure and End of Life Care*, 2005
- *Organs for Transplants a Report from the Organ Donation Taskforce*, January 2008
- *The Potential Impact of an Opt-out System for Organ Donation in the UK: an Independent Report from the Organ Donation Taskforce*, November 2008.

Human Tissue Authority (HTA) website. Available at: ℞ <http://www.hta.gov.uk>

- Human Tissue Act (England, Wales and Northern Ireland), 2004
- Human Tissue (Scotland) Act, 2006
- HTA Codes of Practice 1 (Consent) & 2 (Donation of Solid Organs for Transplantation)
- *HTA Guidance for Transplant Teams and Independent Assessors.*

NHS Blood and Transplant (NHSBT) website. Available at: ℞ <http://www.nhsbt.nhs.uk> and <http://www.odt.nhs.uk>

General website and clinical microsite for access to/information about:

- Patient educational resources
- Milestones in transplantation
- Latest statistics and transplant activity
- Research and presentations
- National standards for organ retrieval from deceased donors
- Transplanting centres
- Organ allocation system
- National living donor kidney sharing schemes (NLDKSS)
- Organ donor register
- Organ donor enquiry line-telephone and email
- Links to patient association/charity websites.

UK Donation Ethics Committee (UKDEC). Academy of Medical Royal Colleges website. Available at: ℞ <http://www.aomrc.org.uk/donations-ethics-committee.html>

- *An Ethical Framework for Controlled Donation after Circulatory Death*, 2011.

Transplantation: patient choice, recipient selection, and surgery

Choices for transplantation

Access to Tx as a treatment of choice for suitable patients is embedded in the Renal National Service Framework (2004–2005). The range of choices available for potential kidney transplant recipients makes the decision-making process complex. Patients and their families rely upon the knowledge and expertise of healthcare professionals to guide them and they can only be fully involved in the decision to choose Tx if they are appropriately informed. Referral to another centre for a second opinion should be offered if a patient's preference is not available locally.

Pre-emptive transplantation

The best option for both patient and transplant outcome is a transplant before the commencement of alternative RRT (i.e. dialysis). The availability of kidneys from the DD pool is unpredictable but timely listing on the NTL, i.e. within 6 months of the commencement of RRT, helps some patients to receive a kidney transplant pre-emptively.

The role of living donor kidney transplantation (LDKT)

Planned LDKT allows more scope for effective pre-emptive Tx. In the UK, the average rate of pre-emptive LDKT is 30% per annum but some centres achieve up to 50% and offer this option to patients routinely. In North America, some centres transplant 70% of their LDKT recipients pre-emptively. The keys to success are:
- Enthusiasm from patients and their families
- Shared philosophy of care across healthcare teams in transplant 'hub' and referring nephrology 'spokes'
- Effective clinical pathways for timely donor and recipient evaluation
- Consistent patient information in a variety of formats (DVD, web-based, written, verbal (face-to-face & information groups))
- Information about transplant options discussed with all recipients at an eGFR of 20ml/min/1.73m^2 for early identification of LD options and donor and recipient assessments tailored to recipient decline in kidney function. NB: optimum time for Tx avoids the recipient becoming symptomatic of ESKD; suggested eGFR of 10–15ml/min/1.73m^2
- MPT approach with clinical leads in the advanced kidney care clinic (AKCC) setting and LD teams with responsibility for donor and recipient assessment through agreed clinical care pathways.

Special considerations in pre-emptive transplantation

The following aspects are important considerations:
- Logistical aspects—early referral and timely completion of donor–recipient assessments; scheduling surgery before the recipient starts to feel unwell
- Educational aspects—prior to the transplant operation, the recipient will not have experienced dialysis and may not have had previous surgery; medical management of CKD will have involved adjustment to diet and medication regimens with periodic clinic visits. The transplant operation marks the start of RRT as well as major surgery and expectations about the impact of surgery, postoperative recovery,

frequency of clinic attendances, and long-term rehabilitation must be managed in advance
• Managing expectations—not all patients will have a LD and/or may not be suitable for Tx. Alternative dialysis options should be considered in parallel with planning for Tx.

Living donor vs deceased donor transplantation

If pre-emptive Tx from either a LD or DD cannot be achieved, it is important to minimize waiting time on dialysis and consider transplant options as soon as possible for suitable patients. The benefits of LD vs DD Tx are:
• Improved patient and graft outcomes (Table 14.1)
• Planned event; accommodating donor–recipient lifestyle commitments and preparation of clinically complex recipients (e.g. HIV +ve, pro-thrombotic conditions, complex anatomy ± previous surgery, anaesthetic risk)
• Offers recipients with higher risk of mortality, co-morbidity, or graft failure (i.e. those who may not be suitable for DD listing) the opportunity for Tx
• Reduced risk of delayed graft function (DGF); allows timely monitoring and intervention
• Increases the donor pool and reduces competition for DD kidneys
• Health economics; high-quality, cost effective treatment for ESKD
• In children and young adults, a well HLA matched LDKT reduces the frequency/need for re-Tx and risk of future sensitization.

Table 14.1 Outcome data: LDKT vs DDKT

	Living donors	Deceased donors
Graft half-life	± 20yrs	± 10yrs
1yr graft survival	95%	89%
5yr graft survival	80%	67%
5yr patient survival	95%	86%

The role of deceased donor kidney transplantation (DDKT)

Although 38% of all kidney transplants in the UK are from LDs, most patients wait on the NTL to receive a kidney from either a DBD or DCD donor. DCD activity has ↑ since the implementation of the ODTF and kidney transplant outcomes are now considered to be equivalent to those from DBDs (see 🕮 p. 434, Sources of organs). Timely listing on the NTL is key to ensuring equity of access for patients to DDKT but there are significant differences in timeframes for recipient evaluation and listing practices across the UK.

HIV and transplantation

Historically, being sero-positive for human immunodeficiency virus (HIV) was an absolute contraindication to kidney Tx. Since the use of highly active antiretroviral therapy (HAART) for HIV has become established, life expectancy is ↑ and the opportunity for Tx for patients with CKD caused by HIV-associated nephropathy (HIVAN) is now considered feasible and safe (see 🕮 p. 19). To be eligible, potential recipients must meet the following criteria:[1]

- Undetectable plasma HIV-1 RNA levels (viral load) for 3 months
- CD4+ T-cell count of >200 cells/μL, for 6 months
- No history of auto-immune deficiency syndrome (AIDS) defining conditions, e.g. opportunistic infections; neoplasms.

Standard immunosuppression, includes prednisolone, mycophenolate mofetil, and Calcineurin inhibitors (CNIs) (ciclosporin and tacrolimus). ►HAART therapy has potent enzyme inhibition and the dose of CNI required to maintain adequate IS is usually very low; many patients require a once wkly dose. IS trial during pre-transplant preparation is recommended to establish a therapeutic dosing regimen and individual transplant plan. LDKT is preferable to DDKT in terms of planning, minimizing DGF, ± monitoring IS effectively (see 🕮 pp. 457–8, Recipient pre-transplant assessment and preparation).

Recent evidence shows no significant HIV progression ± adverse effect of HIV on allograft function post Tx. ⚠There is the possibility of ↑ risk of rejection and poorer outcomes in hepatitis C virus-co-infected patients.

Diabetes and transplantation

Evidence confirms that patients with DM and kidney disease benefit from Tx with a positive impact on patient survival, QOL, and diabetic complications. For suitable recipients, choices include:

- Kidney transplant alone (KTA) (remain on diabetic medication)
- Pancreas (alone) after kidney (PAK)
- Simultaneous kidney and pancreas (SPK)
- Pancreas transplant alone (PTA)
- Islet cell Tx.

The choice of transplant is individual to the patient but, SPK (~80%) is preferred for patients with ESKD and insulin-dependent diabetes (Type 1 or II) or PAK (~15%) rather than KTA. PTA and islet cell Tx are used when very unstable diabetes leads to life-threatening complications. Organs for SPK Tx are typically retrieved from younger donors to maximize outcomes. Consequently, SPK recipients are listed separately from the kidney alone recipients on the NTL and do not wait as long for their transplant. Diabetic recipients have a narrow window of opportunity to benefit from a transplant and are more likely to die waiting if they are not prioritized (see 📖 p. 440, Allocation of organs). With the success of LDKT, PAK has increased in popularity. The patient needs to understand the 'pros and cons' of each transplant option:

- SPK is major surgery; in comparison with KTA it is associated with ↑ mortality and morbidity
- Younger recipients are more suitable for SPK
- PAK involves 2 recipient operations
- PAK is historically associated with poorer graft survival but may improve with experience
- Survival benefits associated with pre-emptive and LDKT may outweigh the benefit of SPK for some recipients.

- Specialist nurses have a key role in the education, preparation, and support for potential recipients, living donors, and their families prior to Tx
- An MPT approach and a clinic-setting dedicated to patients with advanced CKD is the most effective model; facilitating pre-emptive LDKT and timely listing for DDKT.

Incompatible transplantation

A recipient may be incompatible with a potential donor because of the presence of antibodies in the recipient against the donor's blood group (ABOi) and/or human leucocyte antigens (HLA-type) (HLAi). The risk of rejection usually prevents a direct transplant between the two. Blood group antibodies are inherent, whilst antibodies against HLA are acquired by exposure to another person(s) HLA through:

• Blood transfusion
• Pregnancy (♀)
• Previous transplant.

The strongest 'immunological memory' is usually associated with antibodies from a previous transplant, followed by pregnancy and then blood transfusion. Even with antibody removal, it is usually preferable to avoid a transplant across a repeat HLA mismatch from a previous graft. Women who have had pregnancies from a number of partners or patients who have had multiple blood transfusions may have been exposed to a broad spectrum of HLA antigens, which makes antibody removal challenging.

Organ allocation from the DD pool is based upon identifying compatible transplants so most incompatible transplants are LDKTs. Historically, incompatible donor–recipient pairs would not have been considered for Tx but advances in antibody removal treatments, changes in the legal framework (see 🕮 pp. 428–9, Legal framework (UK)), and patient choice have facilitated change. ABOi alone, HLAi alone and both ABOi and HLAi in the same patient, present different clinical challenges.

Helpful hints when discussing options for Tx with incompatible donor-recipient pairs (Table 14.2)

• Initial discussion with both donor and recipient to enhance understanding about complex issues and encourage shared decision-making
• Provide supporting written/web-based information for reference
• A compatible transplant is always preferable. The option of alternative compatible donors should always be explored at initial discussion; even if it is to 'positively' exclude them
• In the absence of a compatible donor, an option appraisal, suitable for the individual patient, should be discussed. E.g.:
  • Do nothing ± remain on NTL
  • Remain open to alternative donor offers, especially if compatibility may be improved
  • NLDKSS—PPD/ADC options (see 🕮 p. 434, Sources of organs).
  • Antibody removal with direct LDKT.

▶It is possible for a recipient to remain active on the NTL whilst registered in the NLDKSS and, if suitable, to consider antibody removal if not 'matched' in the scheme.

Table 14.2 Treatment options: PPD (NLDKSS) vs antibody removal

PPD (NLDKSS)	Antibody removal
Compatible living donor transplant	Incompatible living donor transplant
Multiple donors can be registered for a single recipient	More complex clinical scenario
Clinically more straightforward	↑ intervention for the potential recipient
Logistically challenging	Higher risk of failure (spectrum of risk dependence on degree of incompatibility)
Uncertainty about timing of transplant/likelihood of being matched	Planned date of transplant
'Indirect donation' between donors & recipients	Donor known to recipient (direct donation)

The roles and responsibilities of healthcare professionals and donors–recipients in streamlining the registration and transplant processes through the NLDKSS has been defined by the HTA (legal aspects) and NHSBT (administration) and is reflected in the *BTS/RA UK Guidelines for Living Donor Kidney Transplantation*.

Antibody removal

Antibody removal (desensitization) is the removal of pre-existing antibodies to either donor HLA or ABO blood group antigen to facilitate a direct transplant between a donor and recipient. The purpose of a 'pre-conditioning' protocol, which is usually planned prior to a scheduled LDKT, is to:

- To reduce the antibody titre (level) and ↓ the risk of acute rejection
- In HLAi—to create a negative flow crossmatch between donor and recipient
- In ABOi —to ↓ antibody level in the recipient to a dilution of 1:8 (subject to centre differences) or less against the specific donor blood group.

ABOi and HLAi antibody incompatibility are very different clinical scenarios and treatment protocols are tailored accordingly, based upon global and national expertise. Local protocols vary because the evidence does not strongly support a single approach. Suggested protocols are outlined in The British Transplantation Society (BTS) *Guidelines for Antibody Incompatible Transplantation*. Outcomes are improving, suggesting equivalent or slightly better patient and graft survival than compatible DDKT. ABOi Tx is established in more transplant centres than HLAi because ABOi is considered to be more clinically straightforward. Both are relatively expensive treatment options and require infrastructure and expertise to support them. The best outcomes are achieved with:

- *A critical mass of suitable patients*—to develop experience and develop the 'learning curve'
- *A collaborative MPT approach*—to facilitate decision-making, planning and pre-transplant preparation; short- and long-term post-transplant monitoring. This includes clinical and scientific expertise, e.g. H&I, haematology
- *Vigilant post-transplant monitoring*—to optimize long-term outcomes
- *Accurate National Registry*—held by NHSBT as part of the National Transplant Database for the recipients of incompatible transplants.

Patient selection

Appropriate patient selection is key because of the impact of treatment. In general, the lower the titre levels, the less intervention is necessary but the following points should be considered:

- Alternative transplant options
- Extent of incompatibility (e.g. ABOi/HLAi alone, ABOi and HLAi together, ABO antibody titre level or degree of HLA sensitization)
- Antibody removal for HLAi and ABOi in the same recipient is only performed in exceptional circumstances (e.g. highly-sensitized recipients on long-term dialysis with no other transplant options). Challenges include:
  - HLA crossmatching in the presence of pre-transplant
  - IS
  - monitoring both HLA and ABO antibody titres in the same patient
  - managing maintenance IS.
- Existing co-morbidities including length of time on dialysis, previous transplants and outcomes, current health profile
- Donor and recipient expectations of success
- Recipient understanding of intervention required and how it differs from routine Tx
- Balance of risk vs benefit for the recipient between antibody removal and alternative treatment options (including dialysis if no other feasible transplant option).

Methods of antibody removal

Antibody removal/pre-conditioning protocols are tailored according to the type of antibody to be removed, recipient-specific factors, and centre preference but typically include a combination of:

- Pre/post-transplant regular antibody titre monitoring
- Pre-transplant oral IS
- Pre-transplant IV IS ± immunoglobulin (e.g. anti CD20, IVIgG)
- Pre-transplant plasma antibody removal treatment (e.g. immunadsorption (IA), double filtration plasmapheresis (DFPP), plasma exchange (PEX) (see 📖 p. 416, HD)
- Post-transplant plasma treatment PRN and adjustments to IS according to antibody titre levels and transplant function.

Special considerations

- Excellent communication across outpatient and inpatient MPTs to plan, co-ordinate, and deliver transplant plan
- Dedicated antibody removal nurses to co-ordinate and implement recipient protocol
- Recipients without vascular access (e.g. pre-emptive/peritoneal dialysis) require insertion of temporary dialysis access for plasma treatment; extra counselling may be needed
- For recipients who are HD dependent, plan plasma treatment regimen so that they can tolerate regimen
- Impact of pre-conditioning treatment varies. Pre-transplant preparation to include management of symptoms/side effects and education and support for recipients and their families
- Surgery may be delayed if antibody titres do not fall to expected level by planned date and further treatments are required
- Postoperative course can be less predictable than routine Tx with extended length of recipient stay
- Antibody removal significantly ↑ the cost of a kidney transplant.

Specialist nurses play a pivotal role in the management of the recipient undergoing pre-conditioning for antibody removal through:
- Ongoing education and support throughout the decision-making process for donor, recipient, and family members
- Effective co-ordination within the MPT
- Donor and recipient assessment and preparation
- Performing antibody removal techniques
- Administration and monitoring of IS
- Pre- and post-Tx antibody monitoring.

See 📖 p. 483, Further reading.

Transplantation surgery and recipient management: recipient selection and consent

Not all patients are suitable for Tx and there is a limited supply of DD kidneys. Careful selection and decision-making processes ensure that best outcomes are achieved, both for the individual and for the benefit of all potential recipients on the NTL. The following considerations must be discussed with patients and their families prior to listing for Tx as part of the assessment and consent process:

• Recipient diagnosis, age, and co-morbidity
• Choices available ± feasible for Tx and recipient preference (see 📖 pp. 446–7, Choices for transplantation)
• Source and uncertainty about characteristics of donor kidney (e.g. DBD/DCD/LD, age, complex anatomy).
  Other important aspects include:
• A realistic understanding about expected outcomes; over-optimism can lead to problems adjusting to life with a transplant in the future
• The recipient of a pre-emptive transplant is likely to underestimate the impact of Tx, having never experienced dialysis; he/she may feel worse initially
• Tx is usually the best treatment for ESKD but the risk of complications and failure must be balanced against the risks associated with alternative treatment options (i.e. dialysis) for the individual patient
• Any decision, for or against Tx, must be well informed and discussed fully with the patient, i.e. planned LDKT for an older recipient with other co-morbidities may be more appropriate than waiting for a DDKT and unplanned surgery.

Clinical complexity and logistical considerations complicate the recipient consent process. Guidance published jointly between NHSBT and the BTS recommends a 2-stage approach (see 📖 p. 430, Ethics of organ donation and transplantation).

• Prior to listing on the NTL
• On admission for transplant surgery, with annual confirmation of consent to ensure that the decision is still valid.

There are a range of professional standards and guidelines that are published on the BTS website at ✍ <http://www.bts.org.uk> and which offer guidance to clinicians for both DD and LD Tx.

It is difficult to ensure that a potential recipient fully understands the implications of his/her decision and that information is comprehensive. Educational materials must be presented in various formats and discussed and revisited in different ways, e.g. face-to-face consultations, education patient meetings, and peer support settings (see 📖 pp. 604–7, Appendix 4).

An MPT approach, in which nurses play a 1° role in leading and delivering effective education and support to facilitate the consent process for potential transplant recipients, is essential during the preparation for Tx. This should be started at an early stage to maximize the opportunities and minimize delays.

Recipient pre-transplant assessment and preparation

The principle of assessment prior to Tx is to establish:
- If the recipient is suitable to receive a transplant, i.e. the risk/benefit analysis is accepted by the patient and the clinical team
- What type of transplant is most suitable, e.g. DD/LD/SPK
- Where possible, initiate appropriate interventions to ensure that the patient is suitable to receive a transplant
- The recipient can give valid consent for Tx (see 📖 p. 430, Ethics of organ donation and transplantation).

Clinical assessment and preparation

Local investigations and assessment protocols vary but should be based upon published standards and guidelines and include timeframes for frequency ± repeat testing whilst the patient remains on the waiting list without being transplanted. Typically, the following is included:

General health
- Regular nephrological review and referral to specialist colleagues within the MPT in preparation for Tx (e.g. dietitian, clinical psychologist, social worker, specialist nurses, specialist consultant opinions)
- Detailed PMH and FH to establish cause of kidney failure, absolute and possible contraindications to Tx, further investigations ± intervention required (e.g. previous/current cancer, BMI >35, cardiovascular disease, current/chronic infection, current pregnancy in ♀, previous surgery and anaesthetic record)
- Current medications and history (to establish existing regimen, exclude possible interactions, allergies, and adverse reactions with future IS)
- Current and previous modality of treatment (pre-emptive/failing transplant/dialysis dependent)
- Transplant history (type of organ, number, causes of failure)
- MRSA skin screen ± treatment if +ve
- PAP smear test (all ♀ of reproductive age)
- Mammogram (♀ >50yrs, FH Ca breast)
- Bowel screening (>60yrs)
- Pregnancy screening if indicated (NB: urine/serum LH and FSH if anuric)
- Upper GI endoscopy if indicated (exclude peptic ulcer)
- Dental review (treat active disease and pre-empt future sources of infection).

Blood
- Routine blood chemistry (kidney function, liver (LFTs), bone profile) haematology (FBC) and clotting screen
- Blood group (2 samples required for verification)
- HLA type (2 samples required for verification)
- HLA antibody screen (repeat 3-monthly or post blood transfusion, failed transplant ± change in IS, pregnancy/miscarriage)

- Virology screen (repeat 3-monthly) HIV, HTLV (if indicated), HBV (surface antigen and core antibody ± HBsAb check if previously vaccinated)
- Virology screen (single sample but repeat annually if previously –ve or possible exposure suspected) EBV, CMV, VZV, toxoplasmosis, syphilis
- Vaccination for HBV and VZV if sero-negative
- Thrombophilia screening (if FH in 1° relative) to include lupus anticoagulant ± other thrombophilia markers PRN in pro-thrombotic conditions
- PSA (>50yrs, FH in 1° relative, abnormal rectal examination)
- Specific pre-transplant profiling, e.g. CD4 count ± CNI levels for IS trial in HIV recipients.

Urine and urinary tract (biennial or change in findings/symptoms)
- Current urine output, if any
- Urine dipstick analysis and MSU (repeat if infection suspected and routinely on admission for Tx)
- Baseline PCR (e.g. in nephrotic patients, FSGS)
- Other if indicated (e.g. cytology, acid-fast bacilli, EMU, pregnancy test)
- US of native kidneys
- Pre-and post-micturition bladder US (urological indication).

Pulmonary/cardiovascular (biennial or change in findings/symptoms)
- Dry weight assessment (see 📖 pp. 588–601, Appendix 3)
- BP control
- CXR
- ECG
- Echocardiogram if indicated (suspected valve disease, cardiac failure, pericardial effusion)
- Exercise capacity testing if indicated (biennial) (e.g. myocardial perfusion scan/dobutamine stress test for >50yrs, DM, ischaemic heart/vascular disease, >3yrs on dialysis, re-transplant)
- Cardiology opinion ± coronary angiography if indicated
- Duplex scanning to include iliac arteries (routine) and iliac veins, peripheral and carotid arteries if indicated
- Lung function tests (lung disease, thoracic wall deformities)
- Anaesthetic opinion if indicated.

Surgical assessment (biennial or as required)
- Detailed examination (abdominal, cardiovascular, pulmonary)
- Identify significance of previous surgery, particularly abdominal ± complications and special considerations
- Review suitability in the context of PMH, current history, and clinical investigations, including BMI, peripheral circulation, exercise tolerance
- Part 1 patient consent (annually) (see 📖 pp. 454–5).

Special considerations
- *Clinical complexity*—special consideration is required when planning Tx for patients with, e.g. HIV disease, risk of recurrent disease, complex haematological/pro-thrombotic conditions, ↑ anaesthetic/CV risk, and antibody incompatible transplantation (AiT). Early identification of

risk, specific pre-transplant monitoring, and involvement of specialist colleagues is recommended to agree a joint Tx management plan. Planned LDKT is often the preferred option for these recipients

- *Pre-emptive Tx*—pre-transplant preparation and evaluation is time-critical and early referral to the transplant MPT is essential to achieve pre-emptive listing for DD within 6 months of RRT or timely LDKT (eGFR between 10–15ml/min/1.73m^2)
- *Logistical aspects*—the organization of transplant services with a central transplant 'hub', which receives referrals from a network of 'feeder' nephrology or dialysis units is logistically and clinically challenging. Agreed clinical protocols, excellent communication, and clinicians who are actively engaged in the process are key to success.

The role of the specialist nurse is integral to:
- Managing an effective recipient transplant pathway
- Promoting access to Tx through ongoing management and review of the patients listed for Tx.

Best practice models include experienced nurses who co-ordinate recipient work-up in collaboration with nephrologists, transplant surgeons, and the wider MPT.

It is the responsibility of every nurse working in CKD and dialysis settings to liaise closely with local recipient co-ordinators, and the transplant team to ensure that potential transplant recipients are identified and assessed in a timely manner, particularly for pre-emptive Tx.

Transplant operation: admission for surgery

The type of admission for the recipient will depend upon the source of the organ and recipient considerations, e.g. clinical complexity:

- Planned—LDKT
- Unplanned—DDKT/SPK.

All patients will have been assessed prior to listing for DD organ(s) or to be considered suitable to receive a LDKT (see 🕮 pp. 454–5). They will all be admitted directly to the transplant centre for surgery. Recipients of a DD donor organ are called in at short notice and time is of the essence in order to minimize delay between retrieval and implantation (CIT), which has an impact on immediate graft function. Pre-transplant assessment and preparation is pivotal to proceeding quickly at this stage. If the chosen recipient is not suitable to proceed with the transplant plan, it must be identified quickly so that the donated organ(s) can be re-allocated to another recipient on the NTL as soon as possible.

Recipients of a LDKT will usually be admitted the day before surgery with an individual transplant plan in place. The recipient and donor usually attend a pre-admission clinic for immunological crossmatching and final tests (see 🕮 pp. 487 and 476). 1–2wks prior to the planned date to pre-empt any unforeseen problems for LD specific issues.

The potential recipient is assessed on admission to ensure that it is safe to proceed with the transplant as planned, i.e.:

- The donated organ is immunologically compatible
- There is no current clinical problem that would prevent Tx (i.e. infection, recent health issue)
- He/she is fit for major surgery under general anaesthetic (GA)
- Dialysis is not required prior to GA (i.e. ↑ K⁺, ↑ urea, fluid overload)
- All special considerations identified in pre-assessment have been noted and acted upon
- All appropriate clinical investigations have been performed and are up to date; results available
- He/she wishes to proceed with the transplant according to the terms of previous consent and confirms consent in writing with an appropriately qualified surgeon

The recipient assessment should include the following:

Urgent blood tests

- Donor specific flow cytometry crossmatch (H&I lab)
- ABO blood group and save ± crossmatch for blood
- Full blood chemistry (kidney function, liver (LFTs), bone profile), glucose
- FBC
- Clotting screen/INR if indicated
- Check virology.

Urine output

- Dipstick urinalysis and MSU ± PCR if indicated by 1° diagnosis (e.g. FSGS).

Other

- MRSA skin screen
- Full history and physical examination as per pre-transplant assessment (see 📖 pp. 456–8, Recipient pre-transplant assessment and preparation)
- ▶ Check and implement MPT transplant plan for complex recipients (e.g. HIV, AiT, FSGS, pro-thrombotic conditions)
- Review of previous and current investigations
- Current medications, including history of allergies and adverse reactions
- Monitor vital signs: BP, pulse, temperature, and respirations
- Weight and BMI
- CXR
- ECG
- Check pregnancy status in ♀ of child-bearing age
- VTE risk assessment (if not previously considered and planned)
- Immediate psycho-social concerns (e.g. child care/elderly dependents)
- Anaesthetic and surgical review.

Preoperative management

The admission assessment will identify preoperative interventions that are essential before the patient goes to theatre, e.g.:

- Dialysis treatment (fluid balance, correction of ↑ K⁺/ ↑ urea) NB: drain out dwelling fluid if on PD prior to leaving ward for theatre
- BP control (aim to be normotensive)
- Diabetic management (sliding scale IV insulin and dextrose to replace SC insulin/oral agents)
- Anticoagulation therapy.

Tailor according to VTE assessment (oral aspirin ± SC heparin).

If on warfarin, stop, administer IV vitamin K/FFP/prothrombotic agents and manage according to INR. ▶Potential recipients for planned LDKT on warfarin to be converted to heparin 3 days pre-op.

The patient will be prescribed specific medications, according to local protocol, disease-specific considerations, ± individual transplant plan (see 🕮 p. 489, Immunosuppression), including:

- Pre-op/induction IS and IV prophylactic antibiotics
- Pre-medication (usually oral temazepam PRN)
- Maintenance IS (to commence post-op)
- Prophylactic maintenance medications to cover early phase of IS, e.g. co-trimoxazole/pentamidine (PCP), valganciclovir (CMV donor +ve, recipient −ve), oral nystatin (anti-fungal), ranitidine/omeprazole (gastro-protective)
- Maintenance medication as indicated (e.g. BP control, anticoagulation therapy).

The role of the nurse from admission to theatre

Activity from the DD pool is unpredictable, time critical (to minimize CIT), and often occurs out of hours on emergency theatre lists. Several organs may become available for different recipients within a short timeframe and the inpatient team may be dealing with multiple admissions and elective LDKT activity simultaneously. It is important that the roles and responsibilities of each member of the MPT are clearly defined so that patient safety is safeguarded and the best transplant outcomes are achieved.

> Nursing has a pivotal role in terms of leadership and co-ordination in both ward and outpatient environments. The organizational skills of nurses are well suited to
> - Ensuring that processes are in place to streamline patient pathways
> - Essential documentation is completed
> - Lines of communication are clear.

Since the ODTF, many transplant centres have designated in-house nurse recipient co-ordinators who are responsible for managing the local transplant waiting list and co-ordinating pre-transplant assessment and recipient admissions. In LDKT, living donor co-ordinators (LDCs) will work alongside the recipient co-ordinators, taking responsibility for donor assessment, preparation, and admission in order to keep donor and recipient pathways running in parallel. Admission for LDKT is planned electively on routine theatre lists (see 📖 pp. 476–7, Living donor kidney transplantation).

In the interests of patient safety, the preoperative checklist must be completed as for any surgical operation/procedure (see 📖 pp. 60, 62), ensuring that:
- The patient is appropriately prepared for theatre
- The operation site is clearly marked by the surgeon
- All general information and specific preoperative preparation is clearly documented; subject to local protocols.

The inpatient/ward nurse who is responsible for the patient must:
- Sign the operation checklist
- Accompany the patient ± the correct donated organs to theatre (according to local arrangements)
- Handover to the designated theatre nurse or operating department assistant (ODA), who will re-check the information prior to accepting the patient for surgery.

Recipient operations
The following procedures will be discussed:
- Single kidney alone transplant (KA)*
- Simultaneous kidney and pancreas transplant (SPK).**

*Rarely, both donated DD kidneys may be used for 1 recipient if the donor is <5yrs of age (en bloc) or if there is concern about the viability of a single kidney e.g. in older donors and a dual transplant is performed. Recipient selection, surgery and management for these procedures are more complicated and are not discussed in the scope of this chapter.

**The pancreas may also be transplanted after a KA (PAK) or as a pancreas alone (PTA).

Preparation of the donated organs
Donated DD organs are accepted by recipient surgeons on the basis of information collected by the retrieval teams and data entered on to the Electronic Offering System (EOS), usually by SN-ODs (see 📖 p. 438, Procurement). This information allows medical teams to decide whether or not to accept a particular organ for the recipient that has been identified through the national allocation system. Before the recipient is called to theatre, the operating surgeon will examine the organs for injury and perform any 'bench' preparation that is needed to ensure the best chance of success (e.g. preparation of blood vessels, removal of perinephric fat).

In *SPK Tx* the careful retrieval, examination and preparation of the donated pancreas significantly improves outcomes. 'Bench' preparation takes approximately 2hrs and is a crucial part of the procedure to prevent bleeding post Tx and to prepare the tissues and blood vessels properly. This includes preparation of the portal vein, which provides the main venous drainage for the pancreas and anastomosis of an iliac Y graft to the superior mesenteric artery (SMA) and the splenic artery of the pancreas graft to create a single 'artery'. This helps to increase blood flow to the pancreas after it has been transplanted into the recipient.

In *LDKT* the donated kidney is usually transplanted into a recipient within the same hospital where there is direct communication between donor–recipient surgeons and 'bench' preparation can be planned if required (e.g. removal of a stone, preparation of multiple arteries). When donated organs travel (i.e. to paediatric recipient hospitals or as part of the NLDKSS), clear communication between operating surgeons ± LDCs is essential to ensure that accurate information is transferred between donor and recipient team, CIT is minimized, and potential problems pre-empted. 'Bench' preparation may be performed in the retrieval centre so that the kidney can be implanted without delay on arrival in the recipient centre.

Recipient preparation in theatre

The patient will be admitted to the anaesthetic room first for:

- Induction of GA (including medications as prescribed) (see 📖 p. 489, Immunosuppression)
- Placement of venous access (i.e. peripheral cannulae, CVP line)
- Insertion of urethral bladder catheter, and drainage bag.

Once in the operating theatre, the patient will need:

- To be positioned on the operating table (supine)
- To be shaved and topical povidone iodine skin preparation applied
- To be 'draped' to create a sterile field
- Diathermy applied
- IV fluids (prepared ready for infusion)
- Patient-controlled analgesic (PCA) pump (IV fentanyl prepared).

Implantation

Kidney

The kidney transplant operation has been standardized over the last few decades (Figure 14.1). The transplanted kidney is placed in a heterotropic (distant site) extraperitoneal location, usually in the iliac fossa (the right side is the site of choice for 1st transplants). A curvilinear incision in the lower quadrant of the abdomen (Gibson's incision) is used to expose the iliac vessels and the bladder. Using non-absorbable sutures and end-to-side anastomoses, the donor renal vein is attached to the recipient external iliac vein and the donor renal artery, with its patch of aortic vessel (in the case of DD) is attached to the recipient iliac artery. In some circumstances the common iliac vessels or 'great vessels' (aorta and inferior vena cava (IVC)) are used instead and if the donor renal artery is 'very short', occasionally an end-to-end anastomosis to the recipient's internal iliac artery is chosen. All blood vessels must be handled and dissected carefully to avoid injury to the lining (intima), which can cause thrombosis and graft loss.

Ureteric anastomosis

The ureteric anastomosis (ureteroneocystostomy) is as important as the vascular anastomoses and requires careful attention to minimize complications. The technique used to implant the ureter into the bladder must prevent:

- Ischaemia caused by damage to the uretric blood supply (necrosis)
- Stenosis at the point of anastomosis with the bladder
- Prevent pulling or twisting of the ureter.

A ureteric, double J stent, which extends from the pelvis of the kidney into the bladder, is routinely used to maintain the patency of the ureter in the early stages of postoperative healing and to prevent urinary leaks. The stent is removed by flexible cystoscopy 4–6wks after Tx. Ongoing research is looking at the option of removing the stent with the removal of the urinary catheter within days of surgery to see if there is an impact on reducing urinary infection post-transplant.

The kidney may function immediately and produce large volumes of urine, encouraged by induction medication, and IV fluids. The bladder catheter is placed on monitored, free drainage from the outset to measure urine output accurately and avoid bladder distention. A bladder lavage may be performed intraoperatively to remove any residual blood/clots or debris (particularly if previously anuric). The catheter is usually removed 5 days postoperatively (see 📖 pp. 470–1, Immediate postoperative management).

Wound closure

The wound is usually closed with SC, dissolvable sutures. A vacuum drain is inserted to prevent collection of lymph/blood, which may cause compression and injury to the newly transplanted kidney.

Simultaneous pancreas and kidney implantation

The pancreas is implanted before the kidney because it is less tolerant to prolonged ischaemia. It is usually placed in an intraperitoneal position, although it can be implanted extraperitoneally. The graft portal vein is usually anastomosed to the recipient lower IVC but the portal circulation (graft superior mesenteric vein) can be used as an alternative, which is thought to reduce hyperinsulinaemia and vascular damage (atherogenesis). The Y graft (see Figure 14.1) is anastomosed to the lower aorta or the common iliac artery. The management of exocrine secretion is controversial. The donor duodenum can be anastomosed to a Roux-en-Y loop of recipient small bowel (enteric drainage) or alternatively this can be anastomosed to the recipient's urinary bladder (bladder drainage).

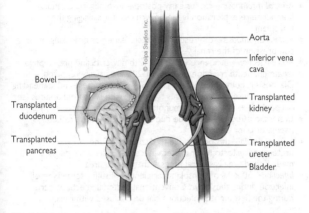

Fig. 14.1 Implantation of kidney ± pancreas. © Tolpa Studios, inc, reproduced with permission.

Early complications

Kidney

- *Acute tubular necrosis (ATN) and delayed graft function (DGF)*—some degree of ATN occurs in 5–30% of all transplants from DBD kidneys, >80% of DCD kidneys, but is uncommon in LDKT because of the planned nature of the surgery and ↓ CIT. Evidence suggests that DGF may be associated with a ↓ 5yr graft survival by up to 10%
- *Primary non-function*—the kidney never functions
- *Arterial thrombosis*—causes early postoperative oliguria or anuria. Immediate re-exploration is the only chance for salvaging the transplant
- *Venous thrombosis*—can result from technical error or kinking or compression of the renal vein
- *Acute rejection*—incidence varies but with newer IS and pre-emptive treatment acute rejection rates of 10–20% are usually reported. Diagnosis requires biopsy (see 📖 p. 62) and treatment and, depending upon the cause, usually involves treatment with IV steroid boluses (see 📖 pp. 502–4, Transplant immunology and Immunosuppression)
- *Ureteral obstruction*—could be due to blood clot in the catheter, haematoma, or oedema
- *Urinary fistula*—this occurs due to disruption of the ureteroneocystostomy or ureteral necrosis. Differential diagnosis is made if fluid urea is several times ↑ than serum urea
- *Infection*—30–60% of transplant recipients will suffer some type of infection during the 1st yr. Conventional bacterial infections occur during the first month. Infections can be confused with rejection.

Pancreas

- *Vascular thrombosis*—the most common non-immunological cause of graft loss
- *Allograft pancreatitis*—this occurs in 10–20% of all pancreas graft recipients. In its most severe form it can result in necrosis of the graft and arterial thrombosis. It is difficult to detect and can be confused with rejection and pancreatic fistula
- *Pancreatic fistula*—more common in enteric drained than in bladder drained grafts
- *Rejection*—hyperglycaemia caused by islet damage is a late sign of rejection. One of the benefits of SPK Tx is that rejection of both organs tends to occur at the same time. Serum creatinine level, which is monitored closely post-kidney transplant, is a sensitive surrogate marker for rejection of the pancreas in SPK recipients.

Immediate postoperative management

Vigilant postoperative monitoring and careful management of the transplant recipient is essential, particularly in the immediate period post transplant to:
- Optimize patient and graft outcome
- Identify and treat early complications

Maintain haemostasis

Perform hrly for minimum 24hrs:
- Check for signs of haemorrhage (outward bleeding/bleeding into wound drain, ↓ urine output, ↓ BP, ↓ CVP, shock)
- Volume and nature of output from bladder catheter and wound drain, e.g. blood stained, excessive wound drainage, changes in urine output
- Replace all output 100% with crystalloid fluid, then orally
- Measure CVP, BP, pulse, respirations, temperature
- Administer colloid/blood as required to maintain CVP within prescribed parameters
- Wound check and venous access sites (pain, oozing, swelling)
- Observe for signs of fluid overload (dyspnoea, tachycardia, peripheral oedema, productive cough). ⚠ Differential diagnoses for chest infection, haemorrhage (see 📖 p. 60).

Monitor for potential complications

Observations and vital signs as previously listed for:
- Haemorrhage
- Infection
- Wound dehiscence
- Primary non-function/DGF (anuria/oliguria)
- Acute rejection
- Disease-specific considerations, e.g. proteinuria in FSGS, clotting in pro-thrombotic conditions.

The role of the nurse in the postoperative management of the recent transplant recipient is to:
- Maintain haemostasis
- Monitor signs and symptoms closely and report changes in condition to ↓ complications
- Recognize that signs and symptoms may be indicative of >1 diagnosis/clinical problem.

General postoperative nursing care
- Care and hygiene, including oral hygiene and care of venous access sites, drain sites, and bladder catheter
- Pain control (PCA *in situ* from theatre for 24hrs)
- Oxygen as prescribed (until awake-mask/nasal specs.)
- Thromboprophylaxis as prescribed (see 📖 p. 61, Clinical assessment)
- Management of nausea (PRN)

- Management of constipation (PRN but max. 3 days if BNO)
- Accurate administration and monitoring of medicines as prescribed ±
  according to individual transplant plan (NB: alternative routes may be
  needed if unable to tolerate orally)
- Early physiotherapy and mobilize day 1 post-op
- Encourage oral intake of fluids and food day 1 post-op (►check for
  ileus first)
- Remove wound drain at surgeon's request (<20ml/24hrs)
- Remove CVP and other venous access as no longer required (3–5
  days)
- Remove wound dressing 3 days and re-dress as required
- Remove bladder catheter 5 days post-op and send MSU
- Education/support of recipient and family (e.g. if difficult postoperative
  course/further investigations required)
- Discharge planning for 5 days (may be extended and longer for SPK).

Investigations/imaging

- Transplant US in recovery ± any change in urine output to ensure
  transplant is perfused and to exclude obstruction/thrombosis
- CXR (post CVP insertion ± fluid overload)
- Immediately postoperatively and then daily/as indicated: full U&Es
  (kidney, liver, bone), FBC, trough CNI level, blood glucose (initially
  2hrs post SPK), amylase (SPK)
- Transplant kidney biopsy (see ⬚ pp. 62–3, Clinical assessment) as
  indicated for differential diagnosis if kidney/SPK non-functioning.

Late complications and long-term follow-up

Kidney

- *Graft rejection and immunosuppression*—with the exception of identical twins, the organ donor and recipient are genetically different. Without IS, a transplanted graft will be rejected within days. Understanding the rejection process is a prerequisite to understanding the principles of IS medication (see 📖 p. 486, Transplant immunology).
- *Renal artery stenosis*—patients present with hypertension and ↓ kidney function. Can be confused with rejection. Renal artery stenosis is often caused by a technical (surgical) problem. It can usually be treated with percutaneous transluminal angioplasty
- *Ureteral obstruction*—late presentation could be due to ureteral stenosis
- *Lymphocele*—manifests wks or months postoperatively with swelling of the wound, oedema of scrotum or labia and lower extremity, and urinary obstruction from pressure on the collecting system or ureter. The treatment of choice is fenestration of the cyst into the peritoneal cavity. External drainage should be avoided as this puts the kidney at risk of infection
- *Infection*—the period 30–180 days postoperative is the usual time for opportunistic infections as this coincides with the period of maximal IS. Viral infections are the most significant (e.g. CMV). Other pathogens include aspergillosis, blastomycosis, nocardiosis, toxoplasmosis, cryptococcosis, *Candida*, and *Pneumocystis jiroveci*
- *Hyperglycaemia*—this is generally attributed to corticosteroid administration and previously normoglycaemic patients may become diabetic. New onset diabetes (NODAT) can also occur with tacrolimus administration
- *Hyperparathyroidism*—patients could suffer from tertiary hyperparathyroidism with significant hypercalcaemia and ↑ parathyroid hormone levels despite a functioning transplant. This is treated by total parathyroidectomy
- *Cancers*—in kidney transplant recipients an incidence of 6% is reported for *de novo* malignancies. This is related to the duration and degree of IS rather than to any particular agent. More prevalent tumours are skin cancers (squamous cell Ca), lymphomas, renal cancers, Kaposi's sarcoma, Ca of the vulva, uterus, and cervix. Post-transplant lymphoproliferative disease (PTLD) is the name given to the spectrum of diseases from benign hyperplasia to malignant lymphomas. EBV is the most important factor in PTLD
- *Chronic allograft nephropathy*—characterized by a progressive ↓ in kidney function, which is not attributable to a specific cause. Chronic changes to the kidney are mediated by both immune and non-immune factors (see 📖 pp. 486–8, Transplant immunology)
- *Recurrent disease*—glomerulonephritides (e.g. FSGS, mesangiocapillary glomerulonephritis type 1, IgA nephropathy) (see 📖 pp. 8–9,

Pathophysiology) are most likely to recur; however, with the exception of FSGS, where graft loss can be early and aggressive with rapid onset proteinuria, loss of the kidney generally occurs late. These diseases are not contraindications to Tx. Patients with DM have poorer outcomes following Tx than patients without diabetes; nearly all patients have evidence of diabetic nephropathy on histology (kidney biopsy) within 4yrs of TX. Hence the treatment of choice for diabetics with ESKD is SPK Tx where possible.

Pancreas

- *Urological complications*—haematuria, urethritis, recurrent urinary tract infections (UTI) and bicarbonate loss are common in bladder-drained recipients. Enteric conversion may be necessary if it cannot be managed conservatively.
- *Autoimmune recurrence*—the autoimmune response to native islets can cause loss of transplanted pancreatic beta cells.

The role of the nurse in long-term follow-up

Tx is a treatment not a cure; the surgery is an acute event but long-term management of the transplant is a chronic illness model. Clinical outcomes are influenced by early detection of:

- Post-transplant complications
- Intercurrent illnesses
- Non-adherence to medications.

As time elapses from the transplant operation, recipients spend relatively little time in the hospital setting and more time in their own environment. Most interaction with post-transplant recipients is in busy outpatient clinics where time is limited and continuity of care is a challenge. Long-term follow-up may take place in the transplant centre or in a DGH nephrology centre, according to local arrangements. Effective long-term management includes:

- Multiprofessional input
- Continuity of care; ongoing education and support
- Partnership between transplant recipient and healthcare professionals
- Strong links between transplant centre ± local DGH nephrology centres and 1° care.

Immediately following discharge post-Tx, regular outpatient appointments are essential. Frequency varies from daily to twice wkly; reducing to wkly according to clinical course in the first few wks/months. Most clinics are both nurse and medically led, and frequent appointments allow for changes to be noted and acted upon and IS to be monitored. Same-day, MPT results review informs treatment/management changes. Recipients understand that they may need to return the next day for urgent repeat blood tests or further investigations if indicated. A typical clinic visit includes:

- Health history, general well-being, concerns/problems
- Vital signs—TPR, BP, and weight
- Blood tests—renal function, liver (LFTs), bone profile, CRP, FBC, and IS levels (e.g. CNIs). Additional tests may be performed according to clinical indications, e.g. disease-specific considerations ± individual transplant plan (see 📖 pp. 456–8, Recipient pre-transplant assessment

and preparation), lipid levels, glucose, further infection markers, blood cultures
- Fluid balance—intake vs output from patient self-assessment record, weight ↑↓, peripheral oedema, dyspnoea, hypertension
- Urinalysis—dipstick glycosuria, signs of infection e.g. nitrites, leucocytes. ▶Microscopic blood and protein are common post Tx due to presence of stent but frank haematuria needs further investigation. MSU for MC&S if indicated
- Wound healing—inflammation, redness or swelling. ⚠Can be confused with signs of rejection
- Signs of rejection—pyrexia, pain over graft, oliguria
- Signs of systemic illness/infection/other health issues—pyrexia, general malaise
- Current medications reviewed; dose adjustments (e.g. protocol changes to IS ± prophylactic medicines, BP control, commencement of antibiotics, changes for poor tolerance) (see 📖 p. 492).
- *Initiate further investigations if indicated:*
  - CXR, ECG (general health/chest infection ± pain)
  - transplant biopsy (graft dysfunction) (see 📖 pp. 62–3)
  - transplant US scan (graft perfusion, blood flow, fluid collection, obstruction)
- *Initiate MPT referrals PRN,* e.g. surgical, medical, nursing, psycho-social.

After the first 3 months post-Tx appointments ↓ in frequency and long-term stable patients will usually attend clinic 3–4 times/yr.

Annual health review

Many transplant centres offer an annual health review for all recipients in addition to routine 'monitoring' appointments. These are particularly helpful for long-term patients who attend less frequently. Consultations focus on overall health and well-being; screening for modifiable risk factors is key, e.g. smoking, obesity, hypercholesterolaemia, hypertension, new onset diabetes, non-adherence, cancer, other co-morbidities, as well as psycho-social and lifestyle factors (see 📖 pp. 84–5, 553).

> The role of the nurse in long-term management of the transplant patient is to promote best transplant and patient outcomes by:
> - Developing the appropriate knowledge and skills to work effectively within the MPT
> - Recognizing potential risks to health and well-being
> - Referring appropriately for specialist opinion/input
> - Providing continuity of care in the outpatient setting
> - Ongoing support for patients and their families
> - Contributing to educational initiatives
> - Developing nurse-led initiatives to improve quality of care.

See 📖 p. 483, Further reading.

Living donor kidney transplantation

LDKT is the treatment of choice for many patients, particularly for recipients who are at higher risk of death or graft failure and/or for planned pre-emptive kidney Tx (see 📖 p. 446, Choices for transplantation). Recipient and donor evaluation, using agreed clinical pathways and central nurse-led co-ordination, is successful in achieving timely Tx. All abdominal transplant centres have at least one LDC who is responsible for co-ordinating the LD pathway and will often work in conjunction with other LDCs/transplant nurses/recipient co-ordinators across regional networks to facilitate LDKT (see Figure 14.2). Donor safety and welfare is paramount; to promote consistent best practice across all transplant centres in the UK, local protocols should be based upon the BTS/RA *UK Guidelines for living Donor Kidney Transplantation*, at 🌎 <http://www.bts.org.uk> which are evidence-based and cover all aspects of the donor evaluation and selection process. The success of the NLDKSS depends upon LD kidneys being shared between transplant centres and the scheme highlights the need for consistent donor assessment and preparation.

Living donor evaluation

Key principles

- Early education and discussion with all potential transplant recipients and their families; identify LD options and optimize timing for Tx. For pre-emptive LDKT, start discussion at recipient eGFR ~20ml/min; tailor donor and recipient evaluation according to ↓ in recipient kidney function to allow for donor attrition.
- Early assessment and investigation of recipient suitability for LDKT prior to commencement of significant LD evaluation
- Central co-ordination of recipient and donor pathways; responsibility for each with separate clinical teams; 'map' progress of both pathways to one another through regular MPT meetings and revise donation/Tx plan as necessary
- Donor assessment using MPT, evidence-based protocol with a logical progression of testing; tailored to local resources and donor requirements/convenience if possible
- Emphasis on donor safety; physical and psychological welfare; early triage of unsuitable donors and provision for appropriate follow-up
- Prospective LDs must feel able to withdraw from the process at any time, supported by the clinical team.

Rationale

- Maximize donor safety
- Achieve a timely transplant
- Manage donor and recipient expectations
- Avoid unnecessary inconvenience and investigations for the prospective donor
- ↓ simultaneous evaluation of multiple donors; optimize use of resources
- Appropriately support unsuitable donors
- Ensure both donor and recipient can give free and valid consent for surgery and meet the legal requirements under the HT Act for LDKT.

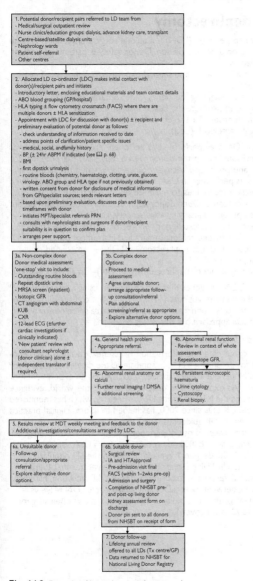

Fig. 14.2 Example of living donor evaluation pathway.

Donor nephrectomy

Living donor nephrectomy (LDN) is a unique surgical procedure because it is performed on a healthy person. Donor safety is paramount and can be safeguarded by:

- Careful donor evaluation and surgical expertise to ↓ the risk of death and complications
- Retrieving and implanting the kidney under optimal, planned circumstances to promote the best transplant outcome
- Ensuring that consent for surgery is truly 'free and valid' (see 🕮 p. 428, Legal framework (UK)).

Traditionally, LDN was performed as an 'open' procedure via a left or right flank incision, leaving the donor with a long scar; the potential for ↑ morbidity, and prolonged recovery. Since 1995, when the first laparoscopic LDN was performed in USA, surgeons have developed and refined minimally invasive techniques to minimize donor complications and optimize recipient outcome. Open donor nephrectomy is still performed but most donors opt for minimally invasive surgery, i.e.

- Hand-assisted laparoscopic donor nephrectomy (HALDN)—small abdominal/Pfannenstiel incision; camera and instrument ports
- Total laparoscopic donor nephrectomy (TLDN)—camera and instrument ports only
- Mini-incision open donor nephrectomy (MODN)—small flank incision.

HALDN and TLDN, on either the right or left side, using a transperitoneal approach is the standard approach in most transplant centres, allowing for easier access and dissection. Laparoscopic LDN can also be performed via a retroperitoneal approach but this is less common.

Mortality and morbidity

Accurate outcome data and information is essential to inform the consent process for prospective LDs. In some areas the data/evidence is poor because healthy people are not subjected to LDN on an experimental or research basis. As expertise has developed around the world, evidence has improved and the NHSBT Living Donor Registry, which has monitored outcomes from UK LDs since 2000, has helped to inform clinical practice and development of UK guidelines (see Table 14.3).

- *Mortality*—the accepted risk of perioperative mortality, based on good retrospective data, is 1:3000 and recent data from USA suggests that the risk is 1:10,000, despite ↑ age and obesity in the LD population
- *Morbidity*—the UK Living Donor Registry demonstrates that there is no significant difference in major morbidity, e.g. PE, infection, bleeding, re-operation, between open LDN and laparoscopic LDN (4.5% vs 5.1%) but that general morbidity is ↓ in laparoscopic vs open surgery (10.3% vs 15.7% respectively).

Table 14.3 Complications: open donor nephrectomy vs LHALDN vs TLDN.

Complication	Open nephrectomy (5,660) %	Laparoscopic hand assisted (2,239) %	Full laparoscopic nephrectomy (2,929) %
Re-operation	0.4	1.0	0.9
Complications not needing re-operation	0.3	1	0.8
Bleeding	0.15	0.18	0.45
Bowel obstruction	0.05	0.27	0.1
Bowel injury	–	0.1	0.14
Hernia	0.18	0.5	0.03
DVT/pulmonary embolus	0.02	0.09	0.1
Pnemothorax	0.09	0.05	–
Prolonged ileus	–	0.05	0.06
Rhabdomyolysis	–	0.09	0.13
Readmission rate	0.6		1.6

Reproduced from *UK Guidelines for Living Donor Kidney Transplantation*, Chapter 6, May 2011, with permission.

Lifelong impact of LDN

In the long term, complications directly related to LDN are rare because LDs are selected on the basis of health. Following postoperative recovery, LDs having undergone LDN are at no ↑ risk of:
• Kidney disease or other health problems than anyone in the general population
• Shortened life expectancy
• Complications during pregnancy.

Consent

HTA approval for a LDKT is dependent upon the donor being able to give voluntary and valid consent for donation; coercion or reward is illegal. The independent assessor (IA) makes an assessment when interviewing the donor and recipient to confirm if the donor's interests have been upheld and reports his/her findings to the HTA. In terms of consent, LDN is unique because:
• The donor does not require surgery for their own physical benefit
• There are many reasons why LDs are motivated to donate (the spec trum of altruism (see 📖 pp. 430–3, Ethics of organ donation and transplantation)
• Some information should be shared between recipient and donor, e.g. HLA typing, crossmatching and ABO blood group, recipient diagnosis and transplant as these may be relevant to the decision to donate. Unless it influences the decision to donate, other donor/

recipient-specific information should not be shared. Agreed boundaries of confidentiality must be agreed at the outset between donor and recipient so that both can make a fully informed decision to proceed with LDKT

- The prospective LD must feel free and be supported by the transplant team to withdraw consent at any time until the time of surgery
- The consent process and decision to donate must meet legal requirements, including prior consent from the LD about the destination of the donated kidney if it cannot be implanted into the intended recipient, e.g. transplant to alternative recipient or re-implant back in the donor
- Transplant teams have a right to challenge donor autonomy in the face of unacceptable risk, i.e. where third-party intervention (surgery) is necessary to proceed with donation.

Which kidney?

The choice of kidney to be donated rests on 2 key principles:
- Leaving the donor with the 'best' kidney if there is a choice
- Ensuring the best transplant outcome in the recipient.
  The final decision is made prior to surgery using:
- Cross-sectional imaging, i.e. CT or MRI
- MPT discussion including experienced radiologist
- Full donor assessment and discussion with the donor and recipient
- Other influencing factors.

The left kidney is usually chosen for donation because of the longer renal vein, which facilitates implantation. Other influencing factors include:

Vascular anatomy—single vessels (renal artery and vein) are ideal; multiple vessels, particularly renal arteries, ↑ complexity and the risk of complications, e.g. graft thrombosis, renal artery stenosis, and renovascular hypertension. Evidence suggests that overall patient and transplant survival are not adversely affected and multiple vessels do not preclude donation in most patients.

Differential kidney function—split/single kidney function tests are performed if an apparent anatomical abnormality on imaging may affect individual kidney function. If it is suitable to proceed, the kidney with the lower function is selected for donation.

Simple cyst/kidney stone in one kidney—the kidney with the cyst/stone is generally removed for donation. In some cases, small stones may be removed 'on the bench' prior to implantation with specialist urological expertise.

Management of the LD undergoing donor nephrectomy

LDN is major surgery and management of the LD should reflect this. Particular emphasis is placed upon:
- *Donor and family support*—often anxious, particularly if recipient is also family member
- *Suitable environment*—donors cared for where there is MPT expertise in LDN care

- **Valid consent**—2-part process with confirmation on admission; including information about which kidney is to be removed
- **Appropriate site marking**—left or right LDN
- **Appropriate positioning on the operating table**—taking into account nephrectomy side and/or previous back injury
- **Monitoring of vital signs**—TPR, BP
- **Fluid balance**—first 24hrs: IV hydration; hrly urinary catheter drainage; then oral fluids and urine output measurements after catheter removal
- **Nutrition**—oral fluids and diet as tolerated postoperatively in the absence of a paralytic ileus; anti-emetics PRN
- **DVT prophylaxis**—e.g. anti-emboli stockings; SC heparin; decompression boots in theatre; early mobilization
- **Optimal pain management and early mobilization**—first 24hrs: patient-controlled, opiate-based analgesic (PCA pump) then oral pain management; anti-emetics as required particularly if PCA poorly tolerated. Oxygen therapy maintained until awake; ⚠observe for drowsiness /nausea on PCA if opiate based
- **Wound care**—monitor for bleeding or infection; remove dressing prior to discharge home; home care advice; peri-op antibiotics
- **Discharge planning, advice and support**—3–7 days post LDN (procedure dependent).

Life-long follow-up

Life-long follow-up, at the transplant centre, regional referring centre, or via the GP, is recommended as best practice for all previous LDs to:

- Offer annual 'well woman/man' health review and identify any potential health issues that may impact on the donor/single kidney, e.g. ageing hypertension, ↑ BMI, pregnancy (as required), mental health issues
- Inform the NHSBT National Living Donor Registry within the National Transplant Database and create continuing evidence base.
- ▶LDs returning overseas following donation must be provided with advice for local follow-up care.
  Many annual review clinics are LDC led and comprise the following:
- Update medical and social history—including new health issues and return to normal activity at 1yr review
- Current medications—including changes/new medications
- Monitor BP (diastolic to be maintained <90mmHg, BMI (<30), (± other vital signs if indicated)
- Urinalysis—dipstick (blood, protein, nitrites, leucocytes, glucose). Send MSU for MC&S ± PCR if indicated
- Wound check—hernia; pain
- Serum creatinine (⚠eGFR is not helpful for healthy LDs with a single kidney as it is designed as a measure of CKD, not single kidney GFR)
- FBC may be performed routinely at 1yr but then as required
- Referral for specialist opinion or to GP for, e.g. microscopic haematuria, hypertension requiring treatment, surgical hernia
- Return data to Living Donor Registry years 1, 2, 5, 10, and then every 5 years.

> **Nurses have a key role in all aspects of the LDKT pathway**
> - Donor and recipient education, support, and decision-making
> - Co-ordination and 'mapping' of donor and recipient evaluations
> - MPT liaison
> - Timely scheduling for donation–Tx
> - Inpatient stay; admission to discharge including postoperative monitoring
> - Lifelong follow-up; donor and recipient.

See 📖 p. 483, Further reading.

Further reading

Danovitch GM (ed). *Handbook of Kidney Transplantation*, 5th edn. Philadelphia, PA: Lippincott Williams & Wilkins; 2010.

Ohler L, Cupples S, International Transplant Nurses Society (eds). *Core Curriculum for Transplant Nurses*. St Louis, MO: Mosby Elsevier; 2008.

Torpey N, Moghal NE, Watson E, *et al*. (eds). *Oxford Handbook of Renal Transplantation*. Oxford: Oxford University Press; 2010.

Reference

1. Stock PG, Roland ME, Carlson L, *et al*. Kidney and liver transplantation in human immunodeficiency virus-infected patients: a pilot safety and efficacy study. *Transplantation* 2003; **76**:370–5.

Useful websites

British Transplantation Society (BTS) website. Available at: ℘ <http://www.bts.org.uk>

Access 'Active Standards and Guidelines' for:
• NHSBT/BTS: *Guidelines for Consent to Solid Organ Transplantation in Adults*, March 2011
• BTS/RA: *UK Guidelines for Living Donor Kidney Transplantation*, 3rd edn, May 2011
• BTS: *Antibody Incompatible Guidelines*, 2nd edn, January 2011
• Renal Association (RA): *Guidelines for Assessment for Renal Transplantation*, 4th edn, 2008
• BTS/ICS: *Consensus Guidelines on Organ Donation after Circulatory Death*, December 2010
• BTS: *Guidelines for Donation after Circulatory Death*, 2nd edn, 2012.

Department of Health website. Available at: ℘ <http://www.dh.gov.uk>

Access 'Publications' for:
• *National Service Framework for Renal Services, Part 1, Dialysis and Transplantation*, 2004
• *National Service Framework for Renal Services, Part 2, Chronic Kidney Disease, Acute Renal Failure and End of Life Care*, 2005
• *Organs for Transplants a Report from the Organ Donation Taskforce*, January 2008
• *The Potential Impact of an Opt-out System for Organ Donation in the UK: an Independent Report from the Organ Donation Taskforce*, November 2008.

Human Tissue Authority (HTA) website. Available at: ℘ <http://www.hta.gov.uk>
• Human Tissue Act (England, Wales and Northern Ireland), 2004
• Human Tissue (Scotland) Act, 2006
• HTA Codes of Practice 1 (Consent) & 2 (Donation of Solid Organs for Transplantation)
• *HTA Guidance for Transplant Teams and Independent Assessors*.

NHS Blood and Transplant (NHSBT) website. Available at: ℘ <http://www.nhsbt.nhs.uk> and <http://www.odt.nhs.uk>

General website and clinical microsite for access to/information about:
• Patient educational resources
• Milestones in transplantation
• Latest statistics and transplant activity
• Research and presentations
• National standards for organ retrieval from deceased donors
• Transplanting centres
• Organ allocation system
• National living donor kidney sharing schemes (NLDKSS)
• Organ donor register
• Organ donor enquiry line-telephone and email
• Links to patient association/charity websites.

UK Donation Ethics Committee (UKDEC). Academy of Medical Royal Colleges website. Available at: ℘ <http://www.aomrc.org.uk/donations-ethics-committee.html>
• *An Ethical Framework for Controlled Donation after Circulatory Death*, 2011.

Transplantation: immunology and immunosuppression

Transplant immunology

Introduction

The immune system provides a unique defence against physiological harm. Through a series of complex mechanisms, it is able to identify between molecules that are 'self' and 'non-self'. The immunological response to a transplanted organ is a significant cause of graft failure in the recipient. Understanding it and why it happens makes it possible to develop strategies to overcome the barriers to successful Tx.

Immune responses are defined as:

- *Humoral*—involving the production of immunoglobulins by plasma cells (antibodies)
- *Cellular*—involving lymphocytes and antigen presenting cells (macrophages and dendritic) throughout the reticuloendothelial system (e.g. lymph nodes, thymus, spleen, bone marrow) which act as 'killer' cells, causing intracellular destruction of foreign cells.
  Transplants fall into one of the following categories:
- *Auto-transplantation*—Tx of 'self' tissue, e.g. if a kidney is removed and re-implanted into the same person
- *Iso-transplantation*—donor and recipient are genetically identical, e.g. identical twins
- *Allo-transplantation*—donor and recipient are genetically different i.e. all donor–recipient combinations except those who are identical twins. This scenario is the most common often and the transplanted organ is referred to as an *allograft*
- *Xeno-transplantation*—donor and recipient are biologically different species, i.e. animal (pig/baboon) to human. Currently only in the research phase and considered a high-risk strategy to address organ shortage due to ↑ potential for rejection and transmission of infection.

In all allograft transplants, the immune system will cause the transplant to reject within days without intervention to suppress the immune response (i.e. 'self' vs 'non-self'). The immunological threat can be assessed by pre-Tx screening and crossmatching (see p. 487), including the risk of immediate (hyperacute) rejection. Understanding the process of rejection helps to manage prevention and IS medication.

What is rejection?

A transplanted organ is rejected because the recipient (host) recognizes that the graft is 'foreign'. This process is driven by the major histocompatibility complex (MHC), which is the system within the immune system that is responsible for antigen recognition. The MHC is individual to both donor and recipient and presents antigens for other immunological cells to screen. Minor histocompatibility systems (miH) are less well identified than the MHC and relatively unimportant in solid organ Tx. However, miH may explain why rejection is seen in HLA identical donor grafts.

Human leucocyte antigens

The antigens relevant to Tx are known as HLAs; protein markers present on cell surfaces that define the immunological identity of a person and have a key role in the immune response. HLAs are biologically inherited and each molecule comprises 2 haplotypes; 1 paternal and 1 maternal. There is an infinite variety of HLAs so the chance of 2 people within the general population being identical is very small (e.g. 1: 50,000 within the Caucasian population) but between blood relatives, there is a 1:4 chance that 2 siblings will have inherited the same haplotypes from their parents. This is important because HLA matching between donor and recipient improves outcomes in DDKT and decreases the potential for sensitization (HLA antibodies) against future transplants. When donor HLA molecules are presented to the recipient's immune system, a reaction is initiated to the 'non-self' HLA, initiating a cascade of immune responses to destroy the 'foreign' tissue.

HLA molecules are divided into 2 classes:

- **Class I** (HLA-A, HLA-B, and HLA-C) are found on plasma membranes of most nucleated cells. They are strongly associated with cellular rejection because they present antigen and are recognized by the T-cell receptor (TCR) on T cells bearing the CD8 protein, which causes lysis of foreign cells
- **Class II** (HLA-DR, HLA-DQ, and HLA-DP) are found on B lymphocytes and dendritic cells (antigen presenting cells). They are strongly associated with humoral rejection because they present antigen and are recognized by the T-cell receptor on T cells bearing the CD4 protein. CD4 cells are referred to as 'helper' cells and have crucial specialized functions in the generation of the immune response (and ∴ graft rejection) such as cytotoxic T-cell generation, B-cell maturation.

To stimulate an immune response, immunological cells rely upon the interaction between HLAs and TCRs and other signals to be fully activated. Co-stimulatory factors (e.g. Il-2, the CD28–B7 and CD40 ligand–CD40 family) are important in helping to choose the most effective IS agents to use in any given situation.

HLA matching and crossmatching

The degree of *mis*match between donor and recipient HLAs is identified prior to Tx using DNA technology and 3 major loci, each of which has 2 antigens. The loci are HLA-A, HLA-B, and HLA-DR and matching for HLA-DR is considered most important. A mismatch of 6 HLA antigens presents a higher immunological threat than a lower mismatch. Mismatching has a greater impact in DDKT than in LDKT. Pre-Tx immunological crossmatching reduces the risk of hyperacute rejection—identifying pre-formed donor-reactive HLA antibodies in the recipient. This is particularly important for 'sensitized' patients (i.e. through blood transfusion, pregnancy, or previous Tx). In DDKT, crossmatching is performed immediately prior to Tx, once a recipient has been identified for the donated organ. LDKT allows for earlier crossmatching; during the donor–recipient assessment, but the crossmatch will always be repeated within 1–2wks of surgery to ensure that nothing has changed. Crossmatching is performed by mixing donor lymphocytes (from the spleen or lymph node in DD and peripheral blood in LD) with recipient serum (WBCs). Flow cytometry (FACS) is the most common technique.

Nursing note

Regular screening for HLA-antibody is an essential part of pre-transplant preparation to:
- Assess immunological risk in all transplants
- Register unacceptable antigens with NHSBT for DD allocation.

For all patients on the NTL and/or being prepared for LDKT, regular samples must be sent to the histocompatibility (H&I) laboratory.
- Monthly for patients who are active on the list
- Approximately 10 days after an intercurrent illness (e.g. infection, PD peritonitis) ± blood transfusion to screen for possible antibody activity by stimulation of the immune system.

See 📖 p. 509, Further reading.

Immunosuppression

To prevent rejection of the transplanted organ the recipient is required to take IS medications. These can be split into 3 levels:
• Induction IS
• Maintenance IS
• Treatment of acute rejection.

⚠ Patients receiving IS therapy are at ↑ risk of developing malignancies, notably skin cancers and uterine cervical cancer. Exposure to sunlight and UV light should be limited and patients should wear protective clothing and use a sunscreen with a high protection factor.

⚠ Special considerations may apply when administering and monitoring IS to clinically complex recipients, e.g. FSGS, HIV recipients on HAART, recipients of AiT transplants. Always refer to the individual transplant plan for IS regimen and dose adjustments (see 📖 p. 457).

Induction immunosuppression

This is given perioperatively or relatively close to surgery.

Interleukin 2 receptor blocker

Basiliximab

Indication: prophylaxis of acute organ rejection in allogeneic renal transplant recipients in combination with other agents.

Adult dose
- IV: 2 doses; 1 given within 2hrs prior to transplant surgery and another dose 4 days after surgery. This is given by bolus IV injection or diluted to a volume of 50ml or greater with normal saline or glucose 5% and given as an IV infusion over 20–30mins.

▶ Basiliximab must not be administered unless it is absolutely certain that the patient will receive the graft and concomitant IS. The 2nd dose should be withheld if severe hypersensitivity or graft loss occurs.

Mode of action and background
- Basiliximab is a monoclonal antibody that prevents T-lymphocyte proliferation.

Examples of adverse effects
- Severe hypersensitivity reactions and cytokine release syndrome have been reported.

Monitoring
- Monitor for hypersensitivity type reactions, e.g. urticaria, pruritus, sneezing, hypotension, tachycardia, dyspnoea, bronchospasm, pulmonary oedema, and respiratory failure.

Polyclonal antibody

Rabbit anti-human thymocyte immunoglobulin (ATG)

Indication: licensed for the:
- Prophylaxis of organ rejection in allogeneic renal transplant recipients
- Treatment of corticosteroid-resistant allograft rejection in renal Tx.

Adult dose
- IV: Tx, 1–1.5mg/kg by IV infusion through a 0.22µm in-line filter over at least 6hrs once a day for 3–9 days.
- Corticosteroid-resistant renal graft rejection: 1.5 mg/kg by IV through a 0.22µm in-line filter, over at least 6hrs once a day for 7–14 days

It should be administered through a high-flow vein but, if administered through a peripheral vein, it is recommended that concomitant heparin and hydrocortisone in an infusion solution of 0.9% sodium chloride may ↓ the potential for:
- Superficial thrombophlebitis
- DVT.

▶ To avoid excessive dosage in obese patients the dose should be calculated using ideal body weight.

Mode of action and background
- ATG is a polyclonal antibody that depletes mainly T cells.

Examples of adverse effects
- Cytokine release syndrome and anaphylaxis
- Fever
- Shivering
- ↑ susceptibility to infection
- Neutropenia
- Thrombocytopenia
- Myalgia
- Pruritus.

Monitoring
- Tolerability is ↑ by pre-treatment with an IV corticosteroid and antihistamine; an antipyretic drug such as paracetamol may also be beneficial Some units advocate daily CD3 counts to monitor treatment and use this to determine whether the next dose is administered.

Maintenance immunosuppression

Maintenance therapy is given for the life of the transplanted organ and often consists of a combination of 2–3 medications, including:
- A CNI
- An antimetabolite
- A corticosteroid.

These are given in as low a dose as possible to ↓ the side effects and are weaned to a stable dose after 6–12 months. There is no universally accepted 'optimal' regimen so each centre uses a locally agreed protocol.

Calcineurin inhibitors

Tacrolimus (FK506)

Indication: prophylaxis and treatment of organ rejection in allogeneic renal transplant recipients.

Adult dose

Initially based on weight then adjusted according to blood trough levels.
- *Oral:* 0.1–0.2mg/kg/day in 1–2 divided doses (depending on preparation). Consult local protocols.
- *IV:* ⚠ the IV dose of tacrolimus is *one fifth of the total 24hr oral dose* and is given as a continuous infusion over 24 hrs.

This infusion should be prepared by diluting the volume of concentrate required for the total 24hr dose to 48ml using sodium chloride 0.9% or glucose 5% and administered at a rate of 2ml/hr. IV administration should be reserved for patients unable to tolerate oral administration. It should be discontinued as soon as oral therapy is tolerated because trough levels cannot be monitored and interpreting treatment during IV therapy is problematic.

Mode of action and background

- Blockade of calcineurin mediated T-cell receptor signal transduction and inhibition of interleukin 2 transcription
- By inhibiting cytokine gene transcription they suppress T-cell and T-cell-dependent B-cell activation.
- Primarily metabolized by the liver by cytochrome p450 3a4
- ⚠ Levels are affected by drugs that induce or inhibit this enzyme, e.g. diltiazem, erythromycin
- Plasma exchange should *not* affect tacrolimus levels as the erythrocytes release tacrolimus and re-equilibration achieved
- Tacrolimus is not removed to any appreciable extent by haemodialysis.

Examples of adverse effects

- Many are dose dependent and responsive to dose reduction
- Nephrotoxicity
- ↑ risk of infection
- Hyperglycaemia and diabetes (occurs in up to 20% of patients)
- Neurotoxicity
- Tremor
- Hyperkalaemia and hypomagnesaemia
- Hypertension
- Nausea, diarrhoea, and headache
- Hirsutism appears to be less of a problem than with ciclosporin.

Monitoring

- Trough blood levels should be monitored and patients must wait until after blood samples have been taken before swallowing their oral dose
- The maximum level occurs around 2–3hrs following oral administration. Spurious levels may occur if blood is sampled soon after the patient has swallowed their oral dose

- Following a dosage change, 3 days should elapse before further alterations in dosage are made or levels measured to allow pharmacokinetic steady state to be attained.
- Switching between different brands and formulations requires careful therapeutic monitoring and substitution should be made only under the close supervision of a transplant specialist. Prescribing and dispensing should be by brand name to avoid inadvertent switching
- △ Care with drug interactions, e.g. clarithromycin, diltiazem, phenytoin, HAART. Consult pharmacist
- △ Food can affect absorption so patients are advised to consistently take it either with or without food
- △ Grapefruit juice should be avoided as this can affect the kinetics of tacrolimus
- Afro-Caribbean patients may require higher doses.

Ciclosporin

Indication: prophylaxis of acute organ rejection in allogeneic renal transplant recipients in combination with other agents.

Adult dose
Initially based on weight then adjusted according to blood trough levels.
- *Oral*: 8–15mg per kg in 2 divided doses. See local protocols.
- *IV*: △ The IV dose is **one third of the recommended oral dose**. This should be diluted 1:20 to 1:100 with normal saline or 5% glucose before use and given by slow IV infusion over 2–6hrs. Reserved for patients who are unable to take it orally (e.g. shortly after surgery) or in whom the absorption of the oral forms might be impaired. Patients should be transferred to oral therapy as soon as possible.

Mode of action and background
- Blockade of calcineurin mediated T-cell receptor signal transduction and inhibition of interleukin 2 transcription
- By inhibiting cytokine gene transcription they suppress T-cell and T-cell-dependent B-cell activation
- Primarily metabolized by the liver by cytochrome p450 3a4
- △ Levels are affected by drugs that induce or inhibit this enzyme, e.g. diltiazem, erythromycin.

Examples of adverse effects
Many are dose-dependent and responsive to dose ↓:
- Nephrotoxicity
- ↑ risk of infection
- Tremor
- Gingival hyperplasia
- Hyperkalaemia and hypomagnesaemia
- Hypertension
- Nausea, diarrhoea, and headache
- Hepatic dysfunction
- Myalgia
- Hirsutism.

Monitoring
- Trough blood levels should be monitored and patients must wait until after blood samples have been taken before swallowing their oral dose
- After commencing or changing a dose of ciclosporin, wait 3 days before measuring levels
- Switching between different brands and formulations requires careful therapeutic monitoring and substitution should be made only under the close supervision of a transplant specialist. Prescribing and dispensing should be by brand name to avoid inadvertent switching
- ⚠ Care with drug interactions, e.g. clarithromycin, diltiazem, phenytoin, HAART. Consult pharmacist
- ⚠ Grapefruit juice should be avoided as this can affect the kinetics of ciclosporin
- Afro-Caribbean patients may require higher doses.

Corticosteroids

Prednisolone

Indication: prophylaxis of acute organ rejection in allogeneic renal transplant recipients in combination with other agents.

Adult dose
- *Oral*: initially 15–30mg daily (according to patient weight) ↓ to a lower maintenance dose over a few weeks and months. See local protocols.
- *IV*: if patients stabilized on prednisolone are unable to take oral medication, they should be converted to IV hydrocortisone (dose equivalent is 4:1 hydrocortisone:prednisolone). Patients on corticosteroids for >2 months will require a bolus of hydrocortisone if 'stressed' by an acute illness, operation, etc.

Mode of action and background
- Act as powerful anti-inflammatories
- Inhibit interleukin 1
- Prevent proliferation of t lymphocyte
- Alters lymphocyte response to antigen at an intracellular level.

Examples of adverse effects
- ↑ risk of infection
- Hypertension
- Na^+ and H_2O retention
- Diabetes
- Osteoporosis
- ↑ appetite
- Cushingoid face ± truncal obesity
- Skin thinning
- Bruising
- Acne
- Poor wound healing
- Cataracts
- Depression
- Psychosis
- Osteoporosis
- Peptic ulceration.

Monitoring
- Monitor for side effects including bone marrow density scans after 6–12 months of treatment
- ⚠ Patients should carry a steroid card
- ⚠ Patients should avoid people with chickenpox or shingles and tell a doctor if they come in contact with people with these conditions. Pre-transplant screening for VZV immunity ± vaccination is advised (see 📖 p. 456, Recipient pre-transplant assessment and preparation).

Antimetabolites

Azatioprine

Indication: prophylaxis of acute organ rejection in allogeneic renal transplant recipients in combination with other agents.

Adult dose
- *Oral*: 1–2mg per kg once a day to a maximum of 150mg. The dose needs to be rounded to the nearest tablet strength (available as 25mg and 50mg tablets)
- *IV*: the IV formulation may be assumed to be dose equivalent to the oral formulation. Azathioprine solution is very alkaline and irritant, and should therefore be given slowly.

⚠ The IV preparation should be made in a cytotoxic unit.

Mode of action and background
- Azathioprine is an imidazole derivative of 6-mercaptopurine (6-MP)
- 6-MP readily crosses cell membranes and is converted into thioguanine nucleotides, which interfere with RNA and DNA synthesis.
  This prevents mitosis and the proliferation of activated T and B lymphocytes
- Thiopurine methyltransferase (TPMT) catalyses the metabolism of thioguanine nucleotides to inactive metabolites.

Examples of adverse effects
- ↑ risk of infection
- Neutropenia
- Occasionally, cholestasis and deterioration of liver function:
  - usually reversible on withdrawal of therapy rare, but life-threatening hepatic damage associated with chronic administration of azathioprine has been described in transplant patients
  - in some cases, withdrawal of azathioprine has resulted in either a temporary or permanent improvement in liver histology and symptoms.

Monitoring
- Regular monitoring for neutropenia. If neutropenia develops it may be appropriate to interrupt or discontinue treatment
- ⚠ Azathioprine is a cytotoxic drug, so it should be handled with caution. The manufacturer of azathioprine advises that as long as the film-coating of the tablet is intact, there is no risk in handling film-coated azathioprine tablets. The injection should be prepared by a cytotoxic unit
- Individuals with an inherited deficiency of the enzyme TPMT may be unusually sensitive to the myelosuppressive effect of azathioprine and prone to developing rapid bone marrow depression following the initiation of treatment. Some units measure TPMT levels prior to starting treatment.
- ▶ Patients should be instructed to report immediately any evidence of infection, unexpected bruising or bleeding or other manifestations of bone marrow depression.

- △ Allopurinol inhibits the breakdown of azathioprine so the dose of azathioprine should be ↓ to 25% of the original dose. Even when the dose of azathioprine is ↓ to 25% of the original dose, concomitant use of allopurinol and azathioprine still carries a significant risk of pancytopenia so the combination is very rarely used.

Mycophenolate/mycophenolic acid

Indication: prophylaxis of acute organ rejection in allogeneic renal transplant recipients in combination with other agents.

Adult dose
- *Oral* : up to 2g in 2–4 divided doses depending on preparation
- *IV:* the IV and oral doses are equivalent. Since the oral bioavailability of mycophenolate mofetil is 94%, IV administration should be reserved for patients unable to tolerate oral administration and should be discontinued as soon as oral therapy can be given.

Mode of action and background
- Mycophenolate mofetil is metabolized to the active compound mycophenolic acid (MPA)
- MPA inhibits guanosine nucleotide synthesis which is required for T- and B-lymphocyte synthesis.

Adverse effects
- ↑ risk of infection
- Cases of GI ulceration and haemorrhage have been reported
- Diarrhoea and vomiting
- Neutropenia
- The gastric side effects can be managed by dividing the daily dose into 4 separate doses.

Monitoring
- MPA serum levels are not routinely measured
- Regular monitoring for neutropenia. If neutropenia develops it may be appropriate to interrupt or discontinue treatment
- △Ciclosporin reduces the MPA AUC by about 30%. This is not seen with tacrolimus or sirolimus so patients on regimens that include these drugs may be more susceptible to mycophenolate toxicity. If this is suspected a dose reduction may be considered
- △ Drugs that undergo renal tubular secretion such as acyclovir, ganciclovir, valaciclovir, and probenecid may compete with mycophenolate resulting in ↑ concentrations of both drugs. Patients should be monitored closely
- △ Antacids, colestyramine, and sevelamer reduce the absorption of mycophenolate and their concomitant use should be with caution
- NICE states that mycophenolate should only be used where there is proven intolerance to CNIs or where there is a ↑ risk of nephrotoxicity requiring ↓ CNIs.

Inhibitors of mammalian target of rapamycin (mTOR)

Sirolimus

Indication: non-calcineurin inhibiting IS licensed for prophylaxis of acute organ rejection in allogeneic renal transplant recipients (licensed initially in combination with ciclosporin and corticosteroid, then with corticosteroid only but other regimes are used).

Adult dose
- *Oral:* initially 6mg, after surgery, then 2mg once daily (dose adjusted according to blood sirolimus concentration aiming for a trough level of 4–12 nanograms/ml) in combination with ciclosporin and corticosteroids. Ciclosporin should then be withdrawn over 4–8wks
- *IV:* not available.

Mode of action and background
- Sirolimus is a macrolide antibiotic with IS activity
- Blocks cytokine-driven proliferation of T cells, B cells, and smooth muscle
- Inhibits T-cell activation induced by most stimuli by blocking calcium-dependent and calcium-independent intracellular signal transduction
- Bioavailability = 14% (AUC may be ↑ by up to 35% if taken with a high fat meal)—hence, it is recommended that sirolimus be taken consistently either with or without food
- Should be taken 4hrs after the ciclosporin dose
- ⚠ Due to impact on healing, it is often not treatment of choice immediately post Tx.

Examples of adverse effects
Many are dose dependent and responsive to dose ↓:
- ↑ risk of infection
- Hyperlipidaemia
- Pneumonitis
- Stomatitis
- Haemolytic uraemic syndrome
- Anaemia
- Thrombocytopenia
- Leucopenia, neutropenia, hypokalaemia
- Hypophosphataemia
- Lymphocele
- Acne
- Rash
- Impaired healing.

Monitoring
- Trough blood levels should be monitored and patients must wait until after blood samples have been taken before swallowing their oral dose
- Sirolimus takes 5–7 days to achieve steady state. To measure steady state sirolimus levels, these need to be taken at least 7 days after commencing/changing the dose
- When changing between oral solution and tablets, measurement of serum trough sirolimus concentration after 1–2wks is recommended
- Afro-Caribbean patients may require higher doses
- ⚠ Sirolimus is extensively metabolized by the CYP3A4 isozyme in the intestinal wall and liver so care should be taken with drugs that are also metabolized by these enzymes, e.g. erythromycin, diltiazem.

Treatment of acute rejection

Additional drugs

During episodes of acute rejection, patients are treated with higher doses of immunosuppressants e.g. 500mg IV methylprednisolone once a day for 3 days. The choice of treatment will depend upon the type of rejection (📖 pp. 486–8).

Anti-infectives

Patients receiving IS have an ↑ risk of bacterial, viral, fungal, and parasitic disease and are prone to opportunistic infections. It is ∴ important that, if transplant patients are thought to be septic, they are treated promptly with sufficient doses. Many units use prophylactic antibiotics, antifungals, and antivirals to prevent infection particularly in the immediate post-transplant period.

Pneumocystis pneumonia (PCP)

A long course (often 6 months) of co-trimoxazole is given to prevent PCP to provide prophylaxis during initial maintenance therapy while IS burden is high.

Bacterial urinary tract infections

These are common and trimethoprim as part of co-trimoxazole (see as for PCP) is often used for prophylaxis.

Oral candidiasis

Oral courses of antifungals (e.g. nystatin mouthwash, or amphotericin lozenges) are given to prevent oral candidiasis. Fluconazole is usually reserved for treatment of systemic infection due to its interaction with CNIs.

Tuberculosis

Reactivation of latent TB is a risk, particularly in communities where the infection is prevalent. Patients with a previous PMH of TB or thought to be at risk of infection will be prescribed isoniazid, along with pyridoxine to prevent peripheral neuropathy associated with isoniazid therapy.

Cytomegalovirus

CMV is an opportunistic infection that can cause life-threatening illness in immunocompromised patients. The symptoms include:
• Flu-like symptoms
• Pneumonitis
• Retinitis
• Deranged LFTs.
  Patients who are particularly susceptible are:
• CMV –ve patients who receive a CMV +ve transplant
• Patients who have received an ↑ IS load.

Valganciclovir is used to prevent and treat infection. It is renally excreted so the dose needs to be altered according to renal function.

BK virus (BKV)
BK virus only causes disease in immunocompromised patients. The symptoms include haematuria and cystitis. BKV infection is directly associated with the IS load so treatment is usually to ↓ IS therapy.

Gastroprotective agents
If not already prescribed, H2 receptor blockers (e.g. ranitidine) or PPIs (e.g. omeprazole) are usually given initially post transplant to prevent gastritis associated with corticosteroids and mycophenolate.

Antihypertensives
These are often stopped immediately post transplant and reintroduced according to the patient's blood pressure (BP). ACEIs are usually avoided initially due to the risks of RAS.

Other drugs
Post transplant, if the kidney is functioning well many drugs (e.g. phosphate binders, epoetin, iron therapy vitamin D derivatives) used during dialysis and renal failure can be stopped. However these drugs may need to be recommenced if renal function subsequently ↓.

Novel agents
Alemtuzumab
- An anti-CD52 monoclonal antibody, licensed for the treatment of B-cell chronic lymphocytic leukaemia. CD52 is present on mature lymphocytes
- Produces rapid and profound depletion of lymphocytes providing long-lasting IS
- IV administration; used in research protocols as induction therapy in steroid and/or CNI avoidance protocols with promising results in low immunological risk renal transplant recipients. More research needed in high-risk renal transplant candidates
- The optimum dose and regime has yet to be determined

Examples of adverse effects
- Cytokine release syndrome and anaphylaxis
- Serum sickness
- Fever
- Shivering
- ↑ susceptibility to infection, malignancy, neutropenia, thrombocytopenia, myalgia, pruritus, and rash.

The tolerability is ↑ by pre-treatment with an IV corticosteroid and antihistamine; an antipyretic drug, e.g. paracetamol, may also be beneficial.

Belatacept
- Blocks CD28 co-stimulation which is required for full activation of T cells
- Only available as an IV preparation; administered every 4–8wks as maintenance therapy
- In trials it is used as part of CNI-free regimens with the aim to preserve GFR. If outcomes are good, the challenge will be to provide regular IV administration following Tx.

Rituximab
- Directed against anti CD3 antigen, which is found on the surface of B lymphocytes and inhibits their proliferation
- Long duration of action
- Shown to assist in overcoming positive cross matches in planned LDKT in conjunction with PEX. It has also been used in the treatment of rejection.

Intravenous immunoglobulin (IVIG)
- Used as part of transplant work-up for LDKT patients with a +ve crossmatch
- Also used to treat rejection post transplant as IVIG has significant immunomodulatory properties.

Drug treatment during pregnancy

All ♀ planning pregnancy should be advised to seek expert opinion regarding their medications. Key points:
- Levels of IS drugs should be maintained at pre-pregnancy levels
- Both tacrolimus and ciclosporin are relatively safe in pregnancy
- Ciclosporin dosage ↑ may be needed to maintain stable levels due to the ↑ effects of oestrogen and ↑ volume of distribution in pregnancy
- Corticosteroids cross the placental barrier but analysis of mothers exposed to steroids indicates a fetal malformation rate similar to the general population
- Mycophenolate and rapamycin are not recommended
- Antibody induction/rejection therapy can cross the placental barrier but are rarely used: pregnancy is not advocated until at least 18 months following Tx when acute rejection is uncommon.

Adherence to medications

The transplanted patient is committed to take IS medication for the life-time of the transplant to prevent loss or damage from rejection (see 🔲 pp. 486–8, Transplant immunology). Taking the prescribed dose at the prescribed time is essential for:
• Maintaining transplant function
• Monitoring safety and efficacy of IS regimens, e.g. CNIs, azathioprine, mTORs
• Dose adjustment of IS.

Incidence

Failure to adhere to a prescribed IS regimen varies from 5–43% and there are a variety of definitions. The majority of patients are non-adherent because of side effects (see 🔲 p. 492, Maintenance immunosuppression). Adherence declines over time, with greater compliance in the early years post trans-plant. Non-adherence causes late rejection in ~20% of transplants and graft loss in ~16%. Poly pharmacy, often prescribed to reduce and protect against unwanted side effects of IS, adds to the daily pill burden. Non-adherence may be intentional or unintentional and is influenced by:
• Frequency of dosing
• Multiple tablets per dose
• Complexity of IS regimen
• Organizational skills, e.g. storage of tablets, renewing prescriptions
• Polypharmacy
• Difficulty swallowing tablets
• Communication barriers, e.g. literacy, language, loss of sight/hearing
• Lifestyle and life events.

Management

Prevention is better than cure but predicting non-adherence is difficult. Cues in the pre-transplant assessment period may include:
• Signs of previous non-compliance, e.g. with dialysis/other treatments
• Attendance at appointments
• Age, e.g. children, adolescents, elderly (see 🔲 pp. 538–9, 548–50).

Education and support

Specialist nurses play a key role throughout the transplant process, from pre-assessment and preparation through to long-term follow-up, in devel-oping educational strategies and supporting patients to be adherent to their medications (see 🔲 pp. 604–7, Appendix 4). Educational strategies should include:
• Consistent, comprehensive information delivered in a variety of formats, e.g. bespoke education sessions/packages, one-to-one discussions, written information, DVDs, interactive IT learning packages
• Resources that address language and other communication barriers, e.g. visual aids, materials in braille
• Involvement of the MPT, e.g. pharmacists, counsellors, nurses, doctors

- An ongoing process, initiated in the pre-transplant preparation phase and continuing throughout the transplant process
- Instruction on self-administration and coping strategies
- Involvement of family members/loved ones
- Peer support/befriending programmes, i.e. patients supporting patients.

Post-transplantation surveillance

Long-term follow-up of transplant recipients is essential. Nurses are uniquely placed to provide continuity of care for patients from community to hospital-based care. Patients are more likely to confide in someone with whom they have a rapport when they are not coping with their medicines. Direct and indirect non-adherence may be detected by:
- Patterns of behaviour, e.g. non-attendance at clinic appointments
- Blood tests, e.g. ↑ creatinine, subtherapeutic drug levels
- Clinical signs and symptoms of rejection (see 📖 pp. 472–3, Late complications and long-term follow-up)
- Discussion with patient, e.g. medicine taking history
- 'Pill count'
- Audit tools, e.g. self-assessment questionnaire
- Microelectronic monitoring on pill bottles with patient consent.

Supportive strategies

Best practice suggests that patients who are unintentionally non-adherent due to forgetfulness or disorganization can be helped by:
- Therapeutic relationships within the healthcare team
- Regular clinic visits in a supportive environment
- ↓ the number of medications, frequency of dosing, and timing of dosing
- Once daily/same time of day dosing
- Alternative preparations, e.g. liquids, if swallowing is difficult
- Dosette boxes, labelled with days of the week
- Automatic reminders/prompts, e.g. setting an alarm, mobile text messaging, 'post-it notes'
- Microelectronic monitoring on pill bottles with patient consent.

For patients who intentionally avoid taking their medicines, it is important to establish the cause and tailor support accordingly, i.e.:
- Understanding the most vulnerable groups, e.g. age groups
- Early identification of non-compliant behaviour, e.g. pre-Tx
- Referral to a clinical psychologist
- Motivational interviewing to overcome barriers to non-adherence
- Peer support.

Specialist nurses play a pivotal role in supporting adherence to IS and medications by:
- Engaging with patients and their families
- Continuity of care throughout the transplant process
- Ongoing education and support
- Transplant monitoring and surveillance
- MPT liaison
- Facilitating peer support.

See 📖 p. 509, Further reading.

What next in transplantation?

Tx is a rapidly developing area of clinical practice. What might the future look like? Key areas of development are likely to be:

Expansion of the donor pool

- ↑ in DD activity by 50–60% by 2013 from ODTF initiatives
- NHSBT Strategy for LDKT (launched January 2012) aims to ↑ LDKT activity in line with the best international benchmarks with a focus on donor safety, pre-emptive LDKT, and further development of the NLDKSS
- Xeno-transplantation is unlikely to make a meaningful contribution to expanding the donor pool due to the risks of cross-species transmission of infection (see 📖 pp. 486–8, Transplant immunology).

Surgical techniques

- Minimally invasive recipient transplant surgery (i.e. laparoscopic) to ↓ co-morbidity and improve surgical outcomes.

Immunosuppression

- Development of new agents; 'designer' IS with less toxicity for patient and graft; will help to ↑ adherence and optimize patient and transplant survival.

Antibody depletion

- New agents and techniques for pre-conditioning 'highly-sensitized' potential recipients of incompatible transplants to extend the benefits AiT to more of the most difficult to transplant patients
- Clinical research involving 'domino' left-lobe liver Tx with DDKT to absorb HLA antibody in 'highly-sensitized' adult recipients. The recipient receives a left lobe from the DD and donates his/her left lobe to a suitable child on the NTL. A few hours later, allowing time for recipient HLA antibody to be absorbed by the newly transplanted left liver lobe, the kidney from the same DD is implanted into the adult recipient. In the absence of a LD option, this may offer an opportunity for selected highly HLA sensitized recipients to be transplanted.

Pancreatic transplantation

- Clinical research into the use of mesenchymal stem cells to stimulate/ co-stimulate the production of insulin-secreting pancreatic islet cells may ↑ the efficacy of islet Tx for diabetic recipients.

See 📖 p. 509, Further reading.

Further reading

Danovitch GM (ed). *Handbook of Kidney Transplantation*, 5th edn. Philadelphia, PA: Lippincott Williams & Wilkins; 2010.

National Institute for Health and Clinical Excellence (NICE). *Renal Transplantation—Immunosuppressive regimens (adults)*. London: NICE; 2004. Available at: ℘ <http://www.guidance.nice.org.uk>

Ohler L, Cupples S, International Transplant Nurses Society (eds). *Core Curriculum for Transplant Nurses*. St Louis, MO: Mosby Elsevier; 2008.

Steddon S, Ashman N, Chesser A, *et al.* (eds). *Oxford Handbook of Nephrology and Hypertension*. Oxford: Oxford University Press; 2006.

Torpey N, Moghal NE, Watson E, *et al.* (eds). *Oxford Handbook of Renal Transplantation*. Oxford: Oxford University Press; 2010.

Useful websites

British Transplantation Society (BTS) website. Available at: ℘ <http://www.bts.org.uk>
Access 'Active Standards and Guidelines' for:

- NHSBT/BTS: *Guidelines for Consent to Solid Organ Transplantation in Adults*, March 2011
- BTS/RA: *UK Guidelines for Living Donor Kidney Transplantation*, 3rd edn, May 2011
- BTS: *Antibody Incompatible Guidelines*, 2nd edn, January 2011
- Renal Association (RA): *Guidelines for Assessment for Renal Transplantation*, 4th edn, 2008
- BTS/ICS: *Consensus Guidelines on Organ Donation after Circulatory Death*, December 2010
- BTS: *Guidelines for Donation after Circulatory Death*, 2nd edn, 2012.

NHS Blood and Transplant (NHSBT) website. Available at: ℘ <http://www.nhsbt.nhs.uk> and <http://www.odt.nhs.uk>

General website and clinical microsite for access to/information about:

- Patient educational resources
- Milestones in transplantation
- Latest statistics and transplant activity
- Research and presentations
- National standards for organ retrieval from deceased donors
- Transplanting centres
- Organ allocation system
- National living donor kidney sharing schemes (NLDKSS)
- Organ donor register
- Organ donor enquiry line-telephone and email
- Links to patient association/charity websites.

End of life care in advanced kidney disease

Conservative care

- People with advanced kidney disease (stage 5 CKD) are required to make informed decisions regarding available treatment options:
  - dialysis: HD/PD
  - transplantation (if suitable)
  - maximum conservative management without RRT
- Patients should have access to education and information programmes to enable them to make an informed choice about their treatment
- Reasons why people do not have RRT include:
  - unsuitability due to multiple co-morbidities
  - poor prognosis with dialysis linked to medical condition, i.e. severe HF
  - patient choice
- Dialysis offers no survival benefit to those aged >75yrs with >2 co-morbidities i.e. diabetes, IHD, PVD
- It is important to explain to patients and family that a non-RRT decision is not a non-treatment option
- The aim of conservative care is to relieve the symptoms of CKD where possible and maximize the person's health and QOL for the remainder of their life.

Terminology

- *End of life (EOL) care in advanced kidney disease*—EOL care for people with advanced kidney disease irrespective of treatment modality
- *Conservative kidney management*—full supportive treatment for those with advanced kidney disease, who, in conjunction with carers and clinical team, decide against dialysis
- *Deteriorating despite dialysis*—persons who are struggling to cope with dialysis often with multiple co-morbidities, frailty, and increasing dependency
- *Dialysis withdrawal*—cessation of dialysis treatment. Evident need for EOL care; decision made by patient in conjunction with carers and clinical team. This may sometimes be a clinical decision due to the inability to sustain dialysis
- *Palliative dialysis*—dialysis to align with supportive needs of a person deteriorating despite dialysis. Mainly aimed at preventing and treating symptoms such as fluid overload. Reduced duration and frequency of sessions
- *Preferred priority of care*—preferences and wishes for EOL care including preferred place of death.

Conservative kidney management

- Patients who chose not to have RRT
- Receive all other aspects of kidney care, e.g. anaemia/MBD management
- Pathway commences at the time dialysis would have started.

▶ Once a decision not to have dialysis is made, a plan of care needs to be established.

Care planning

Those approaching EOL care should have their needs assessed, wishes and preferences discussed, and an agreed plan of care documented.

Some people may wish to make an advanced decision to refuse treatment, should they lack mental capacity to make such a decision in the future. Others may want to share their wishes and preferences about how they are cared for and where they wish to die. This should be documented in a patient-held care plan and copies sent to relevant health care professionals involved in their care. The care plan should include:

- Details of a nominated key worker
- Record of preferences and choices they wish to make
- Resuscitation wishes
- Record of ongoing assessments
- Identification of supportive care needs
- Outcomes of MPT meetings
- Communication between 1° and 2° care
- Information for out-of-hrs and emergency/urgent care services.

Advanced directives

- Legal documents with powers and requirements that vary widely with jurisdictions
- Advanced directives mainly fall into 2 categories:
  - instructional, i.e. living will
  - proxy (power of attorney for healthcare)
- Instructional directives specify patients medical care preferences while proxy directives appoint a surrogate decision-maker
- Advanced directives do not necessarily ensure the clinical circumstances, prognosis, patient's values, and goals are discussed
- An advanced care plan involves ongoing discussions, to clarify values and treatment preferences for EOL care and is not the same as an advanced directive.

Key aspects of advance care planning

- Enhance patient and family understanding about illness and EOL issues including prognosis
- Define patient's key priorities in EOL care and develop a care plan to reflect these:
  - respect patient's autonomy and shape future care plans to fit their preferences and needs
  - review patient and family satisfaction with decision-making
  - help patients to achieve sense of spiritual peace
  - ease emotional and financial burdens borne by families and patients
  - strengthen relationships with loved ones.

Co-ordinating care

Co-ordination of care across 1° and 2° care will facilitate high-quality EOL care. Key measures should include:

- Supportive care register for patients in kidney units, i.e. those who require added assistance with care and/or have EOL care needs

- Link patients identified as requiring supportive care with GP palliative care register
- Key worker within renal, palliative care, and community services, each having identified responsibilities for specific aspects of care
- Use of advanced care plans, e.g. preferred priorities of care
- IT links between the different sectors of care
- Identified clinical leads (nursing and medical) for EOL care in kidney units
- Identified member of local palliative care team as lead for EOL care in advanced kidney disease
- Generic EOL care leads in commissioning, 1° care, and community care
- Local group to oversee development and implementation of EOL care in advanced kidney disease.

Conservative care

- Patients should be able to access relevant members of the MPT team which should be led by a nephrologist or specialist nurse. Dietetic, anaemia, social work, psychological, and spiritual care should also be provided
- Integration with 1° care and specialist palliative care is essential
- Care should be delivered as close to home as possible and unnecessary hospital visits should be avoided
- Nephrology services may have designated MPT who oversee the care of these patients and consist of:
  - nephrologist
  - renal nurses
  - specialist palliative care nurses
  - dietitians
  - social worker
  - counsellor/psychologist
  - occupational therapist
  - community hospice nurses
  - dedicated renal palliative nurses.
▶ Not all teams will have dedicated renal palliative nurses

- Communication is key between all agencies involved and the patient should possess a record of their decision not to have dialysis:
  - a patient-held record can prevent unnecessary interventions and admissions if seen by an unfamiliar medical team out of hrs
  - a 'not for cardiopulmonary resuscitation' (CPR) order should be in place in both 1° and 2° care if this is the patient's wish/medical decision.

End of life care

It is important to recognize that the patient has EOL needs and support mechanisms are put in place in a timely manner. The key focus of EOL includes all aspects of the conservative model of care plus:

- Symptom relief
- Preparation for death—place of care
- Care and support after death for families and carers.

Liverpool Care Pathway (LCP)

The LCP is an integrated care pathway for the care of those in the last days/hrs of life. Emphasis is on symptom control, communication, and spiritual/religious needs. Regular reviews are carried out frequently. The LCP has been adapted for use in hospital, hospice, home, and care homes. Modifications have been made so it can be applied to those with advanced kidney disease, with treatment algorithms for pain control, dyspnoea, agitation, respiratory tract secretions, nausea, and vomiting.

Symptom control

Symptom control

The most common symptoms, associated causes, and recommended treatments can be seen in Table 16.1.

Many symptoms may not be recognized as often the focus is on the management of the disease itself rather than the symptoms which may be related to co-morbid factors and not the kidney disease. To aid the identification of symptoms, specific symptom questionnaires such as the Dialysis Symptom Index (DSI) and a modified version of the Patient Outcome Scale-symptom (POS-s) module can be used These can be given to patients prior to clinic or home visits and used to focus the consultation on the management of those symptoms which include:

• Pain
• SOB
• Weakness/lack of energy
• Nausea
• Vomiting
• Poor appetite
• Constipation
• Mouth problems
• Drowsiness
• Poor mobility
• Pruritus
• Difficulty in sleeping
• Restless leg syndrome
• Feeling anxious
• Changes in skin
• Diarrhoea.

These symptoms are measured on a scale from not at all to overwhelming. Regular assessment of symptoms should take place rather than waiting for the patient to report a symptom which may result in crisis management.

⚠ Caution should be taken when prescribing medication for those with ↓ eGFR and consideration of excretion of drugs and build-up of metabolites is required. See 📖 p. 569.

The underlying cause of each symptom should be considered:
• Ischaemic pain from PVD
• Neuropathic pain from polyneuropathy (diabetes)
• Bone pain from osteoporosis
• Specific pain related to kidney disease, i.e. bone pain, cyst pain from polycystic kidney disease.

Table 16.1 Symptom control

Symptom	Cause	Treatment (World Health Organization analgesic ladder)
Pain	Co-morbid factors, e.g. diabetic nephropathy, bone calciphylaxis, neuropathy	Stage 1: paracetamol Stage 2: mild to moderate pain: opioids (tramadol at ↓ doses). ► Avoid codeine and dihydrocodeine Stage 3 & 4: moderate to severe pain: morphine/diamorphine in ↓ doses and ↑ intervals. ► Monitor as accumulates and causes toxicity Stage 5: fentanyl/alfentanil
Nausea Vomiting	Gastropareisis, ↓ gastric motility, uraemia	↓ dose metoclopromide depending on eGFR* Haloperidol 0.5–1.5mcg SC Levomepromazine 6.25mcg Ondansetron Omeprazole/lansoprazole
Pruritus	↑ Ca^{2+}, PO_4 Mg^{2+}, PTH levels (hyperparathyroidism)	Antihistamines Topical creams for localized itching, e.g. capsaicin Phosphate binders One alfacalcidol
Respiratory tract secretions	Excess fluid in lungs, fluid overload	Glycopyrronium 200mcg SC Hyoscine butylbromide 20mg
Agitation	Uraemia	Midazolam 2.5mg SC
Dyspnoea	Fluid overload Heart failure	Fentanyl 25mcg SC Oxycodone 1–2mg Morphine 1.25–2.5mg Use of diuretics
Restless leg syndrome Sleep disturbance	↑ K^+ and Ca^{2+} levels cause muscle spasm	Avoid caffeine and alcohol in the evenings. Use of hypnotics: zopiclone, clonazepam

* Doses are reduced depending on level of eGFR (Check with BNF).

Withdrawal from dialysis

Introduction

The mortality rate for those with ESKD is around 23% per annum. Coexisting cardiovascular, cerebrovascular, and peripheral vascular disease make life on dialysis more difficult. Statistics show that 40–50% of patients aged >75yrs will die in the first yr after commencing dialysis. Dialysis withdrawal is an increasing cause of death as these patients do not do well on dialysis and often have difficulty with access.

Withdrawal of dialysis may be precipitated by symptom burden, significant reduction in QOL, or a medical decision that dialysis is no longer of benefit to the individual. Not all symptoms are relieved by dialysis, e.g. pruritus, anorexia, fatigue, lethargy, and they can continue to cause discomfort.

Factors influencing the decision to withdraw from dialysis

- Older age
- Living alone
- Social isolation
- Recent loss of life partner
- High symptom burden
- Increasing co-morbidity
- Poor QOL
- Cultural/religious reasons
- Dialysis no longer possible due to medical complications/ ↑ severity of associated co-morbidities.

Many of these factors are social rather than medical. The impact of dialysis on QOL should not be underestimated and healthcare professionals should be aware of the social factors which influence patients' decision-making.

Survival

The average survival following dialysis withdrawal is 7–10 days with a range of 1–46 days. The time from cessation of dialysis to death will be dependent on RRF and the patient's general condition. Those who stop dialysis due to general ill health and are dying from other co-morbidities may survive for a shorter period of time, i.e. average 2 days.

Failing transplant

Patients whose transplant has failed are faced with the decision of whether or not to return to dialysis. Those who have received a pre-emptive transplant are likely not to have ever dialysed, and have no idea what dialysis entails. They may find the prospect daunting which could influence the decision not to have dialysis. In some circumstances the patient may not be clinically stable to undergo dialysis and will ∴ need to be managed conservatively.

Care planning

- Caring for patients who withdraw from dialysis is different to those who are managed conservatively as there is a defined period of time (7–10 days) in which to plan and implement EOL care
- Any request by a patient to stop dialysis needs to be discussed fully with the medical and nursing teams
- The patient must be considered to have mental capacity to make such a decision
- A referral to a counsellor or psychologist should be made to discuss how they are feeling and why they wish to stop dialysis. They may change their mind following discussion about their feelings or confirm their decision
- Once a clear decision has been made a clear and realistic plan of care needs to be agreed and implemented. This should include the following:
  - document decision to stop
  - agree date to cease dialysis
  - plan and agree place of care: home, hospice, acute hospital, cottage hospital
  - referral to specialist palliative care team
  - referral to community palliative care team
  - referral to district nursing team
  - inform GP
  - chosen place of death
  - cessation of medication
  - do not attempt CPR order
  - symptom relief
  - bereavement support for family/carer
- Expectations of length of time of survival should be discussed with the patient and their family/carers
- There is a high symptom burden in this group of patients and symptoms experienced during dialysis will increase in severity once dialysis has been withdrawn. The most common symptoms in the last 24hrs of life are:
  - pain
  - agitation
  - myoclonus (involuntary muscle jerks)
  - dyspnoea
- A clear plan for symptom control (see Table 16.1) should be implemented and the renal LCP can assist with this.

Supportive care registers

- A supportive care or 'cause for concern' register identifies both patients 'deteriorating despite dialysis', and those deteriorating during conservative management, as potentially approaching the EOL phase
- Regular assessments help identify signs and symptoms which are becoming too burdensome and trigger conversations with patients/carers to aid advanced care planning

- Answering no to the 'surprise question', i.e. would you be surprised if this person died in the next 6 months, is an indication that EOL care planning should be discussed
- It promotes a consistent and proactive approach in supporting patients and links with the palliative care registers held by GP practices.

Advanced care planning

- Dialysis patients should be given the opportunity to discuss their wishes regarding cessation of dialysis in advance
- Many die unprepared despite being on RRT for many yrs. Such topics as resuscitation wishes should be openly discussed and documented
- Communication in relation to advanced care planning is essential although many healthcare professionals find it difficult to discuss EOL with patients
- Timely discussions and provision of appropriate information has been proven to enhance rather than diminish a patient's hope
- Where possible, avoid patients reaching the end of their ability to tolerate their symptoms/burden of dialysis and withdraw/cease dialysis without any forward planning.

Co-ordinating care

- Once the decision has been made to stop dialysis, transition of care needs to be co-ordinated depending on the setting
- If an advanced care plan or directive is in place this should be reviewed and preferred priority of care considered and where possible adhered to
- In some circumstances the patient's medical condition will dictate where they are cared for, e.g. the patient may not be tolerating dialysis and be too sick to be transferred to the hospice or home and will have no choice but to remain in the acute hospital.

Place of care

Acute hospital

- Many patients chose to die in the renal ward because they feel comfortable in this environment and have built up a relationship over the yrs with the ward staff
- Once dialysis has stopped the patient is admitted to the renal ward and the renal LCP initiated
- Advice and support may also be provided by the hospital palliative care team, renal palliative care nurse, renal counsellor, and hospital chaplain.

Cottage hospital

- Palliative care beds are often available in cottage hospitals and patients are cared for by their family doctor
- If the patient has a valued relationship with their GP and wishes to be nearer to home and not in an acute hospital or hospice environment then this is a good choice
- The community hospice teams are available for advice and guidance if required.

Hospice

- If the patient has an advanced care plan their preferred place of care may be the hospice
- Referral to the hospice team with patient consent should be made before dialysis stops so that the team can meet the patient and discuss their plan of care
- Many patients chose to die in a hospice as they do not wish to be a burden to their loved ones at home.

Home

- Most patients chose to die at home and this requires co-ordination of care between 1° and 2° care
- Equipment such as a hospital bed, specialist mattresses, hoists, and commodes may be needed
- A social needs assessment is required to ensure any equipment is in place when the patient stops dialysis.

Psychological, social, and spiritual needs

Psychological

Patients

- The psychological and social impact of advanced kidney disease are known to be considerable with extensive demands on both patient and family/carers
- The majority of conservatively managed patients are elderly and will have increasing care needs
- The advancing disease brings changes in appearance, social roles, financial challenges, and physical dependency
- Resources need to be identified to support these changes and provision of social and family support is required
- Patients mostly want family members to be actively involved in their care but this can present many challenges
- Patient and family preferences may differ and it is often difficult for the family to care for those closest to them in the last days of life. The expectation of the patient that their family can care for them may not be a realistic one
- Transferring care to home can be stressful for the family and the fear that they may not be able to cope is common
- Family and carers need as much support as possible and should have access to counselling services
- The death of a dialysis patient can also impact on other patients in the dialysis unit as they are used to seeing each other up to 3 times a wk:
  - staff should be aware of the effect a patient withdrawing from dialysis has on other patients
  - advice and support from the renal counsellor may be required.

Staff

- Bereavement support for staff should be available as they tend to have a longstanding relationship with their patients and the death of a patient can have a considerable impact on them.

Social

- The community nurses and social work team play a key role in assessing patient needs
- Care packages many need to be initiated and reviewed regularly
- Financial support may be required and those patients with palliative needs are entitled to certain benefits. These can be identified and claimed on the patient's behalf by the social worker/case manager
- If the patient wishes to die at home it is essential that adequate care is in place. However, if 24hr nursing care is required it may not always be possible for the patient to remain at home. It will depend on the availability of resources such as hospice at home teams or Macmillan nurses.

Spiritual

- Spiritual care is often left until very near the time of death which makes provision of help or resolution of issues difficult
- Spiritual care should become part of usual practice to effectively deliver holistic care. Illness and approaching death in particular the uncertainty associated with death can often raise spiritual issues
- Imminent death can have profound and diverse effects on the patient, family/carers, and healthcare professionals
- Openness and the ability to listen are the most important skills in provision of spiritual care.

Case study

Mary has been having haemodialysis for 8 months, and she wishes to stop dialysis. She didn't really want to have dialysis but pressure from her family influenced her decision. Her husband died 2 months ago and ever since he died she has been asking to stop dialysis.

Mary's wishes are clear and she had been saying for some time that she wants to stop dialysis, but because of the recent loss of another family member and the possibility of her being depressed, the healthcare professionals find it difficult to accept her decision.

She is seen by the renal counsellor in the unit and at home by the renal palliative care team. Her daughter supports her decision, but her son does not as he feels he cannot cope with losing both parents in a short period of time.

What are the main concerns here?

- Patient's wishes
- Family needs
- Conflict between the family
- Psychological factors.

What should happen?

- Discussion with family as a group, if possible at home
- Respect patient's wishes
- Agree a way forward
- Formulate an advanced care plan
- Discuss preferred place of care
- Agree a date to stop dialysis.

How can this be managed?

- Put support mechanisms in place—hospice team, community nurses, GP, care package if required, equipment, follow-up from renal palliative care team
- Agree preferred place of care—in this case Mary wanted to be in the hospice as felt her family couldn't cope with her dying at home
- Continued psychological support for family members
- Support staff in the unit.

Outcome
- Mary stopped dialysis; she was admitted to the local hospice where she died 5 days later
- Her daughter and son stayed in the hospice with her and were present when she died.

Lessons learnt
- Withdrawal from dialysis not an easy subject to discuss amongst healthcare professionals
- Impact of decision on family members
- Clear plan of care needed to ensure smooth transition to EOL care.

Further reading

Chambers EJ, Brown EA, Germain MJ. *Supportive Care for The Renal Patient*, 2nd edn. Oxford: Oxford University Press; 2010.

Jenkins K, Bennett L, Ho TM (eds). *Conservative Management in Advanced Kidney Disease. A Guide to Clinical Practice*. Luzerne: EDTNA/ERCA Publications; 2011. Available at: ℘ <http://www.edtnaerca.org>

NHS. *End of Life Care in Advanced Kidney Disease: A framework for implementation*, 2009. Available at: ℘ <http://www.kidneycare.nhs.uk>

Useful websites

℘ <http://www.bnf.org>

℘ <http://www.dh.gov.uk/en/Publicationsandstatistics/Publications/PublicationsPolicyAndGuidance/DH_085320>

℘ <http://www.endoflifecare.nhs.uk>

℘ <http://www.endoflifecareforadults.nhs/uk>

℘ <http://www.kidneycare.nhs.uk/EndofLifeCare>

℘ <http://www.mariecurie.org.uk>

℘ <http://www.nice.org.uk/guidance/qualitystandards/chronickidneydisease/planningcare>

℘ <http://www.renal.org/Clinical/GuidelinesSection/RenalReplacementTherapy.aspx>

Living with chronic kidney disease and renal replacement therapy

Psychological impact of chronic kidney disease and treatment

People with CKD experience different emotions and face many challenges both physical and emotional, whether it be commencing dialysis or undergoing a Tx. Each individual responds to these situations in their own way and may find it difficult to cope living with a chronic condition that has no cure and to accept a new, more regimented life as a result of medications, dialysis, and other clinical factors, e.g. diet and fluid restrictions. They may experience feelings of loss for their declining kidney function, lack of self-worth, and believe that they are no longer a valuable and contributing member of their family or community. It is common for people to go through a grieving process and express an array of emotions (denial, anger, bargaining, depression, and acceptance) at different stages in their disease: at time of diagnosis, commencing RRT, undergoing a Tx, and at the EOL.

Impact of CKD

- Emotions of loss, stress, anxiety, and depression—overwhelmed and the inability to cope, often mistaken for non-adherence
- Affects employment whether it is current or prospective—job loss, financial hardship, and strains on personal relationships
- Altered relationships in the family home, e.g. role reversal may cause feelings of loss for the previous relationship
- Sexual problems; tiredness and change in relationship with partner
- Inadequate social support; feelings of isolation and loneliness leading to depression
- Interference with normal family routine and social life due to planning around dialysis days → feeling of isolation and loss
- Loss of independence due to immobility, fatigue, and being unable to attend to all normal activities of life
- Concern for partners or family members, particularly if they are ill, elderly, or dependent, e.g. patient may be the main carer
- Inadequate discussion, planning, and/or preparation for EOL care with family and healthcare providers, → anxiety and stress.

Impact on family

- ↑ responsibility and work due to managing a different role within the household, i.e. impact of finances on QOL, financial difficulties as a result of job loss of partner, ↑ work if have to accompany or drive the patient to HD sessions or appointments
- Disturbed sleep as a result of symptoms of ESKD, RRT, and/or home-based treatment, e.g. APD machine alarms
- ↑ levels of stress and tiredness, → neglect of their own needs and health
- Anger and frustration for partners if not engaging with healthcare professionals to manage and take control of his/her condition
- Stress and anxiety associated with decision-making/treatment options, e.g. involvement/lack of involvement in EOL decisions; choice of RRT including options for transplantation, ± living kidney donation.

Factors affecting adaptation and coping with a chronic condition

- The perceived degree of intrusion CKD upon his/her life and how much change is required
- Effects on QOL
- The amount of control the patient perceives he/she has over life, i.e. internal or external locus of control
- Past experience—how the person has dealt and managed with illness or loss in the past affects health beliefs and ability to make decisions in the present
- The person's health belief system, what they feel and understand about his/her condition, hospital, and treatment—identify to minimize the risk of miscommunication
- The person's inherent ability to deal with change
- Personality—it has been reported that patients with a good sense of humour appear to having better coping abilities
- Knowledge base and understanding of the different treatment options available for CKD and ESKD
- Degree of involvement in decision-making in treatment choices
- The impact of social and financial support on illness and treatment
- Mental health ± illnesses, e.g. depression and anxiety; character traits, e.g. optimism or a pessimism.

Nursing considerations

- Effective communication skills, e.g. listening and observing for non-verbal cues with both patient and family
- Have a good understanding of coping mechanisms and demonstrate a respect for individuals learning to live with sudden change
- Denial is a good defence mechanism used to block out difficult to manage emotions and situations. May be mistaken as obstructive behaviour and is often expressed until the person feels able to cope and is ready to address the situation
- Develop a partnership with the person; provide information and support to facilitate informed decision-making and patient choice
- Facilitating and foster self-care management—take control of his/her own health
- Review goals and expectations of treatment and of living with CKD with the patient and their family—facilitate them to have set realistic and achievable goals
- Teach the patient problem solving and effective coping techniques to manage their health
- Encourage the patient to continue with normal activities, start a new hobby, join a support group, community activities
- Provide guidance and support on altered body image, fear of dying, changes with personal relationships, financial difficulties, dependence and support issues, and living with new life restrictions and new limitations
- Refer for additional support—counselling, i.e. psychosocial support, social worker, finances, supportive care team, community nursing teams.

Quality of life

QOL is subjective and relates to a person's satisfaction with, and perception of, their position in life. It is drawn from their expectations, goals, physical and psychological well-being, relationships, and concerns. Studies have shown that physical QOL is lower in ESKD patients compared with the normal population and this may affect mortality rates in ESKD, mental QOL components, however, are unaffected. A person's expectations of his/her QOL will vary according to factors such as age and past personal experiences. The main aim of the MPT should be to assist the person to have the best possible QOL.

The benefits of measuring QOL

- Provides a personal dimension to the patient assessment—practitioner is able to gain some insight into personal and social circumstances which cannot be determined from a medical examination
- Early identification of issues or potential problems, enabling strategies to be put in place to assist patients:
  - ↓ in QOL or at ↑ risk, e.g. depression, anxiety, sleep disturbance
  - opportunity to discuss with person the results of the assessment and facilitate communication
- Person's perspective of the efficacy of treatment rather than from clinical outcomes alone
- Identify and monitor changes as a result of changes to clinical practice
- Provide feedback on the impact on QOL of new treatments, i.e. outcome benefits vs cost of treatment
- Clinical governance, audit, and research tools to measure clinical outcomes—results may be useful to demonstrate the need for additional resources, e.g. in commissioning.

Assessment tools

- Ideally be disease specific if assessing a particular population, e.g. ESKD rather than multidimensional as more relevant
- There are various well validated tools available such as Short-form 26 (SF26), HD QOL (HDQOL), Health-Related QOL (HRQL), Nottingham Health Profile (NHP), Sickness Impact Profile (SIP), World Health Organization QOL (WHOQOL).

Potential problems associated with HRQOL assessment tools

- Questionnaires can be time consuming, especially if the person requires assistance to complete them in a clinic environment
- Difficult to administer if there are communication problems, e.g. dysphasic, non-English speaking or if they have a learning disability
- Should not be used to replace clinical assessment and communication
- May raise expectations of the person/family that there is a treatment for the problems identified when in fact nothing can be done:
  - may lead to further disappointment, e.g. poor physical mobility
  - discuss the purpose of the assessment tool prior to use
- Could affect decision-making if used as part of decision-making process by the healthcare professional, e.g. choice of RRT modality.

Altered body image

Body image is a subjective term and describes how people perceive their own appearance, i.e. how they see and feel about their body. Alteration in that perception is very common throughout CKD, different modalities of RRT, and conservative care. Good support from family, friends, and the staff in the renal unit is important for patients to adjust to the physical changes in their bodies.

A person's reaction to a change in their body image is dependent on:

- Individual coping ability to deal with a change in appearance and acceptance of that change
- Level of self-esteem, i.e. those with ↓ self-esteem are more vulnerable
- Pre-existing high level of importance in appearance, e.g. young ♀, low level of optimism, poor interpersonal skills
- Level of family and social support available
- Influence of society (i.e. peer group pressure); religious or cultural beliefs
- Hereditary, genetic/biological factors, e.g. inherent appearance such as large nose.

Specific reasons for altered body image in CKD patients

- Physical/appearance changes:
  - scarring from incision wounds, e.g. abdomen, chest, arms
  - presence of a fistula or PD catheter
  - weight gain, e.g. due to corticosteroids (see 📖 p. 497)
  - change in body shape (e.g. waist measurement) as a result of side effects to medications or carrying PD fluid, catheters, dressings
  - side effects of medications, e.g. hirsutism, acne, nausea, constipation
- Impaired growth, e.g. adolescents.

Effects of body image problems

- Anxiety and depression, ↓ self-esteem and ↓ QOL
- May express feelings of anger, rage, embarrassment, shame, fear of rejection by others
- Depression
- Pre-occupied with the change in their body
- Problems with adherence
- Avoidance of social engagement, increasing isolation.

Nursing considerations

- Development of a good rapport with the patient using effective communication skills
- Provide support and reassurance, listen and observe for any non-verbal cues of distress with the change in body image
- Encourage the patient to discuss their feelings and reassure them that it takes time to adjust and re-integrate their new appearance into how they view themselves
- Providing a culturally sensitive and non-judgemental approach to concerns raised by the patient
- Provide support to partners/family members and discuss what changes to expect
- Awareness of those at risk and observe for signs of anxiety and distress
- Provide information prior to access formation so the patient is aware what to expect (e.g. show photographs, talk with other patients) to reduce anxiety
- Offer ideas on how to dress to avoid their scar, fistula, or PD catheter being visible
- Offer guidance of what types of clothes may be more comfortable if concerned about weight gain, e.g. ↑ waist measurement with PD fluid
- Good explanation of potential side effects of medications:
  - pro-active early interventions such as altering medications that cause external changes, e.g. change of IS can assist in ↓ the associated anxiety especially in younger patients
- Referral to a psychologist may be required as a result of the large impact on a patient's life:
  - may lead to relationship problems
  - ↓ libido
  - poor confidence and self-esteem
  - inability to cope with the 'outside world—become introverted some patients may be offered CBT.

Dementia

As a result of the ageing population, dementia is a problem increasingly seen in CKD. Dementia is defined as impairment of memory and one other cognitive domain, e.g. language comprehension or speech, executive functioning, attention, memory. There must be evidence of decline and be sufficiently severe to interfere with daily activity and function.

- Need to differentiate from other conditions to identify the cause and type and other potentially treatable ± reversible conditions, e.g. depression/anxiety, cognitive impairment, sensory impairment
- Most patients do not complain of memory loss; it is usually insidious with a family member reporting the problem
- Most common type is Alzheimer's disease—accounts for 50–80% in the general population (35–40% >90yrs). Other types include vascular (multi-infarct) dementia (10–20%), Parkinson's disease with dementia.

Potentially reversible causes

Alcohol, side effects of medication, e.g. antihistamine use, depression, sleep disturbance, electrolyte imbalance, anaemia, vitamin B12 deficiency, inadequate dialysis, aluminium toxicity, hypothyroidism.

Implications for nephrology service

- ↑ hospitalization with associated ↑ in healthcare burden and cost
- ↑ disability
- Impact on treatment decisions, ability to learn and retain new information, handle complex tasks, reasoning, spatial ability and orientation, language, and behaviour
- Withdrawal from dialysis—difficulty making a differential diagnosis if present acutely requiring RRT
- A trial of dialysis may be recommended to assess improvement, i.e. whether it is uraemic encephalopathy. In this situation, the family must be made aware that it is a trial, of which may cease at some point if the patient is unable to sustain the dialysis itself.

Nursing considerations
- Vascular causes involve aggressively treating the risk factors
- Medications to slow the progression of the disease—cholinesterase inhibitor or N-methyl D-aspartate receptor antagonists for Alzheimer's disease. ▶ No long-term data available on the safety and efficacy in ESKD patients
- Good communications skills—offer flexibility of timing of procedures where possible, good negotiation skills, use of distractions, e.g. talking with the patient performing tasks
- ↓ anxiety—request the carer attend appointments and dialysis sessions
- Assess whether a home-based treatment may be more suitable if carer able to perform assisted dialysis
- Discussion about advanced directives and EOL care (see 🕮 p. 514)
- Strategies for care and management in the future—liaise with social worker for community assessment, e.g. ↑ social services may be required and respite care.

Adherence

The most common terms used to describe failure to adhere to medical advice and treatment are non-adherence, non-compliance, and non-concordance. Adherence is now the accepted term as it reflects an agreement between two parties, i.e. a partnership between the patient and healthcare professionals leading to collaborative decision-making. There are many reasons why patients choose not to follow advice and it worth reflecting on the impact of living with a chronic condition which prescribes strict diet, fluid and lifestyle changes. The incidence rates vary in study reports from 30–50% (see p. 506).

Factors that affect adherence

- Gender, more common in ♂
- Younger age
- Lack of social support
- Lower socio-economic background, lower level of education
- Depression
- Smoking
- Presence of other co-morbid conditions.

Reasons for non-adherence

- Depression—feelings of disinterest and apathy
- Poor understanding of condition and the consequences of not complying with treatment
- Cultural or language barrier
- Denial that they have a chronic condition
- Defiance due to feeling constantly being told what to do
- Cognitive dysfunction due to uraemia
- Unwanted side effects of medications or the burden of taking large amounts of medications
- Intrusive impact on daily life
- Impersonal nature of renal unit
- Lack of joint decision-making approach when planning treatment.

Common renal-related adherence issues

- Failure to attend scheduled appointment in clinic
- Late to attend appointments
- Late or failure to attend HD session or shortened time on HD
- Failure to undertake prescribed PD exchanges or shortening APD time (usually found on stock taking of fluids)
- Tx rejection ± premature graft failure
- Peritonitis or exit site infections
- Frequently fluid overloaded
- Under-dialysed
- Not taking medications as prescribed, common with phosphate binders or medications that have side effects seen on biochemistry results and/or drug levels, i.e. IS medications
- Do not follow dietary advice, e.g. ↑ K^+ levels, poor diabetes control.

Impact of non-adherence
- Detrimental to the patient's health, well-being, and long-term outcome
- Psychological impact on family and/or carer as result of ↑ support and time management for the patient
- Cost to the health service, e.g. ↑ hospitalization.

Assessment
- Blood results, e.g. K^+ levels, PO_4, Hb, drug levels, e.g. CNIs may indicate if medications are being taken
- Under-dialysed adequacy results—shortening or skipping PD exchange, showing up late or taking themselves off early from HD
- Tx recipient; patterns of non-attendance, ↑ serum Cr, oliguria, sub-therapeutic blood drug levels ± signs of rejection (see 📖 pp. 506–7)
- Not ordering repeat prescriptions
- Not ordering as much PD fluid—the dialysis companies will usually inform the PD unit if this is occurring.

Nursing considerations
- Ensure no physical or psychological reason is the cause of non-adherence, e.g. depression, mental illness, cognitive impairment, too unwell to understand
- Ensure use of good and effective communications skills
- Give patients advice and information to make an informed choice about their care and treatment
- Develop a partnership with the patient and set realistic achievable goals:
  - how best to reach these goals
  - encourage the patient to identify solutions that will work
- Empower patient to take control of their illness/condition
- If the patient has cognitive impairment, involve the support of family members to reinforce the information and advice
- Provide some flexibility, e.g. if rules are not so strict they may cause the patient to be defiant
- Use a non-judgemental and non-confrontational approach when addressing the problem of non-adherence—be empathetic
- Provide education and training at the level that the patient can understand:
  - assess whether they have any barriers to learning, e.g. illiterate (see 📖 pp. 605–6 for teaching assessment)
  - offer re-training programmes to review patient's knowledge and understanding
- Provide support, e.g. patient counselling and support groups
- See also 📖 pp. 506–7, 572 regarding medicines adherence.

Managing challenging behaviour

Work-related violence in the health sector is a serious and growing concern and requires training for all staff to prevent and manage it in the workplace. The UK Health and Safety Executive[1] define violence towards staff as 'any incident in which a person is abused, threatened or assaulted in circumstances relating to their work'. Violence and aggression, in particular verbal abuse towards staff working in the nephrology service, is a common problem in certain areas. This may be physical or verbal/psychological abuse, intimidation, and can involve sexual harassment or racist comments. It may also be made by family members or visitors to the nephrology service.

The impact on staff includes:
- Psychological, e.g. stress, including post-traumatic stress disorder, anxiety, fear, depression, and isolation
- Physical, e.g. pain or disability from assault injury
- ↓ problem-solving ability, poor concentration
- Effect on general health.

Risks to the renal unit include:
- Poor staff retention and recruitment, ↑ sickness with ↑ in overall cost to the unit
- ↓ staff morale
- Poor public image of the organization.

Potential triggers
- Physical—fluid and electrolyte imbalance, pain, medications, confusion, alcohol or substance abuse, mental health issues
- Nephrology service:
  - patient is kept waiting and start of HD session is delayed
  - out-patient appointments run over time; patients are kept waiting
  - poor environment, e.g. seating, lighting, too hot/cold, overcrowded
  - noise, e.g. in HD unit: lack of privacy and space; HD stations too close together
  - behaviour of other patients who are aggressive or abusive
- Healthcare professionals:
  - appear unfriendly, unhelpful, or verbally abrupt
  - patients feel staff members are not listening to them nor interested in their problems
  - patients feel anxious or frustrated due to lack of information ± problems/concerns they have raised have not been addressed, e.g. blood results.

It is very difficult to withhold treatment from patients who require dialysis and the medical staff must be involved in discussions about options ± interventions in order to provide a safe working environment for the MPT. However, to prevent escalation, all staff are required to attend training in methods of prevention, de-escalation techniques, and management of violence and aggressive situations.

Pregnancy

In the earlier stages of CKD, the risks associated with pregnancy vary according to the stage and type of disease. The chance of conception diminishes with declining GFR. Miscarriage is common and pregnancy can lead to irreversible loss of kidney function.

- Pregnancy may not be advised in some pre-existing renal conditions and more intensive management by the obstetric and nephrology teams will be required
- Counselling and support should be provided about the risks for both the fetus and pregnant mother and circumstances where pregnancy is not advised, e.g. lupus nephritis with active disease or antiphospholipid antibodies, scleroderma
- Advice on contraception should be provided to all ♀, e.g. barrier devices (e.g. condoms, diaphragms), implants, depot injections and Mirena® coil. ⚠ Combined oral contraceptive pill, kidney dysfunction relative contraindication, risk of ↑ BP and thrombosis—patient should discuss with medical staff.

Effects of pregnancy

- ↑ proteinuria, oedema (if nephrotic)
- Develop or worsening of hypertension—normally resolves post-partum
- ↑ risk of fetal death, intrauterine growth retardation, and premature delivery associated with hypertension
- ↑ risk of pre-eclampsia
- ⚠ Any ♀ planning a pregnancy should be advised about the risks associated with certain medications to avoid unnecessary exposure of the fetus, e.g. ACEIs which are teratogenic, cytotoxics, and IS.

Pregnancy outcome in CKD

Cr <125µmol/L, eGFR >45 (CKD stage 1, 2, 3A)
- Usually normal pregnancy and good prognosis
- 90–96% successful pregnancy, <3% permanent loss of kidney function.

Cr >125 and <250µmol/L, eGFR 20–45 (CKD stage 3B, 4)
- High-risk pregnancy, e.g. pre-eclampsia, fetal growth retardation, and/or 50–60% chance of premature birth (2° pre-eclampsia and/or growth retardation)
- 90% live births with good BP control
- 25–33% or more will have ↓ kidney function with 10% ESKD.

Cr >250µmol/L, eGFR <20 (CKD 4/5)
- Poor fetal outcome and high risk of progressing to ESKD
- Risk of maternal intraperitoneal haemorrhage and accelerated hypertension
- 50–71% fetal survival in those on dialysis
- 53% permanent loss of kidney function with 35% ESKD and on dialysis within 1yr.

Dialysis

The incidence of pregnancy in ESKD patients is 1–7%, less common in PD than HD. Requires close monitoring and management by both the nephrology and obstetric teams throughout the pregnancy.

- No evidence to suggest that HD is better than PD during pregnancy and patients are not advised to switch to HD
- In the later stages, it can be difficult to achieve dialysis adequacy ∴ switch to HD
- Theoretically, PD may be better i.e. continuous dialysis vs peaks and troughs associated with HD, electrolytes and fluid shifts which may affect fetal circulation
- ↓ blood loss and better control of anaemia, less chance of hypotensive episodes and the need to use drugs such as heparin.

Nursing considerations

- Joint management between obstetric and nephrology services
- Birth arrangements—premature delivery common and may be organized as elective caesarean
- Liaise to arrange dialysis, especially if in another hospital
- Review and model prescription—↑ dialysis dose aim for: Kt/Vurea >2.5, Ur <16–17mmol/L
- Fluid balance
  - wkly weight assessment >4 months (estimated weight gain is 0.3–0.5kg/wk for a normal pregnancy)
- BP—avoid episodes of hypotension or hypertension:
  - if antihypertensive required, follow-up of BP to prevent any ↓ BP
- Medications—liaise with pharmacist as some drugs contraindicated, e.g. ⚠ ACEI or ARB are teratogenic and should not be used, particularly in the 1st trimester. β blockers are associated with growth retardation
  - heparin—use LMWH as anticoagulant
- PD—better infant survival with RRF (80% compared to 40% without RRF):
  - ↑ number of exchanges with a total daily volume of 12L, e.g. CAPD with smaller volumes, e.g. 1.5L and 5 exchanges ~4–5 months
  - APD with smaller volumes, ↑ number of cycles + day CAPD exchange or exchanges
  - tidal PD, leaving a small residual volume *in situ*
- Advise patient not to bypass a slow drain alarm and re-fill without checking that the correct amount has been drained
- Contact the PD unit immediately if blood present in PD effluent. May be caused by retrograde blood flow from the uterus and requires urgent investigation, e.g. problem with the placenta or spontaneous abortion. ▶ Need to rule out peritonitis
- Infection—peritonitis should be treated the same way (see 🕮 pp. 312–13), more prone to CMV, herpes viruses, and toxoplasmosis

(Continued)

(Continued)

- HD:
  - 1st trimester—20hrs/wk over 4/5 sessions
  - 2/3rd trimester—daily HD
- Investigations—more frequent FBC, U&E, Ca^{2+}, PO_4:
  - in the later stages will require wkly bloods to assess for signs of ↓ K^+, PO_4, and ↑ Ca^{2+} levels
- Anaemia management—aim for Hb 10.5–12g/dl
- ↑ ESAs and iron supplementation, ensure taking folic acid supplements
- Nutrition—refer to the renal dietitian for dietary advice, i.e. ↑ protein intake to 1.5g/kg/day:
  - review diet and may require additional vitamin supplementation.
- Transplantation:
  - As the effects of uraemia are reversed after a successful kidney Tx, women of child-bearing age must be advised not to conceive for the first yr. This allows the graft to stabilize and lower doses of IS. Education regarding pregnancy risk and birth control is required pre and post transplantation.
- Many nephrology services offer a joint obstetric and nephrology pregnancy clinic to support patients planning a pregnancy and maximizes the health and well-being of mother and fetus, e.g. no teratogenic medications (see 📖 p. 504).

Infertility

Infertility is a common problem for ♂ and ♀ CKD patients, which generally improves following a kidney transplant. The psychological impact of infertility can be devastating and lead to stress, feelings of worthlessness, depression, and relationship problems.

Male infertility
- Uraemic toxins and altered hormone levels:
  - ↑ FSH and ↑ oestrodiol levels → impaired spermatogenesis, azoospermia or severe oligozoospermia, and ↓ sperm viability
  - usually reversed post transplantation.

Female infertility
- Anovulation due to the lack of an oestradiol-stimulated LH surge particularly those on RRT—menstrual irregularity or amenorrhoea
- Usually reversed in premenopausal ♀ post transplantation.

Nursing considerations
- ♂—referral to a reproductive clinic for a sperm count, assessment and treatment. Zinc therapy may improve sperm characteristics.
- ♀—treat hyperprolactinaemia and anaemia to restore normal menstrual cycle. Medical staff may refer to reproductive clinic for assessment and treatment if appropriate
- Referral for counselling and support for infertility issues

Transition to adult care

Introduction

Adolescence is a period of personal growth and development in which risk-taking and experimentation are key characteristic behaviours. The burden of a chronic condition such as ESKD on young people can have a devastating impact on lifestyle and typically enhances challenging behaviours:

- Denial
- Poor social interaction with peers
- Breakdown of family relationships
- Blatant non-adherence with treatment plans.

Without appropriate help and support, the health and well-being of the young person is threatened. Young people with CKD and/or on RRT from childhood are required to transfer from a paediatric to an adult care setting in adolescence, usually at 18yrs of age, for ongoing care and management. The way in which this process is managed and understood by healthcare professionals has a direct impact on clinical outcomes and the future welfare of the young person. Significant work has been done to identify key barriers and to develop systems of care that are 'young people' friendly.

Definitions

Transition is a planned, seamless process that facilitates the movement of young people with chronic illness from child-centred to adult-centred care during their adolescence; continuing beyond the point of transfer to adult services. For transition to be effective and therapeutic it must be guided and evidence based; acknowledging the wider needs of the young person as well as his/her clinical requirements.

Transfer is the point when clinical responsibility for the young person moves from paediatric to adult services from an operational/administrative perspective.

Effective transition

All have a role to play:

- *The young person*—needs to feel involved and exercise autonomy in decision-making about his/her own care and service improvements
- *The parents/carers*—need to allow the young person to feel empowered and withdraw from the historical 'parental relationship'
- *Healthcare professionals*—need to acknowledge and support the roles of young people and parents in 'letting go'; appropriately involve young people in planning transition; work across professional boundaries and different care settings.

Healthcare professionals have some specific responsibilities to facilitate the transition process:

- Establish agreed local policy on transition care that can be audited against quality indicators, e.g. *You're Welcome quality criteria* (DH, 2011[2]), with the involvement of young people and families to ensure that it is fit for purpose

- Recognize that the needs of adolescents are different from those of younger children and older adults to drive change in provision of services and resources
- Develop specialist knowledge and skills within both adult and paediatric teams to understand and respond appropriately to the needs of young people
- Provide services tailored specifically to young people, e.g. dedicated clinics, independent, confidential appointments, engagement through social networking, peer support
- MPT collaboration with local champions for young adults to strengthen clinical leadership
- Maintain accurate records and individual plan for each young person that can form a hand-held personal record
- Plan transition and transfer well in advance to achieve the best outcome for the young person.

Transition—making it happen

The process of transition can be started with the young person from 12yrs of age with a view to transfer at 18yrs of age, although exact timing will be influenced by individual cognitive and physical development. The process should include the following elements:

- Individual transitional plan and care pathway, tailored to treatment plan, e.g. timing of transplantation, planned modality of treatment at time of transfer
- Consideration of complex special needs requiring an amended pathway, e.g. learning difficulties, social/mental health needs
- Education and support (young person and parents)
- Increasing autonomy for the young person, e.g. clinic attendances, self-management, decision-making
- Streamlined medication regimens, e.g. reduce frequency of dosing, dosette boxes, mobile phone reminders
- Joint clinics between adult and paediatric services in adult care setting/ young person friendly setting, e.g. sports club, community centre
- Ongoing support from both adult and paediatric services with named contacts/key-workers
- Peer support/buddy system with other young people; matched by age and modality of treatment, e.g. timing of planned living donor kidney transplant/start of dialysis therapy.

Transition can be divided into 3 key stages (ages are a guide only):

- *Early stage (12–14yrs)*—introducing the young person and their family to the concept of transition; development of autonomy with family support and checking young person's understanding and implications of his/her medical condition. The young person will start to see healthcare professionals in clinic independently
- *Middle stage (14–15yrs)*—the young person becomes more autonomous in decision-making; improves knowledge and understanding about the process of transition and gains insight into how adult services are delivered

- *Late stage (15–16yrs)*—maximum autonomy achieved in the young person with parental confidence in the transfer to adult services.

At each stage, there are 6 areas for consideration/discussion which can be used to create an individual transitional plan:
- Self-advocacy
- Independent healthcare behaviour
- Sexual health
- Psychosocial support
- Educational and vocational planning
- Health and lifestyle.

A useful tool for interviewing adolescents is the **HEADSS psychosocial screening tool**[3] which stands for:
- **H**ome
- **E**ducation/Employment
- **E**ating
- **A**ctivities (peer group)
- **D**rugs
- **S**exuality
- **S**uicide/depression
- **S**afety.

HEADSS comprises a range of questions which are categorized according to the level of importance; depending upon the depth of screening that is required.
- 'Essential' questions should be used in all cases
- 'Important' questions should be used with most teenagers and the remaining questions may be used time permitting.

Health promotion

Health promotion activities empower individuals to improve health and well-being by taking control of their health. There are various models and theories of health promotion, e.g. heath belief, social learning theory. A good understanding and knowledge of health behaviour and the change process enables healthcare professionals to gain insight into:
- What affects a person's decision to change a particular behaviour, e.g. smoking cessation, weight loss, exercise
- How to facilitate people to self-manage
- How to work with and help people to understand and accept the preferred treatment for their condition.

The factors that affect a person's health and well-being
- Inherited disease
- Modality of RRT ± co-morbidity
- Age, e.g. elderly
- Lifestyle choices, e.g. smoking, excessive alcohol intake, poor diet
- Socioeconomic—level of education, presence/absence of supportive partner/family, peer group pressure, social deprivation, e.g. unemployment and poverty are linked to poorer health
- Health access inequality
- Environment—housing, healthy food, clean air and water
- Ethnicity, e.g. diabetes more common in the Asian population.

Factors that can affect health behaviour include:
- Age of onset of disease/RRT, e.g. adolescence
- Person's expectations and prior experiences
- Self-confidence
- Risk/benefit ratio
- Seriousness of the condition
- Incentive/reward
- Perceived/actual potential difficulties/barriers
- Influence of other people
- Socio-economic, i.e. poverty
- Cultural/religious—e.g. belief in predestination.

Other factors that contribute to successful change in behaviour
- Self-efficacy—a person's self-belief in their ability to take the necessary actions which will lead to a difference in the outcome, e.g. may be influenced by observing/watching others who have been successful or are performing the action successfully, e.g. self-needling own AVF, exercising
- Self-regulation—actual processes involved in undertaking the change in behaviour. Set realistic attainable goals and review them regularly, provide information about how and when they can perform the action and identify the barriers that the person will need to overcome:
- Monitor performance by using a diary, e.g. food diary; identify and acknowledge both achievements and failures, provide feedback on performance.

Healthcare professionals' barriers
- Using paternalistic techniques to persuade the person
- A confrontational approach, i.e. critical rather than supportive
- Using scare tactics to force the patient to change
- Labelling the person as non-adherent when they are unable to develop a partnership with the person i.e. justify failure to change.

Chronic kidney disease health promotion activities

RRT is costly but, by providing interventions for the prevention, early detection and subsequent delay of progression, of CKD, the overall cost burden can be reduced.

Aims of CKD health promotion activities
- Promote health and well-being—living a healthy lifestyle, e.g. smoking cessation, ↓ salt intake, exercise, maintaining a healthy weight
- Development and implementation of educational programmes:
  - for the early detection of CKD
  - prevention of CKD where possible, e.g. complications associated with smoking
  - minimizing the effects of other conditions/diseases, e.g. diabetes, CVD, ↑ BP
  - care and management of CKD for other healthcare professionals in 1° and 2° care
  - working with patient associations to provide education and support in the community
- Development and implementation of health reforms and policies to promote health and well-being, e.g. national working groups and associations who have developed policies, e.g. RA, NICE, NSF for Renal Services:
  - ensure healthcare access equity and all people have access to RRT
  - work with and involve community groups.

CKD health promotion programmes include:
- 1° *prevention programmes*—aimed at healthy individuals in the community in whom lifestyle changes will improve health and prevent long-term kidney damage
- 2° *prevention programmes*—aimed at early detection of kidney disease and delay in progression. The goal is to prevent early CKD progressing to ESKD by early interventions and management of co-morbid conditions
- 3° *prevention programmes*—aimed at people with the late stages of CKD, RRT from developing associated long-term complications, e.g. anaemia, metabolic bone disease, malnutrition
- Educational programmes within the renal setting are aimed at all levels of health promotion and include in-house programmes facilitated by:
  - MPT input
  - expert patients, patient groups, and peer support (buddy systems)
  - community healthcare professionals.

Rehabilitation

Many people with CKD lead active and healthy lifestyles. Rehabilitation in the context of CKD should focus on enhancing and restoring emotional and physical well-being, adjustment and coping with CKD, employment ability, and QOL to the best possible level achievable for the individual patient.

Assessment of the patient should include:

- Physical ability, long-term or short-term disability, level of exercise/fitness
- Day-to-day functioning—employment, social activities, normal daily activities
- Social, e.g. living conditions, support network
- Psychological, e.g. coping with CKD, depression, anxiety
- Satisfaction with QOL
- Modality of RRT.

Aspects of rehabilitation include:

- Day-to-day functioning—maintain normal activities:
  - employment or training/educational courses
  - finances
  - holidays
  - driving
- Psychological
- Physical fitness and exercise.

Employment/educational institutions

Many patients experience problems either maintaining or attaining a job/attending college as a result of psychological problems, physical symptoms (e.g. lethargy, SOB, reduced exercise tolerance and ability to concentrate) and/or practical aspects of accommodating dialysis. It is important to provide support to maintain as normal life as possible for the person and their family. Many people are employed when they become unwell and require the support of the nephrology service to liaise with their employer/educational institution to explain their condition and special requirements.

Employer/educational institution issues
- Potential ↑ number and frequency of sick days
- Ergonomic adjustments in the workplace
- Flexible working hrs to allow person to attend dialysis sessions
- Providing space in the workplace to attend to PD exchange
- Inability to meet deadlines for work submissions if unwell
- Organizing to attend classes around dialysis times.

Nursing considerations
- Liaise with medical staff to provide sickness certificates and letters of support for the employer/educational institution
- Refer to the social worker—provide person with information on employment rights and responsibilities. Liaise with the employer regarding flexibility of working hrs to maximize the chances of remaining in employment
- PD staff to visit the workplace/educational institution to assist in finding and assessing suitable areas for undertaking a PD procedure
- Switch to APD for overnight dialysis freeing the day for work
- HD staff to review home HD/overnight home HD is a possible option to free up the day for work or transfer the person to a satellite unit to ↓ travelling time.

Finances
There may be financial issues as a result of lost income, inability to work, or loss of employment. This can cause additional anxiety and stress further exacerbating health and well-being. All people with CKD should be offered referral to the renal social worker to discuss any financial issues, e.g. problems with mortgage/loan/rent repayments. The renal social worker is the most appropriate to discuss options and advise on resources and benefits available.

Driving
The DVLA must be advised if the person's medical condition has worsened since obtaining a UK driver's licence.

Holidays and overseas travel

Travelling and holidays are an important part of normal life.
- A letter from the hospital for customs clearance and contact details for the local nephrology unit in the destination country will be needed
- Appropriate immunization (see 📖 p. 557)
- Travel insurance for overseas travel is essential, especially to the USA. The NKF[4] provides excellent travel advice and information about companies that insure people with a pre-existing medical condition
- European Health Insurance Card (EHIC)[5] required if travelling to EU countries and Switzerland for reciprocal medical cover. Insurance required for emergency transfer home if required and dialysis sessions still need to be organized separately.

Haemodialysis

Allow time to organize—arrangements can be complex and time-consuming.
- Overseas HD units must be assessed for suitability, i.e. low risk of hepatitis B, C, or HIV infection with acceptable virus surveillance and infection control policies in place
- On return, check viral status and segregate until results clear conversion
- If listed for Tx, will usually be suspended from the NTL whilst overseas. Depending upon local arrangements and level of risk associated with travel destination, status on the NTL may be affected on return—reactivation on the NTL often delayed until viral surveillance is completed, e.g. up to 6 months
- Discuss on an individual basis prior to overseas travel so that they are fully aware of the implications for them should they decide to travel abroad.

Peritoneal dialysis

Delivery of PD dialysate in developed countries is usually straightforward to organize. There is more risk of dialysate not arriving or being held up in customs and not reaching the person in more remote or less developed countries.
- Fluid/supplies can be organized via the PD staff and they will require a delivery address and a minimum of 8wks' notice
- Take supplies in hand luggage, i.e. in case of delays/lost luggage and if an exchange is required during travel to destination
- Check compatibility of electrical voltage for APD machine and adaptor
- Education on signs and symptoms of peritonitis and action to take, administration of antibiotics, and be provided with a course of antibiotics.

Transplantation

- Local policies vary but overseas travel usually not advised during 1st yr post transplantation due to frequent follow-up appointments and close monitoring. Short trips may be possible but must be discussed on an individual basis

- Provide a larger supply of medication than required for the length of the trip to avoid interruption to IS, e.g. if return to UK is delayed
- Medications to be carried in both hand and hold baggage in case luggage is lost or stolen
- Provide information about the closest Tx centre to planned destination(s) and how to make contact if needed in non-urgent and emergency situations.

Key points on vaccinations and CKD

- People with CKD have impaired immune response but immunizations should be offered as per the area they are travelling to:
  - *no live vaccines* should be given to people with CKD/on IS, e.g. yellow fever, measles, mumps and rubella, oral polio (Sabin), oral typhoid. If polio vaccination required, the dead (Salk) polio vaccine should be given
  - *safe vaccinations* include diphtheria, hepatitis A and B, influenza, immunoglobulins, meningococcus, pertussis, pneumococcal rabies, tetanus, typhoid
- Prior to travelling, check status—if −ve, immunoglobulin may be required for high-risk areas:
  - *malaria prophylaxis*—discuss on an individual basis with the pharmacist as dose adjustments are required depending on kidney function
  - *special consideration must be given to Tx recipients* receiving vaccinations as IS can interfere with efficacy
- ↑ non-response rate in the early months post Tx when IS doses are typically ↑.

Physical fitness and exercise

Physical fitness and functioning is significantly affected in the advanced stages of CKD and for people on dialysis or with failing/poorly functioning transplants. Muscle weakness, decreased muscle strength, and atrophy are common problems which impact on a person's ability to carry out even normal day-to-day activities, e.g. shopping, gardening, and housework. The physical and psychological effects include:

- Cramps
- Restless leg syndrome
- Sleep disturbances
- Depression
- Anxiety
- Decline in HRQOL.

As a result of the reduced functional capacity, there is a tendency to become even more inactive which is associated with ↑ cardiovascular risk.

Associated causes

It is not fully known what the underlying causes of reduced physical fitness are; however, there are associations with the following:

- The accumulation of uraemic toxins
- Insulin resistance and defects in insulin and insulin-like growth factor (IGF-1)
- Metabolic acidosis
- Vitamin D deficiency
- Hyperparathyroidism
- Poor nutritional state, i.e. protein-energy malnutrition (PEM)
- Anaemia
- Systemic inflammation associated with CKD
- Decline in kidney function and the effects of dialysis itself.

The benefits of regular exercise

- ↑ exercise capacity
- ↓ cardiovascular risk and improve cardiovascular outcome:
  - improve BP control ∴ ↓ need for antihypertensive medications
- Improved diabetes control
- Improved HRQOL
- ↑ physical functioning and independence
- ↑ psychological well-being:
  - improvement in depression, stress, anxiety
- ± assist to attain desired weight reduction
- ↑ dialysis efficacy
- Improve neuromuscular symptoms, e.g. restless leg syndrome.

Barriers to exercise

Patient or healthcare professional barriers may influence how effectively a patient takes up an exercise programme. These are outlined in Table 17.1.

Table 17.1 Possible barriers to exercising

Patient perspective	Healthcare perspective
Usual lifestyle and choices	Management of other medical problems >priority
Previous experience with exercising—may not like/enjoy it	Non-exercise culture:
Time constraints	• Lack of commitment, enthusiasm, knowledge and skill
Health beliefs—adoption of 'sick-role':	
• Should not exercise with chronic condition; may exacerbate their condition, impact on dialysis treatment/Tx	Time constraints
	Resources:
• Cultural/religious belief, e.g. accept their 'fate'	• Lack of suitably trained staff
Physical/medical problems:	• Not an appropriate environment, e.g. space
• Lethargy, fatigue, pain	• No access to exercise equipment
• Osteoarthritis, back pain, musculoskeletal, obesity	• Overall staffing levels
Poor motivation and commitment	
Altered body image	
Postoperative recovery period, e.g. post Tx/PD insertion	

Contraindications

Absolute contraindications

- Uncontrolled cardiovascular disease:
  - unstable angina or cardiac event within last 6wks, e.g. MI
  - severe cardiac arrhythmia, possible or known aneurysm
  - uncontrolled BP
  - SBP >200mmHg and DBP >105mmHg
  - Uncontrolled resting tachycardia pulse ≥100bpm
- Acute infection/pyrexia >38°C
- Hyperkalaemia
- Uncontrolled diabetes
- Uncontrolled psychiatric condition
- Hypervolaemia, e.g. SOB, evidence of oedema
- Haemodynamically unstable during dialysis, e.g. ↓ BP
- Recovering from recent surgery/procedure, e.g. abdominal operation, recent Tx.

Relative contraindications

- Weight gain >5% of IBW in between HD treatments
- Symptomatic anaemia, arteriosclerotic CVD
- Symptomatic metabolic bone disease.

Exercise recommendations

KDOQI[6] and the UK Renal Association[7] recommend CKD and those people on dialysis should be encouraged to exercise for 30mins, 3–5 times/wk and where possible enrolled in a formal exercise programme. The Swedish National Institute of Public Health[8] has also produced guidance on the physical activity in the prevention and treatment of disease with reference to CKD. Tx recipients with well-functioning grafts should be able to return to normal exercise tolerance, other co-morbidities permitting, as part of a healthy living regimen. Weight gain due to immunosuppressant regimens and cardiovascular risk are significant risks to long-term post Tx outcomes.

Consideration should be given to:
- Referral to physical/occupational therapists, cardiac rehabilitation specialists, or clinical exercise physiologists who are specifically trained to manage chronic conditions where possible and appropriate
- Where possible the inclusion of exercise physiology/physiotherapy expertise in dialysis units
- Individualize exercise programme:
  - take in to consideration the diversity of fitness levels amongst older adults, other co-morbidities and modality of treatment, e.g. moderate intensity may for some be a slow walk, but for others, a brisk walk.

Physical exercise recommendations
- Include muscle strengthening, flexibility, and balance exercise:
  - *low level*—↑ physical activity by walking
  - *moderate intensity aerobic*—minimum of 30mins 5 days/wk
  - *vigorous intensity aerobic*—minimum of 20mins 3 days/wk
  - gradually increase to patient's ability, e.g. walking 10mins/day increasing to ≥30mins/day ≥3 days/wk
- A fitness programme should include any or all 3 types of these exercises:
  - flexibility exercise, e.g. gentle muscle stretching to improve flexibility and balance
  - strengthening exercise, e.g. resistance training (such as weights, elastic bands)
  - cardiovascular exercise, e.g. sustained, rhythmic movements of arms and/or legs (such as a stationary bike).

Nursing considerations

Physical exercise is only contraindicated in ~25% of those with CKD. If there are no medical contraindications, the person is not unwell or unwilling to exercise the following should be considered:

- Liaise with MPT team, e.g. physiotherapist, exercise physiologist, occupational therapist, dietitian, and social worker if support required
- Assess current fitness level and level of physical activity
- Liaise with GP to see if able to refer the person to an exercise programme or for cardiac rehabilitation programme if appropriate:
  - GPs also provide brief interventions such as verbal advice, counselling, use of pedometers, and walking and exercise programmes in the community
- Identify any barriers and address where possible
- Provide education and information on types of exercises in a variety of formats, e.g. leaflets, DVDs, posters
- Plan exercise programme with the person:
  - may require gradual increase in intensity and duration of exercise
  - set realistic goals and expectations with the person
- Advise the person to stop exercising if they develop any of the following and seek medical advice:
  - SOB, dizziness, nausea, leg cramps, excessively fatigued
  - chest pain and/or an irregular pulse/heart beat/pain or pressure in neck or jaw, blurred vision
- Assist those with diabetes to plan exercise around the right time of day, review of diabetes agents and BGLs, meal times and regular foot care
- Risk of tendonitis, preventative measures include:
  - extend the warm up and cool down period, include flexibility and stretching exercises
- Those with polycystic kidney disease should not do exercises that causes ↑ IAP exercise which may put them at risk of a mechanical injury to the kidney
- Exercise on dialysis should be low and moderate in intensity:
  - undertake during the 2nd or 3rd hr into treatment, close to IBW and less haemodynamic instability
  - aim to exercise for 30mins/dialysis treatment (may require gradual build-up to desired time)
  - monitor for signs and symptoms of over-exertion
- Assess people on dialysis for any alteration in body composition:
  - may need adjustment of IBW
- People on PD who undertake exercise that involves and ↑ IAP should:
  - exercise with an empty peritoneum if it is too uncomfortable with fluid *in situ* or causing SOB or those at risk or history of at hernia/have weak pelvic floor muscle
- Tx recipients—aim to initiate an exercise regimen to encourage a gradual ↑ to maximum exercise tolerance and independence.

Further reading

Castledine G, Close A (eds). *Oxford Handbook of Adult Nursing*. Oxford: Oxford University Press; 2009.

Kidney Research UK. *Living with kidney disease*. Available at: ℅ <http://www.kidneyresearchuk.org/health/living-with-kidney-disease-dvd.php>

Dementia

Tamura MK, Yaffe K. Dementia and cognitive impairment in ESRD: diagnostic and therapeutic strategies. *Kidney Int* 2011; **79**(1):14–22.

Pregnancy

Davison JM, Lindheimer MD. Pregnancy and chronic kidney disease. *Semin in Nephrol* 2011; **31**(1): 86–99.

Piccoli GB, Attini R, Vasario E, et al. Pregnancy and chronic kidney disease: a challenge in all CKD stages. *Clin J Am Soc Nephrol* 2010; **5**:844–55.

Transitional care

Department of Health. *Transition: moving on well*, 2008. Available at: ℅ <http://www.dh/gov/uk>

Department of Health. *Transition: getting it right for young people*, 2006. Available at: ℅ <http://www.dh/gov/uk>

Royal College of Nursing. *Adolescent Transition Care, Guidance for Nursing Staff*, 2004. Available at: ℅ <http://www.rcn.org.uk>

Violence and aggression

Burns T, Smyth A. Reducing aggression in the haemodialysis unit by improving the dialysis experience for patients. *RSA J* 2011; **7**(2):79–89. Available at: ℅ <http://www.rcn.org.uk>

Exercise

Bennett PN, Breugelmans L, Barnard R, et al. Sustaining a haemodialysis exercise program: A review. *Semin Dial* 2010; **23**(1):62–73.

Johansen KL. Exercise in the end-stage renal disease population. *Am J Kidney Dis* 2007; **18**:1845–54. Available at: ℅ <http://jasn.asnjournals.org/content/18/6/1845.full> (accessed 22 April 2012).

Johansen KL, Painter P. Exercise in individuals with CKD. *Am J Kidney Dis* 2012; **59**(1):126–34.

References

1. UK Health and Safety Executive (HSE). *Work related violence*. Available at: ℅ <http://www.hse.gov/violence/index.htm>

2. Department of Health. *You're welcome quality criteria: making health services young people friendly*, 2011. Available at: ℅ <http://www.dh/gov/uk>

3. Goldenring JM, Rosen DS. Getting into adolescent heads: an essential update. *Contemp Pediatr* 2004; **21**:64–90.

4. UK NKF. *Travel tips*. Available at: ℅ <http://www.kidney.org.uk/holidays/tips.html>

5. European Health Insurance Card. Available at: ℅ <http://www.nhs.uk/NHSEngland/Healthcareabroad/EHIC/Pages/about-the-ehic.aspx>

6. KDOQI. *Clinical Practice Guidelines for Cardiovascular disease in dialysis patients*, 2005. Available at: ℅ <http://www.kidney.org/professionals/kdoqi/guidelines_cvd/guide14.htm> (accessed 22 April 2012).

7. UK Renal Association. *Cardiovascular disease in CKD*, 5th edn. 2010. Available at: ℅ <http://www.renal.org/Libraries/Guidelines/Cardiovascular_Disease_in_CKD_-_FINAL_DRAFT_26_May_2010.sflb.ashx> (accessed 22 April 2012).

8. The Swedish National Institute of Public Health. Physical activity in the prevention and treatment of disease. Östersund: Professional Associations for Physical Activity; 2010. Available at: ℅ <http://www.fhi.se/en/Publications/All-publications-in-english/Physical-Activity-in-the-Prevention-and-Treatment-of-Desease> (accessed 23 April 2012).

Patient information websites

Dialysis freedom. Available at: ℳ <http://www.dialysisfreedom.co.uk>

EdRen Information: Available at: ℳ <http://www.edren.org/pages/edreninfo/pregnancy-and-contraception-in-renal-disease.php>

European Health Insurance Card. Available at: ℳ <http://www.nhs.uk/NHSEngland/Healthcareabroad/EHIC/Pages/about-the-ehic.aspx>

Global dialysis. Available at: ℳ <http://www.globaldialysis.com>

National Kidney Foundation. *Staying fit with kidney disease*. Available at: ℳ <http://www.kidney.org/atoz/pdf/stayfit.pdf>

Painter P. *A guide for people on dialysis*. Available at: ℳ <http://lifeoptions.org/catalog/pdfs/booklets/exercise.pdf>

The British Renal Society. *TIME programme: Exercise programme information for healthcare professionals*, 2007. Available at: ℳ <http://www.britishrenal.org/TIME/EXERCISE.aspx>

UK NKF. *Travel tips*. Available at: ℳ <http://www.kidney.org.uk/holidays/tips.html>

Renal pharmacology

Basic pharmacology

Drugs exert their therapeutic and toxic effects by acting on cells within the body. When a drug interacts with a cellular receptor, it initiates the chain of biochemical events leading to a drug's effects.

- An agonist is any substance that switches a receptor on and initiates cellular activity
- A substance that turns off a receptor is an antagonist or blocker.

Drug metabolism

The kidneys play a large role in the elimination of many drugs from the body, and as kidney function declines, the amount of drug excreted can reduce dramatically. In addition, the way drugs are handled within the body can be markedly affected, which is also affected by dialysis.

- Patients with renal impairment (includes both CKD and AKI) can therefore require different doses of certain medications compared with the general population
- How the drug is absorbed, distributed, metabolized, and excreted can all be affected in renal impairment and dialysis, so each of these factors need to be taken into consideration
- An accurate assessment of kidney function is required prior to making a decision about drug dosage.

Absorption

Drug absorption may be affected in renal impairment. The doses of drugs are not routinely altered to take absorption into account, but if quick onset is required, the dose or route of administration may need to be changed.

Causes of poor absorption

- Nausea (and resultant non-adherence) and vomiting 2° to uraemia
- Diarrhoea
- Medication that alters the pH of the gut
- Fluid overload causing GI tract mucosal changes ('boggy-gut').

Distribution

Drug distribution varies and drugs may:

- Remain free (unbound) in the plasma
- Bind onto plasma proteins, e.g.:
  - Alb: ↓ serum Alb → ↑ free drug and ↑ side effects, particularly a problem if a drug is >80% protein bound, e.g. phenytoin or warfarin
  - uraemia: ↓ drug binding of drugs to plasma proteins → ↑ free drug which may cause toxicity
  - ⚠ care must be taken when interpreting drug blood levels to take account of the ↑ in free drug, which can cause toxicity since total (bound + free) drug concentrations are often reported and not active free drug levels
- Bind on to other tissues:
  - tissue binding can also be affected, and these alterations may affect the volume of distribution of a drug

- e.g. digoxin as in uraemia → ↑ displacement of digoxin from skeletal muscle sites by metabolic waste, ∴ ↓ volume of distribution and ↑ amount of free drug available to cause toxicity
- Absorbed into fat deposits around the body.

Effects of extracellular fluid volume

Marked oedema or dehydration may affect levels of certain drugs.
- The excess fluid present in oedema will tend to dilute drugs
- In dehydration, drugs will become more concentrated
- In practice this only affects drugs with a small volume of distribution (vd <50L), e.g. gentamicin.

Metabolism

Many drugs are metabolized in the liver by a series of enzymes, for example, the cytochrome P450 monooxygenase system, and this process is generally unchanged in CKD. The kidneys metabolize a few drugs and this may be slower in CKD leading to increased drug levels and toxicity. Consideration should be given to vitamin D supplementation (see 📖 p. 194) or insulin requirements.

- The kidney converts 25-hydroxycholecalciferol to the active form of vitamin D 1α,25-dihydroxycholecalciferol:
  - vitamin D supplementation—either the active drug (calcitriol) or a preparation requiring metabolism by the liver, i.e. 1α-hydroxycholecalciferol (alfacalcidol).

Elimination

The kidneys are responsible for the elimination of many drugs and their metabolites. As kidney function declines the amount of drug or metabolite that is eliminated is reduced and will accumulate in the body, possibly causing side effects. With some drugs, it is the pharmacologically active metabolite which accumulates and causes side effects, e.g. pethidine → norpethidine causing CNS stimulation or seizures.

Prescribing in renal impairment

When deciding on drug dosage it is important to take into consideration that most drug companies use CrCl and not eGFR for advice on drug doses. For most drugs there is guidance giving a range of doses according to the level of kidney function.

Ideal characteristics

Ideally, drugs with the following characteristics should be used in patients with renal impairment:
- Large therapeutic index
- Low adverse effect profile
- Not highly protein bound
- Non-nephrotoxic
- Unaffected by fluid balance
- No renal excretion of active drug or metabolites
- Action unaffected by altered tissue sensitivity
- Can be given in a small volume if given IV.

Drug dosage

Once a drug has been chosen that meets as many of these criteria as possible, guidance on dosing should be sought from the drug's summary of product characteristics and from one of the widely available renal drug dosing reference sources.[1,2]
- If loading dose required, may be lower in CKD
- Maintenance doses and the dosing frequency will depend on the level of kidney function
- The alterations required tend to be drug specific, depending on the therapeutic effect desired, and the toxicity profile of that drug.

Examples of dose adjustments:
- Allopurinol:
  - ↓ drug dose from 300mg to 100mg daily
- Vancomycin:
  - dose tends to remain the same at 500–1000mg
  - adjust in time between doses from 12hrs to once every 2–3 days.

Drugs removed during dialysis

Some drugs are removed from the body during dialysis.
- If a drug is removed by dialysis, the drug should be given post dialysis
- If the drug is to be given during dialysis, the dose should be administered as close to the end of dialysis as possible or during washback
- The type of dialysis used will also affect how much drug is removed:
  - vancomycin is removed by HDF and high-flux HD, but not by low-flux HD or CAPD
  - metronidazole is not removed by CAPD but is removed by low-flux and high-flux HD and HDF

Drugs administered intraperitoneally (IP)

Some drugs can be administered IP, e.g. antibiotics to treat peritonitis, or heparin to prevent or reduce fibrin. Information on giving drugs in this way can be found in the *Renal Drug Handbook*.[1]

⚠ Doses of drugs may vary according to local protocols.

Dose alterations and caution

Drugs with the following features require caution in renal impairment:
- Excreted by the kidney
- A narrow therapeutic index
- Nephrotoxic:
  - ⚠ with reduced kidney function, the use of drugs which are nephrotoxic should be avoided if at all possible
  - using a nephrotoxic drug in an anuric patient with ESKD receiving dialysis, will not cause any further damage to the kidneys
  - ⚠ need to be aware of other side effects e.g. gentamicin is nephrotoxic but is also ototoxic. Incorrect dosing in a patient with no kidney function can still lead to irreversible loss of hearing and vestibular damage
- Possess toxic side effects.

Drug-induced kidney damage can be caused by:
- ATN: aminoglycosides, NSAIDs, ciclosporin, digoxin, phenytoin, quinolones
- Interstitial nephritis: allopurinol, azathioprine, ACEIs, vancomycin
- Crystaluria: methotrexate, aciclovir
- GN: ACEIs, NSAIDs, penicillin.

Drugs that require monitoring

ACEI and ARB

- ACEI and ARB can cause a decline in kidney function which should be measured before commencing therapy and with dosage increases (see 🕮 pp. 92–3 for side effects, monitoring, and management).

NSAIDs

- Avoid NSAIDs if at all possible
- Particularly avoid in combination with ACEI because of the ↑ risk of nephrotoxicity and hyperkalaemia:
  - check kidney function 48–72hrs after starting and discontinue therapy if ↑ serum Cr >30%, or ↓ eGFR >25%
- NSAIDs should be used with caution in uraemic patients who are predisposed to GI bleeding.

Analgesics

- Avoid compound analgesics
- Weak opioids (e.g. tramadol or dihydrocodeine), observe for side effects and notify medical staff
- Stronger opiates, e.g. hydromorphone or oxycodone —commence on low dose and titrate as they have a prolonged half-life.
  ⚠ Observe for any adverse effects, e.g. nausea, vomiting, constipation,

itching, sweating, dry mouth, drowsiness, hallucinations, respiratory depression, myoclonus, and notify medical staff.

Antibiotics

With antibiotic therapy, a high dose is generally required to achieve effective bactericidal blood levels but, at the same time, it is important to avoid potentially toxic side effects. It is necessary to be aware of those antibiotics that are excreted via the kidneys and likely to have toxic side effects.

- Amoxicillin is excreted via the kidneys, but is generally used in normal doses because it is not particularly toxic. However, ceftazidime can readily cause seizures, so the dose interval must be ↑ from 8hrs to 24hrs to avoid accumulation and toxicity

Awareness of polypharmacy

Patients with renal impairment often take many drugs, e.g. 2–3 of antihypertensives, diuretics, phosphate binders, aspirin, PPI, statins, iron tablets. It is important to be aware of potential drug interactions.

- E.g. phosphate binders will tend to bind to iron tablets in the gut and prevent the iron from being absorbed into the body. They should be taken at least 1hr apart
- Alternatively, a patient may be stable on a given drug regimen, and then another drug is added which may affect the drugs they are already taking:
  - e.g. kidney Tx recipient who is already taking IS drugs ciclosporin, azathioprine, and prednisolone, then develops gout and is prescribed allopurinol There is an interaction between allopurinol and azathioprine → large ↑ in blood levels of azathioprine which can cause severe bone marrow suppression.

Generic medicines

A generic medicine contains the same active ingredient and has the equivalent efficacy of the original brand which no longer holds the patent. These medicines still undergo all of the safety and quality requirements as the original product. These drugs may be substantially cheaper to purchase than the original.

- For the majority of drugs, the generic version produces exactly the same clinical effect, and is ∴ fully interchangeable with the original, e.g. antihypertensives, prednisolone, azathioprine, mycophenolate mofetil
- For some drugs, where there is a narrow therapeutic range, the generic drugs are not interchangeable, e.g. ciclosporin, tacrolimus, epileptic medicines.

⚠ Those drugs that are not interchangeable should be prescribed by brand.

Biosimilar medicinal products

Biosimilars are biological products which are similar, but not exactly the same as the original product on the market, e.g. subsequent versions of erythropoietin, growth hormone, that are made by a different company.

▶Not necessarily interchangeable as may have different therapeutic effect.

Herbal medicines

There are many herbal remedies available which are not subject to the same vigorous testing as pharmaceuticals. Some of these have been proven to be harmful to the kidney and some interact with other medications patients may be taking. When looking at the drugs that patients are taking, they should be asked if they take any OTC products or herbal remedies. There are numerous herbal remedies which have adverse effects for those with CKD. For example:

- Aristolochia is commonly used in Chinese herbal remedy and has been proven to cause irreversible damage to kidneys
- St John's wort is a herbal remedy for depression that can interact with medications, reducing their efficacy, e.g. simvastatin, ciclosporin.

The UK Medicines Health products Regulatory Authority (MHRA) have developed a certification process with the aim of regulating herbal remedies. If a traditional herbal remedy (THR) carries a MHRA certification mark, it indicates the herbal medicine has been registered and met with the required safety and quality standards (however, the remedy may still be nephrotoxic or interact with other medications).[4]

⚠ Patients should be advised not to take any herbal remedy unless they have discussed it with their pharmacist or doctor. There are some useful websites which have information on many herbal medicines, however they do not cover all those available.[5–7]

Key points

- Avoid nephrotoxic drugs in CKD and AKI:
  - if these drugs are necessary, keep the course as short as possible
  - monitor kidney function closely.
- Choose a drug with the characteristics listed on 📖 p. 568 if possible
- Assess the degree of renal impairment and adjust the dose accordingly; refer to the *Renal Drug Handbook*[1]
  - ▶ the drug companies' information is based on renal function calculated using Cockcroft and Gault formula rather than MDRD
- For a patient on RRT, time administration of the drug after dialysis, depending on the type of dialysis and the extent to which the drug is removed
- For the majority of drugs, the general principle is to start with a low dose and ↑ slowly to obtain the desired response whilst monitoring the patient for side effects
- Avoid drugs that interact with drugs that the patient is already taking
- For drugs with a narrow therapeutic range, take blood levels after an appropriate time and interpret the levels carefully to ensure that dose adjustments are made correctly
- The prescriber should use the simplest regimen possible
- Keep the number of drugs prescribed to a minimum
- Use once-daily dosing wherever feasible to aid adherence.

Medicines adherence

In 2005, a report from the National Co-ordinating Centre for NHS delivery and organization of research and development (R&D) suggested that between a third and half of medicines prescribed are not taken as intended for long-term conditions.[3] This has both an effect on the patient's health and well-being and the healthcare provider's costs (see 📖 pp. 540–1 for adherence issues). This can be for a variety of reasons and can be intentional or unintentional.

Interventions to promote medication adherence

- Patient-centred care:
  - individualized approach and involve the patient in decisions about their medication to the level they prefer, provide the aims, side effects, risks and benefits of the medicine
  - assess the patient's ability to make decisions regarding their health, e.g. cognitive impairment, mental health problems
  - effective communications skills supported by educational materials at a level appropriate for the patient. Involve the family/carer where the patient agrees, to enable them to be involved in the decision-making process and support management and administration if required
  - non-judgemental approach and accept that some patients will not accept advice on taking a medicine
  - review the patient's knowledge, understanding, and concerns on their medicines regularly
  - provide positive feedback and encouragement to those who are adherent
- Assessing adherence:
  - ask questions about their medicines using a non-blame approach and provide an explanation of why you are asking, e.g. have they missed any doses in the last week?
  - review repeat prescription record liaising with the pharmacy to identify those patients who require additional support
- Interventions to increase adherence:
  - discuss with the patient the reason/s for not taking their medicines, e.g. concerns about side effect, health beliefs (intentional non-adherence), or impracticalities of taking the medicine (unintentional adherence)
  - individualize interventions, e.g. discuss their concerns, offer appropriate support and education, minimize complexity if possible, use of multicompartmental systems, adjust dose or drug where possible if causing unwanted side effects, alter timing of medicines, diary to monitor taking their medicines
- Good communication between healthcare professionals regarding patients medicines, e.g. transfer between health services.

Non-medical prescribing

Non-medical prescribing refers to specially trained nurses, optometrists, pharmacists, physiotherapists, podiatrists, and radiographers who work within their competence as either an independent or supplementary prescriber.

Three types of non-medical prescriber

Independent prescriber
- Autonomous, prescribes independently from the *British National Formulary* (BNF)
- Other than medical personnel, only nurses, pharmacists, and optometrists can currently train to become independent prescribers:
  - may prescribe any licensed medicine; however, it must be within their training and clinical competence
  - restrictions include prescribing some controlled drugs and blood products
  - may prescribe blood clotting factors, albumin, and antibodies as they are considered to be medicinal products
- Nurse prescribers may give directions for the administration of drugs for a condition which is within his/her competence:
  - the provision is that the nurse is satisfied that the person they are giving the instructions to is competent to administer the prescribed medicine.

Community practitioner nurse prescriber (CPNP)
E.g. district nurse, health visitor, or school nurse.
- Independently prescribe from a limited formulary called the Nurse Prescribers' Formulary for Community Practitioners found in the BNF.

Supplementary prescriber
- Involves the prescribing of medicines in line with a clinical management plan which has been agreed between the supplementary prescriber, doctor and patient
- Medicines can be given by another professional with the instructions of an independent prescriber or via a local arrangement.

Benefits of non-medical prescribing
- Utilize the skills and expertise of a group of professionals
- To improve patient access to medicines, advice, and treatment across the NHS
- Enhance patient care; improve patient choice without compromising patient safety
- Provide a flexible service for patients
- To contribute to more flexible team working across the NHS
- Nurses working with CKD patients have autonomy to manage patients more efficiently and in a timely manner.

Further reading

Beckwith S, Franklin P. *Oxford Handbook of Nurse Prescribing*. Oxford: Oxford University Press; 2007.

References

1. Ashley C, Currie A. *Renal Drug Handbook*, 3rd edn. Oxford: Radcliffe Medical Press; 2009. Available at: ℛ <http://xa.yimg.com/kq/groups/16749867/1032282199/name/Renal+Drug+Handbook.pdf> (accessed 29 April 2012).
2. Bennet WM, Aronoff GR, Berns JS, et al. *Drug Prescribing in Renal Failure*, 5th edn. Philadelphia, PA: American College of Physicians; 2007.
3. NICE. *Medicines adherence: involving patients in decisions about prescribed medicines and supporting adherence*. Clinical guideline CG79. London: NICE; 2009. Available at: ℛ <http://www.nice.org.uk>
4. MHRA. *Herbal medicine advice for consumers*. London: MHRA; 2012. Available at: ℛ <http://www.mhra.gov.uk/Safetyinformation/Generalsafetyinformationandadvice/Herbalmedicines/index.htm> (accessed 29 April 2012).
5. British Herbal Medicine Association. Available at: ℛ <http://www.bhma.info/resources/links.html> (accessed 6 May 2012).
6. National Kidney Foundation. *Use of herbal supplements in chronic kidney disease*. Available at ℛ <http://www.kidney.org/atoz/content/herbalsupp.cfm> (accessed 6 May 2012).
7. Patient.co.uk. *Alternative/complementary therapy*, 2012. Available at: ℛ <http://www.patient.co.uk/showdoc/6/> (accessed 26 April 2012).

Useful websites

British National Formulary. Available at: ℛ <http://www.bnf.org>

Department of Health. *Non-medical prescribing programme*. Available at: ℛ <http://www.dh.gov.uk/en/Healthcare/Medicinespharmacyandindustry/Prescriptions/TheNon-MedicalPrescribingProgramme/index.htm>

National Prescribing Centre. *Non-medical prescribing*. Available at: ℛ <http://www.npc.nhs.uk/non_medical/>

Nursing and Midwifery Council (NMC). *Medicines and prescribing*. Available at: ℛ <http://www.nmc-uk.org/Nurses-and-midwives/Prescribing>

Nursing admission and discharge

Nursing admission and discharge

Ward admission

In addition to routine admission procedure, all kidney patients admitted to the ward should have the following undertaken:

- Baseline haemodynamic observations including lying and standing BP to identify any postural drop, hypo- or hypertension
- Weight and height—calculate BMI:
  - ⚠ not as accurate if patient is fluid overloaded
- Urinalysis and normal urine volume if still passing urine (see 📖 pp. 52–6)
- Identification of special dietary requirements e.g. diabetes, low protein, and referral to the renal dietitian
- List of current medications
- Cancel social services if required
- Referrals to MPT, e.g. renal social worker, dietitian, renal specialist nurses (anaemia, PD, HD, CKD, Tx/AKC nurse, nurse consultant, access etc), pharmacist, renal counsellor, CMT.

  Additional requirements dependant on renal status: AKI, CKD stage, RRT modality.

Routine investigations on admission

Bloods

- FBC and ESR:
  - If Hb <11g/dl, check haematinics (% TSAT, ferritin, or % HRC, B_{12}, folate)
- U&Es/eGFR, HCO_3, Alb
- Lipid profile (preferably fasting), glucose, LFTs, TFTs, CRP, HbA1c (if known diabetic)
- Bone profile, i.e. Ca^{2+}, PO_4, PTH if stage 4 or 5 if no prior result available <6 months.

Urine

- Urinalysis:
  - MSU if UTI suspected to exclude UTI or inflammation
  - ACR may be requested if proteinuria present
- Kidney US
- MRSA swabs
- Other investigations that may be required:
  - Serum and urinary electrophoresis
  - Urine electrolytes
  - CRP
  - ANA, anti-GBM antibody, ANCA, cryoglobulins, Rh factor
  - Hepatitis B, C, and HIV testing if requires RRT
  - Kidney biopsy (see 📖 pp. 62–3).

Ward discharge

It is important to ensure adequate discharge planning and preparation is commenced on the day of admission. Involve a discharge co-ordinator and/or social worker if available. Prior to discharge ensure the following are completed:

- Adequate supply of medications/prescriptions/dressings (if required)
- Education about fluid allowance/target weight/care, medications and management of access
- Anaemia team notified of discharge and supply of ESAs organized
- District nurse/social services referral sent and organized if required
- If supportive care or withdrawal from dialysis decided as management plan, ensure renal palliative care team are notified and have seen the patient prior to discharge:
  - if DNACPR in place ensure patient has a copy to take home
- Liaise with care managers/renal social worker if required
- Notify social services if required to resume services
- Liaise with family/carer regarding discharge date, follow-up, and support in place
- Liaise with other nursing teams who have ongoing responsibility for the patient (i.e. dialysis unit/Tx clinic) and ensure appropriate follow-up arrangements/outpatient appointments if required are in place
- Transport booked for HD or follow-up appointments if required
- Patient has a copy of the discharge summary/updated list of medications:
  - copy has been sent electronically to the GP.

Specific issues

- HD unit notified of discharge and next dialysis session booked—transport booked if required
- PD fluid ordered and delivery confirmed if required and confirmed discharge with PD nursing staff
- Nursing home or interhospital patients have a discharge transfer letter
- Community renal home visit organized, e.g. PD patient/palliative patient
- Suspended from Tx list if required and Tx team notified of discharge.

Renal pathophysiology

Pathophysiology

Acquired cystic disease (ACD)
Occurs in people on long-term dialysis; multiple small cysts in kidney cortex and medulla. ↑ risk of renal cell carcinoma (RCC) (5–30x).

Acute post infectious
Group B-haemolytic streptococcal infection post URTI or skin infection is more common in children (<7yrs of age), though now uncommon in developed countries. Presents ~2wks post infection and causes diffuse proliferative GN with children usually going on to have a full recovery. Causes of non-streptococcal GN include toxoplasmosis, syphilis, influenza B, schistosomiasis and plasmodium, viral infections, e.g. Epstein–Barr, Hepatitis B, coxsackie viruses.

Alport's syndrome
X-linked disease mainly in ♂ usually presents in early adulthood, → ESKD by the age of 40yrs. ♀ tend to be carriers and have asymptomatic microscopic haematuria. Abnormality in basement membrane collagen IV → glomerulosclerosis and tubulo-interstitial scarring. Thin GBM seen on kidney biopsy. Present with microscopic haematuria, ↑ BP, proteinuria (± nephrotic), progressive renal impairment, sensorineural deafness, lenticonus, platelet dysfunction, and hyperproteinaemia.

Analgesic nephropathy (AN)
Previously, one of the most common causes of ESKD in Europe, Australia, and the USA due to the availability of OTC phenacetin (withdrawn ~30yrs ago). Mostly affecting ♀ aged 30–70yrs on regular analgesics, e.g. for headaches/lower back pain. Mechanism not completely known—vascular and toxic effects → papillary necrosis and chronic interstitial nephritis. Also caused by aspirin ± paracetamol usage. May be asymptomatic, NAD urinalysis or sterile pyuria and/or mild proteinuria, flank pain, or microscopic haematuria.

Fabry's syndrome
X-linked disorder, presents in early childhood. The enzyme galactosidase is either deficient/ineffective which affects glycoprotein metabolism → build-up of the glycolipid ceramide trihexoside in the kidneys, skin, and vascular system. May present with pain and paraesthesia of the extremities, ↑ BP, cardiomyopathy, angiokeratomas (dark reddish/purple skin lesions), anhidrosis (inadequate sweating), proteinuria, and renal impairment.

Goodpasture's syndrome (anti-GBM disease)
Rare disease, involves IgG anti-GBM antibody production to the antigen in the GBM → rapidly progressive crescentic GN. May also cause pulmonary haemorrhage as it affects the pulmonary capillaries → poor prognosis. Affects ♂ aged 20–30yrs and ♀ >60yrs. Specific diagnostic investigations include biopsy, lung function tests, and the presence of ANCA and anti-GBM antibodies. Presentation may be acute (few days)/months to yrs with fever, weight loss, dyspnoea, cough, haemoptysis, respiratory failure,

anaemia. proteinuria, haematuria and AKI. May recur in a transplanted kidney.

Haemolytic uraemic syndrome (HUS)

This is the most common cause of AKI in children (usually in the summer) who present with flu-like symptoms or a GI infection (70–80% caused by *Escherichia coli*). In children, damage develops in the vascular endothelium 2° to an inflammatory reaction. In adults, deposits of fibrin attach to the capillary walls → narrowing of the blood vessels and thrombi formation in the capillaries and small blood vessels. Presents with:

- Microangiopathic haemolytic anaemia, intravascular haemolysis
- Renal impairment, sudden onset of oliguria, haematuria, ↑ BP
- Diarrhoea, ± melaena, fever
- ↓ platelets with normal clotting
- Other organs may be affected, e.g. heart, brain.

Causes include:

- Pre-eclampsia, infections e.g. typhoid, *Escherichia coli*, salmonella (food poisoning), campylobacter, drugs (e.g. ciclosporin, ciprofloxacin, tacrolimus, heparin, combined OCP)
- Associated with cancer, with a mortality rate of 16–25%
- Rare inherited type which is related to a deficiency on factor H (glycoprotein) and known as atypical HUS.

Henoch–Schönlein purpura (HSP)

One of the most common childhood vasculitides seen is HSP post URTI (common in winter) with 2♂:1♀ affected. It is usually lasts a few months presenting with a purpuric rash. Immune complex deposits of IgA which cause inflammation to small vessels. Adults tend to have kidney involvement and require long-term follow-up of kidney function whereas children usually make a full recovery. Presents with abdominal symptoms of colic (e.g. vomiting, abdominal pain), GI bleeding (bowel vasculitis), polyarthralgia, purpuric rash to legs, buttocks, and arms, haematuria, proteinuria, renal impairment, ↑ BP (related to IgAN).

Infective endocarditis

Most commonly left-sided heart valves (mitral valve). Right-sided infections associated with IV drug users (tricuspid valve). Can occur in native/ prosthetic valves; pre-disposing factors include:

- History of rheumatic fever, recurrent bacteraemia, valvular heart disease, prosthetic valves, IV drug use and invasive procedures, e.g. dental
- Common organism: acute endocarditis—*Streptococcus viridans* (post dental), chronic endocarditis—*Staphylococcus aureus*, *S. epidermis* or coagulase −ve staphylococci
- Associated complications include post-infectious immune complex-mediated GN, aminoglycoside-induced ATN, renal emboli from an infected valve and drug-induced AIN, presenting with ↑ Cr, NAD urinalysis, fever/rigors, rash, flank pain (indicate emboli), ± haematuria.

Malaria

Various plasmodium species are responsible and cause 1–3 million deaths per year. *Plasmodium falciparum* (Indian) and *P. malariae* (Africa) are the 2 species of parasite that can cause kidney disease:

• Present with post-infectious GN affecting up to 18% of cases
• Treatment usually results in full recovery.

Acute malarial nephropathy

Associated with *P. falciparum*; occurs in 1–4% of cases in endemic regions, more commonly in non-immune travellers. Presents with fever, headache, confusion, nausea, vomiting, diarrhoea, hepatosplenomegaly, anaemia, jaundice, myalgia (± progress to rhabdomyolysis, see 📖 p. 102), ↓ BP, peripheral vasodilation, oliguria, haematuria, proteinuria. ATN >50% require acute HD; mortality rate of ~10%.

Pelvic–ureteric junction (PUJ) and vesico-ureteric junction (VUJ) obstruction

Common congenital abnormalities present with flank pain after drinking alcohol, coffee, or taking diuretics, i.e. anything that promotes diuresis.

• PUJ obstruction—mostly affects both kidneys due to abnormal flow of urine from the pelvis to the ureter → 'baggy pelvis'; usually diagnosed antenatally
• VUJ obstruction—urine cannot pass from the ureter into the bladder → enlarged ureter 'megaureter'
• PUJ and VUJ have the same symptoms.

Renal amyloidosis

A multi-organ disease involving the deposition of amyloid (a variety of protein aggregates) causing organ failure and death.

• Deposits in the kidney occur in glomeruli, tubules, and vasculature.
• Range from asymptomatic proteinuria to nephrotic syndrome ± renal impairment
• Lethargy, weight loss
• Prone to bleeding/bruising (e.g. GI bleed)
• Heart failure, cardiomyopathy, and neuropathy

There are 3 types:

• 1° (AL): glomerular deposits: twice as common in ♂ >50yrs with a poor prognosis, presenting with heavy proteinuria or nephritic syndrome, monoclonal gammopathy serum ± urine
• 2° or reactive (AA): associated with inflammatory diseases e.g. rheumatoid arthritis (~40%), ankylosing spondylitis, psoriatic arthritis, inflammatory bowel disease, familial Mediterranean fever, TB, and some neoplasms
• Hereditary/familial: autosomally dominant; occurs in middle age/later. Less common than AA or AL (10%). Variable levels of severity.

Renal cell carcinoma (RCC)

RCC (adenocarcinoma) accounts for 80–85% of 1° renal cancer (5♂:3♀). Usually an incidental finding affecting one/both kidneys; strong association with smoking. 25% of cases have metastases at first diagnosis, e.g. bone, lung, nodes, liver, brain. May be asymptomatic or have flank or back pain radiating into the groin (with large tumour), ↑ BP, microscopic haematuria, palpable mass, varicocoele in ♂, ± paraneoplastic syndrome which includes fever (± night sweats), cachexia, anaemia, ↑ Ca^{2+}, liver dysfunction (ascites), peripheral oedema, polymyalgia, erythrocytosis, amyloid deposits.

- Complications include haemorrhage, infection, ± kidney obstruction
- Tumours staged according to tumours metastasis nodes (TMN) classification (4 stages), with T1 5yr survival 90%; in metastatic disease 5yr survival is <10%
- Wilms' tumour—common in young children; good prognosis (5yr survival is 90%).

Renal tuberculosis

TB is caused by the *Mycobacterium tuberculosis* organism; commonly affects the lungs. Affects ~8–10 million people/yr, ↑ risk with ethnic minorities in developed countries, the elderly, and HIV sufferers.

- Genito-urinary (GU): caused by 1° infection of GU tract/ 2° infection as a result of military TB:
  - usually affects both kidneys and all GU tract
- Kidney: medulla, pelvis, and papillae → scarring and calcification
- Diagnosis is made on 3 AFB EMU, IVU, changes on CXR ± symptoms
- General symptoms include weight loss, night sweats, and fever. May be ± asymptomatic (incidental finding) or dysuria, frequency, haematuria, urgency or incontinence (bladder fibrosis), flank or back pain, lower abdominal pain and prone to opportunistic UTIs.

Tuberculosis (TB) interstitial nephritis

Chronic interstitial nephritis common (see 📖 p. 23). Seen commonly in south Asians. Diagnosis is made on kidney biopsy. ↑ Cr, NAD urinalysis, −ve EMU for AFBs, TB skin test +ve though remain asymptomatic.

Schistosomiasis

Infection with water-borne fluke (trematodes) affects ~200 million people worldwide. Usually travellers and children living in endemic areas → urinary tract disease or GN. The fluke enters the body via the skin (causes 'swimmer's itch' a localized dermatitis/rash) and the mature worm releases its eggs into the blood vessels → inflammation of localized tissue (granulomatous) → GN (see 📖 p. 8).

Clinical features

- Urinary: caused by *Schistosoma haematobium* can cause ureteric strictures and obstruction (~10% of cases), bladder fibrosis or detrusor muscle problems
- Chronic infection: includes macroscopic haematuria (seen at the end of voiding), dysuria, frequency 2° inflammatory cystitis, opportunistic bacterial infection, bladder calculi and obstruction and there is an associated ↑ risk of bladder cancer
- Renal: caused by σ. *mansoni* or 2° salmonella infections in σ. *haematobium* and is not as common (~10–15%), presenting with

microalbuminuria, ± normal kidney function or renal impairment (MCGN, see 📖 p. 14) and can lead to ESKD in severe cases.

Sickle cell nephropathy

Occurs in ~4–8% of those with sickle cell disease; presents with FSGS, MPGN-like (see 📖 pp. 13–14) predominantly affects patients with sickle cell disease but may occur in sickle cell trait patients. Renal symptoms include nocturia, polyuria, asymptomatic haematuria, macroscopic haematuria, proteinuria, and painful clots → ureteric obstruction, RVT, rhabdomyolysis, AKI 2° volume depletion (see 📖 p. 100).

Thin basement membrane disease (TBMD)

Autosomal dominant familial disease → defect of collagen type IV → thinning of the GBM. Microscopic haematuria in ~5% of the UK population and TBMD accounts for 20–40% of cases. Diagnosis is made on kidney biopsy, may be asymptomatic or have microscopic haematuria with no renal impairment or hypertension.

Thrombotic microangiopathies

Fibrin lines the glomerular capillaries → ischaemia with no immunoglobulin deposit or complement activation.

Causes include:
- Systemic vasculitis
- Haemolytic uraemic syndrome (HUS)
- Disseminated intravascular (DIC)
- Pre-eclampsia
- Thrombotic thrombocytopenic purpura (TTP)
- SLE, rheumatoid
- HIV, malignancy
- Malignant hypertension
- Antiphospholipid syndrome.

Thrombotic thrombocytopenic purpura (TTP)

Clinical features include fever, CNS symptoms e.g. ↓ vision, ↓ consciousness, fits, microangiopathic haemolytic anaemia (often with jaundice), thrombocytopenia, renal impairment, haematuria and proteinuria oliguria, anuria, ±↑ BP, abdominal pain, arrhythmias, vomiting.

Causes include:
- Genetic abnormality of von Willebrand factor → platelet aggregation and fibrin deposits in small blood vessels, → microthrombi formation
- Drug related, e.g. ticlopidine, clopidogrel, ciclosporin, quinine
- Pregnancy
- HIV
- SLE
- Shigella, *Escherichia coli* colitis.

Fluid and electrolytes

Introduction

In terms of weight, 45–74% of the human body is H_2O. Thin individuals ∴ contain a ↑ proportion of H_2O because of ↓ flesh weight. The balance of H_2O and Na^+ content in the body is regulated 'in tandem' to maintain normal osmolality of 285–295mosmol/kg.

Glomerular level

In the glomerulus, H_2O and ions are filtered freely from the blood. The ionic component of the remaining filtrate is reabsorbed within the kidney tubules.

- Rate of H_2O reabsorption is regulated by both the osmotic gradient that is created and the permeability of the tubular epithelium
- Within the highly H_2O permeable proximal tubule, reabsorption of H_2O and filtrate is isotonic
- Energy is used to pump Na^+ across the epithelium out of the tubule; H_2O follows by osmosis
- About 65% of the initial filtrate is reabsorbed at this stage.

Sodium and chloride

- Na^+ and Cl^- are actively transported out of the thick-walled ascending limb of the loop of Henle (LoH) into the interstitium → ↑ interstitial osmolality
- H_2O is drawn from the highly H_2O permeable descending limb of LoH,
- reabsorption rate of Na^+ and Cl^- is > than reabsorption of H_2O within the LoH → in more dilute urine
- Hypertonicity of the interstitium ↑ towards bend in the LoH
- Within the distal tubule more ions, but no H_2O, are reabsorbed
- The resulting ↑ concentrated urine enters the collecting duct; permeability and ∴ reabsorption of H_2O, is controlled by ADH
- ADH secretion is controlled by osmoreceptors in the hypothalamus and baroreceptors (which detect BP) in the major blood vessels.
- ↑ in plasma osmolality (dehydration) → ADH stimulating ↑ H_2O reabsorption in the collecting ducts. Fluid overload and ↓ osmolality has the opposite effect.

Fluid is divided into 3 compartments in the body:
- Intracellular (~45% of body weight)
- Extracellular (17%):
  - interstitial fluid (12.5%)
  - plasma fluid (4.5%).

H_2O is retained in the circulating plasma by the osmotic influence of proteins (e.g. Alb) and other electrolytes (e.g. Na^+).
- If plasma Alb or Na^+ ↓ (e.g. in malnutrition, proteinuria, diarrhoea and vomiting), plasma osmolality ↓ → osmosis of H_2O from plasma → ↑ volume of interstitial fluid → oedema, i.e. person may be fluid replete but H_2O is in the wrong body compartment.

CKD and AKI

Kidney function is disrupted and fluid balance needs to be actively managed. Euvolaemia (correct amount of body fluid) in CKD/AKI is often affected by hypo- or hypervolaemia (dehydration or fluid overload). Euvolaemia in kidney patients is described as IBW or 'dry weight'. Correct assessment of fluid status is a key renal nursing skill.

Assessment of fluid balance

Essential in the management of patients with kidney disease and must be undertaken by an experienced nurse or doctor.

▶ A patient may present with fluid overload despite a ↓ circulating fluid volume, e.g. in nephrotic syndrome; ↓ plasma oncotic pressure → severe oedema but ↓ circulating volume. Assessment of fluid status includes:

- History
- Physical examination
- Haemodynamic state
- Changes detected visually or by touch
- Weight
- Auscultation
- CXR
- Blood tests
- Fluid balance charts.

Assessment characteristics will depend upon the patient, their condition and where they are being cared for, e.g.:

- Nephrology ward: daily assessment of hydration and IBW; may change rapidly
- HD unit: prior to and following HD. IBW is likely to remain constant for weeks at a time (see 📖 pp. 336 and 470 for fluid management).

History

- Identifies possible causes of fluid imbalance, e.g. dehydration 2° to recent diarrhoea and/or nausea/vomiting; diuretic use; fluid overload due to oliguria/anuria
- ↑ thirst may be ≈dehydration; ↑ SOB ≈fluid overloaded
- Dehydration → cramps, muscle weakness and confusion
- ▶ Other causes of signs and symptoms should be excluded
- Fatigue/confusion:
  - uraemia
  - anaemia
  - dementia
- Breathlessness:
  - exacerbation of asthma
  - COPD.

Physical assessment

All signs and symptoms of fluid status must be taken into account to ensure assessment of hydration is accurate.

▶ Haemodynamic status is a good baseline indicator of hydration status.

Blood pressure and pulse

BP is a good indicator but may be misinterpreted when there is a history of hyper-/hypotension. BP *trends* may be more use in these individuals.

> **In fluid overload (not necessarily true in nephrotic syndrome)**
> * BP >140/90mmHg
> * Pulse pressure (difference between systolic and diastolic reading) >60mmHg.
>
> *In dehydration*
> * BP <90/60mmHg
> * ↓ pulse pressure of <25mmHg
> * Postural hypotension: ↓ SBP of >20mmHg when sitting up from lying, or standing from sitting or lying.

▶ The pulse rate should be taken by hand as machines do not register irregular heartbeats; the result of electrolyte disturbance or cardiac disease.
* Slow bounding pulse may = fluid overload
* Rapid weak pulse usually = dehydration.

Jugular venous pressure

JVP is helpful. To measure JVP:
* Observe right internal jugular vein
* Tilt head of bed/back rest so patient is at a 30–60° angle and their neck is straight
* Absent vein may indicate ↓ plasma volume; unreliable in dehydration in some patients with confounding factors (e.g. obesity)
* Distended vein, from top of sternum to the angle of the jaw may indicate ↑ circulating volume
* At ~45° angle, JVP should be <4cm in euvolaemia
* ▶ JVP interpretation requires practice; may be affected by HF and vasodilating drugs (e.g. glyceryl trinitrate).

Capillary refill

* Apply 5secs of pressure to a fingernail, colour should return within 1–2secs.
* Delayed refill may = fluid depletion
* Ensure the digit being tested is marginally higher than the heart
* ▶ Capillary refill is affected by anaemia, ambient temperature, vascular disease, and smoking.

Direct measure of haemodynamic status

CVP can be a good indicator of circulating volume. It is measured using a catheter; the tip of which sits in the vena cava near the right atrium of the heart. Measuring CVP:

- Transducers usually used
- Observe strict adherence to local policy and procedure
- In euvolaemia, normal CVP is 5–10cmH$_2$O.

In ICU, other techniques for measuring cardiac output (which is a product of circulating volume and pulse rate) include:

- Oesophageal doppler, lithium injection dilution curve (LiDCo) calculations and other thermodilution techniques
- ECHO may be but will requires interpretation in myocardial disease.

Visual/touch assessment

Observing and touching the patient may indicate fluid status, prompting further assessment/confirming an original assessment. Trends ± changes are often more useful than 'one off' assessments.

In fluid overload

- Peripheral oedema (e.g. calf and ankle); perhaps pitting
- Sacral and scrotal oedema in bed bound patients
- Peri-orbital oedema
- SOB/Kussmaul breathing
- Orthopnoea
- Copious/frothy sputum
- Warm/moist skin
- ↑ JVP.

In dehydration

- ↓ skin turgor
- Dry, friable skin
- Dry mouth/tongue/lips/mucous membranes
- Sunken eyes
- Cold peripheries.

Weight

Monitoring body weight is an important tool.

▶Weigh individual patients on the same machine, wearing similar clothing, ideally at the same time each day.

- Each litre of fluid ≈1kg. In kidney patients rapid weight ↑↓ invariably relate to fluid ↑↓. Absolute weight is less important than changes and trends in body weight
- IBW changes over time and must be re-assessed regularly, especially after periods of ill health.

Auscultation

Fluid overload can → pulmonary oedema, i.e. fluid in parenchyma and airspaces in the lung. Diagnosis of pulmonary oedema:

- End inspiratory crackles on auscultation, respiratory rate (normal 12–20bpm) and effort ± ↓ oxygen saturations
- Significant involvement of ancillary muscles (e.g. abdominal) in respiration, Kussmaul respirations ± frothy sputum.

Chest x-ray

The presence of pulmonary oedema and pleural effusions on CXR indicate fluid overload in patients with CKD/AKI.

Blood tests

Plasma Na^+ and Alb levels and HCT may indicate fluid status.

- ↑ Alb, ↑ Na^+ and ↑ HCT may = dehydration
- ↓ Alb, ↓ Na^+ and ↓ HCT may = fluid overload.

- ↓ Alb may → oedema ± absolute ↓ in circulating volume
- Nephrotic syndrome may → ↑ IBW and oedema but BP ↓ due to low circulating volume (centrally 'dry')
- ↑ fluid in the circulation can → haemodilution, artificially ↓ levels of circulating electrolytes, Hb, and proteins
- Haemodilution prior to a session of HD is common.

Case study

A man is admitted to the renal ward with SOB, oedema up to his scrotum, eGFR 25ml/min. Initial appearance is fluid overload.
Baseline observations:
- BP: sitting 110/80mm/Hg, standing 90/65mm/Hg
- Complaining of dizziness
- Urinalysis: +++ protein, trace of blood
- Plasma Na^+ 132mmol/L, albumin 24g/L.

Whilst the patient is carrying ↑ fluid, he is centrally dry due to nephrotic syndrome (proteinuria and oedema), ↓ Na^+ and dehydration due to the overuse of diuretics.

Fluid balance charts

Fluid balance recording is not a direct measure of fluid status but, together with body weight measurements, it helps to assess trends in fluid balance and IBW in patients with kidney disease. 24hr fluid balance status may also be used to determine fluid allowances for the next 24hrs in patients with CKD/AKI or in RRT.

▶ The nurse's role in recording fluid balance is vital; requiring a thorough understanding of, and adherence to, local policy and practice. Fluid balance monitoring should account for:
- Oral intake
- IV fluids (including medications, infusions, and parenteral nutrition)
- Fluid loss e.g. urine, diarrhoea, vomit, blood (including any wound drainage), UF in PD

- Insensible loss 500ml/day ($\uparrow$ in pyrexia and hot weather)
- 24hr urine output can indicate ability to self-regulate fluid status
- Daily weight should be recorded on the fluid balance chart as IL fluid $\approx$1kg in weight.

Urinalysis

Urine osmolality rather than specific gravity (SG) may be relevant to assess fluid status in CKD. SG is affected by electrolyte imbalance and low protein diets and $\therefore$ may be misleading. Urine osmolality (normal range 500–800mOsmol/kg):

- Indicates ability to concentrate urine in the kidney, but must be interpreted in context of other measures of hydration and eGFR
- Can help to assess plasma Na^+ disturbance (see 📖 pp. 593–601) as Na^+ is the major contributor to body and urinary osmolality
- If $\uparrow$ in AKI, $\pm$ normal serum Na^+ it is consistent with pre-renal causes whilst renal causes of AKI $\rightarrow$ consistency between both levels.

Long-term effects of fluid overload

CVD and cerebrovascular incident are the most prevalent causes of morbidity and mortality in patients with CKD/ESKD. One of the major causes of CVD in CKD/ESKD is persistent fluid overload $\rightarrow$:
- Hypertension ($\uparrow$ pulse pressure)
- LVH
- Left ventricular dysfunction
- CHF
- Pulmonary oedema.

Assessment and management of fluid status to prevent repeated or persistent fluid overload is a fundamental task of the MPT.

Thirst
- Partly driven by plasma osmolality ($1°$ Na^+)
- Fluid adherence patient education strategies include thirst inducing-effects of dietary salt intake
- In health, excess salt is excreted in urine ($\uparrow$ urinary Na^+ and osmolality). Disrupted in CKD $\rightarrow$ $\uparrow$ impact of salt on plasma osmolality.

Nursing considerations

Engaging patients with fluid management strategies in all aspects of kidney disease is a key role for nurses.

▶ There is no 'one size fits all' strategy; understanding the pathophysiology of the patient's condition is fundamental:
- Anuria/oliguria is common in ESKD/on dialysis. Tx recipients post-tx or with a poorly functioning/failing graft may have altered urine output; ranging from anuria to polyuria

(Continued)

(Continued)

- Ability to manage body H_2O is dependent on underlying pathology, other co-morbidities, RRF, modality of RRT insensible and other fluid losses 📖 pp. 590–1. Fluid intake is adjusted accordingly
- Daily HD fluid restrictions ~1L/day.

▶ In HD patients evidence suggests that ↓ Na^+ diets and ↓ Na^+ dialysis ↓ oral fluid intake ∴ ↓ the need for large amounts of fluid removal on HD and ↓ the incidence of IDH.

Patient education
- Encourage patients to take ownership of their condition and responsibility for day-to-day diet and fluid restrictions
- Involve the MPT (especially the dietitian)
- Use appropriate educational aids
- Regular reinforcement of key messages
- Education re: fluid management:
  - importance of fluid restriction
  - understanding fluid in the diet—H_2O rich foods
  - using weight to monitor fluid intake
  - oral fluid volumes
  - the use of salt/restriction
- Management of thirst:
  - educate patient on dietary salt and various dietary sources/ preparations (see 📖 p. 84)
  - ↓ salt intake
  - using ice instead of cold drinks
  - avoid ↑ body heat → over heating
- Mouth and skin care
- Cardiovascular consequences
- Hypertension
- Pulmonary oedema
- Sources of help and support.

Table A3.1 Electrolyte table

Electrolyte	Causes of imbalance	Clinical features	Management
Sodium (Na⁺) normal range: 135–145mmol/L			
Hyponatraemia Na⁺ <135mmol/L	*Hypovol:* diuretic e.g. thiazide, osmotic diuresis, chronic tubular dysfunction, Addison's disease, diarrhoea, vomiting, bleeding, malnourished *Hypervol:* HF, cirrhosis, nephrotic syndrome, CKD, excess IV fluids *Euvol:* ↑ ADH (SIADH with, e.g. lung disease, neurological disease, medication (e.g. NSAIDs, antidepressants), pains, stress, hormonal (e.g. pregnancy, hypothyroid, adrenal insufficiency)	*Mild:* nausea/ vomiting, headache, anorexia, fatigue *Moderate* muscle cramps/spasms, confusion *Severe:* drowsiness, seizures, encephalopathy, coma	Identify and treat underlying cause, e.g. stop diuretic, IV fluids Managed according to fluid volume: *Hypovol:* ↑ oral fluids or IV NaCl *Hypervol:* fluid restriction to remove excess fluid, stop IV fluids *Euvol:* fluid restriction or NaCl tabs.⚠ Use in HF and liver cirrhosis with oedema, ± loop diuretic, ± vasopressin receptor agonist Dialysis may be considered if conservative measures fail ▲ Check K⁺, Mg²⁺ as may be ↓ ▲ ↑ Na⁺ slowly <10mmol/L/24hrS—prevent osmotic myelinosis
Hypernatremia Na⁺ >150mmol/L	Dehydration—diuretics, diarrhoea, burns, osmotic laxatives Diet Diabetes insipidus Hypertonic fluid ↑mineralocorticoid levels (e.g. aldosterone)	Lethargy, weakness Oedema Irritability Thirst	Oral water IV saline/half strength saline/glucose saline *Dialysis* ▲ Na⁺should be ↓ slowly <10mmol/L/24hrs

(Continued)

Table A3.1 (Continued)

Electrolyte	Causes of imbalance	Clinical features	Management
Potassium (K+) normal range: 3.0–5.0 mmol/L			
Hypokalaemia K+ <3.0mmol/L	Poor intake/anorexia Medications, e.g. digoxin, K+-sparing diuretic, aminoglycosides, glucocorticosteroid, bronchodilators, insulin Acquired tubular disease— tubular acidosis GI: diarrhoea/vomiting/ileostomy Adrenal disorders—1°/2° hyperaldosteronism Syndromes: Liddle's and Bartler's Vitamin B$_{12}$ correction Alkalosis ↓ Na+, ↓ Mg^{2+} HD: dialysed against too ↓ K+	Muscle weakness, ↓ tone, cramps Lethargy Constipation Confusion Cardiac arrhythmias Paralysis if severe <2.5 requires admission— should check Mg^{2+} levels as may need correcting	Identify and treat underlying cause, e.g. medications (e.g. ± switch to K+-sparing diuretic), GI, anorexia Mild: oral K+ supplement, ↑K+ in diet—refer to dietitian Severe: admission with cardiac monitoring, Oral/IV K+ supplement, check Mg^{2+}

Hyperkalaemia K^+ >6mmol/L (see 📖 p. 93)	Diet: non-adherence to K^+ restriction, use of salt substitutes, e.g. LoSalt® Medications: ACEIs, NSAIDs, ciclosporin, tacrolinus, trimethoprim, K^+-sparing diuretic CKD Trauma, rhabdomyolysis Diabetic ketoacidosis Addison's disease Acidosis HD: dialysed against too ↑K^+ ↓aldosterone Haemolysed blood sample	May be asymptomatic if mild Muscle irritability (cramps and twitching) Fatigue Cardiac arrhythmias, palpitations Cardiac arrest	Consider re-checking urgently Review medications and diet—refer to dietitian Calcium Resonium® Fludrocortisone Correct metabolic acidosis—oral/IV HCO_3—if not fluid overloaded Check diet—refer to dietitian Review medications Dialysis if not responding to conservative treatment *Life threatening >6.5 admission and ECG—monitoring* IV glucose and insulin IV calcium gluconate or IV calcium chloride
Chloride (Cl^-) normal range: 98–108mmol/L			
Hypochloraemia; Cl^- <98mmol/L	CKD Excessive sweating Vomiting Adrenal disorders Acidosis	Cramps Apathy Anorexia	IV normal saline

(Continued)

Table A3.1 (Continued)

Electrolyte	Causes of imbalance	Clinical features	Management
Hyperchloraemia Cl⁻>108mmol/L	CKD ↑PTH Diarrhoea Acidosis	Usually asymptomatic Thirst Kussmaul respiration Fatigue	Rehydration Correct acidosis
Calcium (Ca²⁺) normal range: 2.2–2.6mmol/L Corrected Ca²⁺: for every gram of albumin: >40 – 0.02mmol/L <40 + 0.02mmol/L			
Hypocalcaemia Ca²⁺<2.1mmol/L	↓/ineffective PTH ↓/ineffective vitamin D CKD/AKI Diet/malabsorption Acute pancreatitis Alkalosis ↓Mg²⁺	Asymptomatic Pins and needles Petechiae	Oral vitamin D (alfacalcidol) Oral Ca²⁺ IV Ca²⁺/calcium gluconate—requires cardiac monitoring

(Continued)

Hypercalcaemia Ca^{2+}>2.6mmol/L only usually symptomatic when Ca^{2+}>3.0mmol/L	↑PTH Malignancy Ca^{2+}/vitamin D supplements TB, sarcoidosis Thiazide diuretics	Headache/confusion Muscle weakness Nausea/vomiting Thirst Frequent urination Constipation	Review medications Steroids Parathyroidectomy If >3.0mmol/L IV normal saline infusion Loop diuretics Cinacalcet Calcitonin + bisphosphonate Dialysis
Magnesium (Mg^{2+}) normal range: 0.7–1.05mmol/L			
Hypomagnesaemia Mg^{2+}<0.7mmol/L	Medications: diuretics/some antibiotics/PPIs Alcohol abuse GI: diarrhoea, malnourished, pancreatitis Hypercalciuria, ↓ PO_4 ↑Ca^{2+} Diabetes mellitus	Nausea/vomiting Lethargy/weakness/cramps Altered personality Tetany, convulsions	Assess if kidney related—treat underlying cause Asymptomatic—PO, Mg^{2+} supplement Symptomatic—IM or IV Mg^{2+}, then PO

Table A3.1 (Continued)

Electrolyte	Causes of imbalance	Clinical features	Management
Hypermagnesaemia Mg^{2+} >1.05mmol/L	CKD/AKI IV Mg^{2+} Antacids or enemas containing Mg^{2+} hydroxide or carbonate	Nausea/vomiting Facial paraesthesiae Muscle weakness Atrial fibrillation (Mg^{2+}>2.3) Bradycardia Respiratory depression + ↓ BP >3.5	Stop Mg^{2+} preparation IV calcium gluconate if Mg^{2+} >5 and bradycardic Diuretics Dialysis
Phosphate (PO_4) normal range: 0.7–1.5mmol/L			
Hypophosphataemia PO_4 <0.7mmol/L	Kidney transplant Hyperparathyroidism Malabsorption, chronic diarrhoea Alcoholism Diet, re-feeding syndrome Alkalosis Insulin, anatacids	Muscle weakness Confusion Anaemia Seizures WBC dysfunction	Oral/IV supplementation

| Hyperphosphataemia PO_4 >1.8mmol/L | CKD ↓ /ineffective PTH ↓ /ineffective vitamin D | Vascular calcifications Itching Joint pain Fractures Red eye (conjunctival hyperaemia) | PO_4 restriction PO_4 binding medication taken with food Optimize dialysis |

Hydrogen (H⁺) normal range: 7.36 –7.44

| Alkalosis pH >7.45 | Vomiting/NG suction Diuretics ↓ K⁺/ ↓ aldosterone Alkalizing agents Post-hypercapnic compensation Respiratory alkalosis caused by hyperventilation (anxiety, hypoxia (e.g. asthma, pulmonary embolism, pulmonary oedema), pregnancy) | Muscle weakness/spasm Nausea/vomiting Hypoventilation Altered mental state Tingling in extremities Cardiac arrhythmias | Treat underlying cause NaCl/KCl depending if hypochloraemia or hypokalaemia HCL infusion (central line) if urgent correction needed |

(Continued)

Table A3.1 (*Continued*)

Electrolyte	Causes of imbalance	Clinical features	Management
Acidosis pH <7.3	CKD/AKI Rhabdomyolysis Diabetic ketoacidosis CNS suppression Chronic respiratory disease	Chest pain Altered mental state Nausea/vomiting Cardiac arrhythmia Kussmaul respiration	Respiratory support IV NaHCO$_3$ (with caution pH <7.2) Dialysis pH 7.30–7.35 does not require therapy
Bicarbonate (HCO$_3$) normal range: 22–30mol/L			
Hypobicarbonataemia acidosis; HCO$_3$<20 Very rare to see alone usually associated with acidosis	CKD/AKI Rhabdomyolysis Diabetic ketoacidosis CNS suppression Chronic respiratory disease	Nausea/ vomiting/hiccups Altered consciousness Kussmaul respiration Cardiac arrhythmias	PO ▶↑ serum Na$^+$ → fluid retention and ↑ BP IV NaHCO$_3$ (severe) Prevent malnutrition (catabolic state)—refer to dietitian May require correction of ↑K$^+$—check Ca^{2+} levels as may cause ↓ Respiratory support Dialysis NaHCO$_3$ associated with slowing the reduction in kidney function

| Hyperbicarbonataemia alkalosis; $HCO_3 > 30$ mmol/L | Vomiting/NG suction
Diuretics
↓ K⁺/ ↓ aldosterone
Alkalizing agents
Post hypercapnic compensation | Irritability
Muscle weakness/spasms | Rehydration
Treat underlying respiratory condition if respiratory alkalosis
Dialysis |

NB In Tx recipients, fluid and electrolyte imbalances can occur in the immediate and post-transplant period as result of anuria, e.g. in DGF or induced polyuria. Correction with IV fluids, supplements, or dialysis may be required if electrolytes do not correct spontaneously. In failing Tx recipients, the risks of fluid and electrolyte imbalance are similar to those experienced in CKD, depending upon the degree of graft failure.

Person-centred education

Person-centred education

All nephrology and Tx services should have person-centred, structured MPT education programmes in place. Educational material should be standardized to ensure validity, ease of understanding, and to ensure consistency of the information delivered. Education is an integral part of the renal practitioner's role whether they are based on the ward, in the dialysis unit, or in a clinic environment.

- All interactions should be seen as ideal opportunities to teach person/carers, with learning viewed as a continuous process
- Requires well-constructed and planned educational activities which aim to:
  - improve health literacy
  - increase the person's knowledge and understanding of their health
  - equip the person with self-management skills where possible
- People should be offered the choice of individual or group teaching to suit their learning style and needs
- The majority of people prefer face-to-face education sessions, a forum for discussion to have a family member or friend present for support. Group sessions also provide peer support.

Benefits of CKD educational programmes

- Facilitate people to manage their health and make informed choices, e.g. advantages and disadvantages of the various treatment options and lifestyle changes
- Promote self-efficacy, motivation, and empowerment to improve health:
  - identify risk factors and health behaviour
  - ↑ adherence and the ability to self-manage
  - promote and support continued employment
- Provide psychosocial support:
  - ↓ anxiety and stress
  - ↑ ability to cope with living with a long-term condition
- Improve person/family experience and satisfaction with the service
- Clinical benefits:
  - delay progression of CKD and time to RRT
  - ↓ complications and mortality rates of CKD
  - ↓ cardiovascular risk
- Improve efficiency and cost-effectiveness as a result of better informed patients.

Factors to consider when organizing education

- Stage of the CKD—content required
  - CKD stage 2 education will be different from that provided at stage 4—the person will have different learning needs and goals
- Age—younger people will have different learning needs, concerns and skills from older people:
  - older people may find it more difficult to learn new skills as this ability declines with age
  - transition from paediatric to adult services requires specific education needs (see pp. 548–50)

- Gender, e.g. different concerns
- Barriers to learning:
  - physical, sensory, or learning disability
  - cognitive impairment, mental state
  - low literacy level may require alternative educational material and ↑ explanation
  - communication issues, e.g. interpreter if unable to speak or read English
  - overall physical state of the person, e.g. too unwell to teach
  - educational level achieved
  - psychological state as they may be depressed or unable to cope with any information
  - culture/religious beliefs
- Prior experience, e.g. other illness or healthcare professionals
- Presence of other conditions, e.g. diabetes
- Social support and commitments
- Employment/studying
- Motivation, attitude towards learning, and healthcare including their past experience with healthcare professionals
- History of non-adherence, alcohol, or drug abuse.

Prior to teaching

- Requires a systematic approach to planning and implementing
- Develop a teaching strategy which involves the assessment of the person's learning needs, ability to learn, and learning style.

Learning style

This refers to how a person likes to learn which can vary depending on the skill or information to be learnt. There are various models of learning styles available; one of the most common is Honey and Mumford (1986) which used Kolb's theory as a basis,[1] describing learning styles as:

- *Activist*: easy going and enthusiastic about new opportunities—prefer to experience new skill rather than read about it
- *Theorist*: 'thinker' and analytical in their approach—favour reading literature and access to websites to collate information
- *Reflector*: reflect on experiences, gather all the information and then make a decision—prefer to observe
- *Pragmatist*: prefer to experiment and try new skills. Identifying learning style enables the practitioner to focus educational activities that will meet the needs of the individual.

Assessment

- Background, history, and social circumstances
- General health status, e.g. shorter and more frequent sessions if physically unwell
- Identify any potential barriers to learning—organize any special requirements, e.g. interpreter or family member for support
- Current knowledge—identify information to cover in the session:
  - expectations about the treatment

- prior knowledge and understanding about their condition, treatment options
- person's identified learning needs/goals
- Psychosocial:
  - readiness and ability to learn
  - current coping strategy—reaction to their condition
  - motivation and commitment to learning
  - in transition programme for transfer to adult care
- Learning style:
  - usual learning style, e.g. reading, DVD
  - group or individual sessions, e.g. feel intimidated in a group or prefer the company of others and discussion.

Educational tools available

- Written, e.g. leaflets, booklets, posters
- Audio-visual, e.g. DVD, CDs, talking books
- Graphical, e.g. visual for poor literacy level
- Models, e.g. abdomen, kidneys
- Demonstration of technique, e.g. PD exchange, setting up dialysis machine or APD machine, injection technique for ESAs
- Web-based educational tools:
  - recommend accredited sites as some sites may cause more anxiety and stress by providing incorrect information
- Bespoke 'toolkits'/learning aids, e.g. to promote adherence to medications post transplantation
- Peer support ('buddy'), patient support groups, expert patients
- Development of educational material—include patient user groups/ expert patients. The majority of Trusts have patient experience teams who peer review written information to ensure it is clearly written and easily understood.

Planning and delivering education session

- Plan how you are going to deliver the education and evaluate the effectiveness:
  - educator needs to have the underpinning knowledge of the subject
  - information and education needs to be consistent, structured, and well organized
- Consider the following prior to planning the session:
  - aim/goal of the session
  - allocated time
  - content of the session, e.g. dialysis options, fluid balance
  - attendance, e.g. person, person and carer/family
  - group or individual session
- Teaching environment:
  - clinic room, ward, e.g. privacy, noise, interruptions
- Age, e.g. older patient
- If possible, suggest that the person thinks and writes down any questions they have prior to the session

- Use of effective communication skills to put the person at ease and ↓ stress and anxiety, e.g. use humour—always demonstrate respect and a non-judgement approach:
  - verbal and non-verbal skills, e.g. good eye contact and body language (e.g. attentive)
  - use plain language avoiding the use of medical jargon
  - provide opportunity for questions—open and closed
  - listen to the person—pick up on non-verbal cues
  - provide affirmation and opportunity to reflect on feelings
- Provide information in small amounts to avoid overwhelming the person as they may have a short attention span (5–15mins maximum):
  - discuss the most important information first as people tend to retain this longer
  - repeat information by summarizing key points at the end of the session
- Involve family where possible in the learning experience, encourage and facilitate questions
- Provide culturally sensitive information
- Explain practical information, e.g. process of diffusion, use an analogy:
  - use props to demonstrate technique and repeat as required
  - encourage participation
  - relate information to day-to-day life
- Provide reading material/DVDs to take home to consolidate teaching
- Provide follow-up contact numbers of the staff providing the information
- Invite patients already receiving RRT to share their knowledge and experience as the 'expert patient' and for peer support
- Include other agencies such as your local Kidney Patient Association and transport providers.

Evaluating educational session

- Reflect with the patient and identify areas that were more/less successful in order to plan future teaching sessions:
  - identify educational needs
- Document and review goals to enable continuity of educational care using on care plan and/or medical notes
- Liaise with other members in the MPT, e.g. areas identified that may require their advice, support, and input.

Reasons for non-attendance

May be misinterpreted as lack of motivation or interest; however there are often reasons such as:
- Distance to travel/no transport
- Acopia with condition/diagnosis
- Denial—not ready to learn more about their condition
- Uncomfortable with activity's format, e.g. group/individual/lack of interpreter/previous experience.

Further reading

Reference

1. The Experiential Learning Cycle. Available at: <http://www.learningandteaching.info/learning/experience.htm> (accessed 5 May 2012)

Patient information websites

<http://www.kidney.org.uk/> (which also provides details of local KPAs)
<http://www.edren.org/pages/edreninfo/>
<http://www.patient.co.uk/>
<http://www.renal.org/whatwedo/InformationResources/>
<http://www.renalpatientview.org>

Index